# Treatment Strategies in Child and Adolescent Psychiatry

# Treatment Strategies in Child and Adolescent Psychiatry

Edited by

## Jovan G. Simeon
University of Ottawa
Ottawa, Ontario, Canada

and

## H. Bruce Ferguson
Royal Ottawa Hospital
Ottawa, Ontario, Canada

With a foreword by
Daniel Offord

Plenum Press • New York and London

Library of Congress Cataloging-in-Publication Data

```
Treatment strategies in child and adolescent psychiatry / edited by
  Jovan G. Simeon and H. Bruce Ferguson ; with a foreword by Daniel
  Offord.
        p.   cm.
     Includes bibliographical references.
     Includes index.
     ISBN 0-306-43466-0
     1. Child psychotherapy. 2. Adolescent psychotherapy.  I. Simeon,
  Jovan G.  II. Ferguson, H. Bruce.
     [DNLM: 1. Mental Disorders--in adolescence. 2. Mental Disorders-
  -in infancy & childhood. 3. Mental Disorders--therapy.  WS 350
  T7845]
  RJ504.T74  1990
  618.92'89--dc20
  DNLM/DLC
  for Library of Congress                                     90-7429
                                                                  CIP
```

© 1990 Plenum Press, New York
A Division of Plenum Publishing Corporation
233 Spring Street, New York, N.Y. 10013

All rights reserved

No part of this book may be reproduced, stored in a retrieval system, or transmitted in any form or by any means, electronic, mechanical, photocopying, microfilming, recording, or otherwise, without written permission from the Publisher

Printed in the United States of America

# *Contributors*

***Magda Campbell***   Department of Psychiatry, New York University Medical Center, New York, New York 10016

***Vincenzo F. DiNicola***   Division of Child and Adolescent Psychiatry, University of Ottawa; and Family Psychiatry Service and Adolescent Day Care Program, Royal Ottawa Hospital, Ottawa, Ontario K1Z 7K4, Canada

***Denis M. Donovan***   The Children's Center for Developmental Psychiatry, St. Petersburg, Florida 33710

***Michel Dugas***   Service de Psycho-Pathologie de l'Enfant et de l'Adolescent, Hôpital Robert Debre, 75935 Paris CEDEX 19, France.

***H. Bruce Ferguson***   Department of Psychology, Royal Ottawa Hospital, Ottawa, Ontario K1Z 7K4, Canada

***Martine F. Flament***   International Hospital of the University of Paris, 75014 Paris, France

***Barry D. Garfinkel***   Division of Child and Adolescent Psychiatry, University of Minnesota Medical School, Minneapolis, Minnesota 55455

***Christophe Gérard***   Service de Psycho-Pathologie de l'Enfant et de l'Adolescent, Hôpital Robert Debre, 75935 Paris CEDEX 19, France.

***Vivian Kafantaris***   Department of Psychiatry, New York University Medical Center, New York, New York 10016

***S.P. Kutcher***   Department of Psychiatry and Department of Psychology, Sunnybrook Medical Centre, University of Toronto, Toronto, Ontario M4N 3M5, Canada

***Richard P. Malone***   Department of Psychiatry, New York University Medical Center, New York, New York 10016

***P. Marton***   Department of Psychiatry and Department of Psychology, Sunnybrook Medical Centre, University of Toronto, Toronto, Ontario M4N 3M5 Canada

***Deborah McIntyre*** The Children's Center for Developmental Psychiatry, St. Petersburg, Florida 33710

***Nicholas L. Rock*** Department of Psychiatry, Louisiana State University Medical Center, New Orleans, Louisiana 70112

***Walid O. Shekim*** Department of Psychiatry and Biobehavioral Sciences, UCLA Neuropsychiatric Institute and Hospital, Los Angeles, California 90024

***Jovan G. Simeon*** Department of Psychiatry, University of Ottawa, Ottawa, Ontario K1Z 7K4, Canada

***Kai Tolstrup*** University Clinic of Child Psychiatry, Rigshospitalet University Hospital, Copenhagen, Denmark 2100,Ø

***Luis Vera*** Robert Debre Hospital, 75019 Paris, France

# *Foreword*

It is clear that child and adolescent psychiatric disorders impose a heavy burden of suffering. Recent large-scale community epidemiological studies suggest that as many as 20% of children and adolescents in the general population may have clinically important mental disorders. These disorders are accompanied by associated impairments in various domains of the child's life, resulting in lowered life quality for the child and his or her family. In addition, for some conditions, the onset of the disorder in childhood heralds a lifetime of serious psychosocial disturbance for a significant subgroup of affected children. For instance, about 40% of children seen in clinic settings with conduct disorder in late childhood and early adolescence will have serious psychiatric disorders in adult life. Finally, the heavy burden of suffering of these conditions is indicated by the large amounts of both human and financial resources devoted to their assessment and treatment.

There is a pressing need in the field for effective treatments (that is, those that have been shown to do more good than harm) that will result in a significant reduction in the burden of suffering resulting from these disorders. Further, these effective interventions must be readily available and acceptable to clinicians in the settings in which children with mental disorders (and their families) seek care.

This book addresses an important need in the treatment field. It provides a concise description of the treatments currently in use for child and adolescent psychiatric disorders and, more important, presents a critical appraisal of their effectiveness.

The book has a number of laudable strengths. First, it furnishes excellent coverage of the wide diversity of conditions that constitute child and adolescent mental disorders. Second, it makes it clear that advances in treatment for these conditions are dependent to an important extent on progress in other areas of investigation, such as research design, classification, measurement, and etiology. Third, it presents a balanced view of the different treatment modalities from psychopharmacology to individual and family therapy and, further, covers succinctly the advantages and disadvantages of various combinations of treatments. Last, the book continually points out the limitations in our knowledge in the treatment domain and suggests the next steps that are needed to move the field forward.

After reading the manuscript I was left with a couple of strong impressions. There have been a number of important recent advances in the treatment of child and adolescent mental disorders, and this book provides the means for clinicians to be brought up to date on this progress in such a way that they can use the knowledge immediately and directly for the benefit of their patients. In addition, the rigorous evaluation of commonly used and innovative treatments is of prime importance to the child mental health field. This conclusion is supported by the recently released report by the Institute of Medicine entitled *Research on Children and Adolescents with Mental Disorders and Developmental Disorders: Mobilizing a National Initiative.*

Drs. Simeon and Ferguson and their colleagues are to be congratulated on bringing together in one book a summary of existing treatments for child and adolescent psychiatric disorders, an evaluation of their effectiveness, coverage of the limitations of knowledge in this domain, and suggestions for future research. This has resulted in an important contribution, which will be useful to clinicians, teachers, and researchers concerned with children and adolescents with mental disorders.

Daniel R. Offord, M.D.

# *Preface*

> LIFE is short, and the art long; the occasion fleeting; experience fallacious, and judgement difficult. The physician must not only be prepared to do what is right himself, but also to make the patient, the attendants and externals co-operate.
>
> Hippocrates

Of all branches of medicine, Hippocrates' famous aphorism seems to apply most appropriately to child psychiatry. Unlike other medical fields, therapists who work with children and adolescents must take into account complex interactions involving the genetic, physical, and psychological aspects of the patient, the family and social environment, as well as the child's academic and developmental tasks. Thus, when treating children, therapists need to also get involved with their families, social and school environments, and various institutions.

Although child psychiatry is a young science, research has produced rapid advances in theoretical and empirical knowledge. These developments have led to further specialization such as infant, child, and adolescent psychiatry. A variety of approaches have evolved in relation to both diagnosis and therapy, and a number of different "schools" have emerged in the areas of psychotherapy, behavioral therapy, family therapy, and group therapy. This has produced some interesting situations in child psychiatry. For example, children with identical problems may receive different diagnoses as well as very different therapies, depending on who treats them and where.

Not only are there marked differences in the psychiatric management of children and adolescents from country to country, but therapists often seem either unaware of or uninterested in the methods of others. Certain differences in management may be easily understood, since developing countries do not have the same priorities or financial and professional resources as developed countries. In countries where children are exposed to epidemics, malnutrition, starvation, overpopulation, and war, child psychiatry services are obviously a very low priority. It is more difficult, however, to accept the marked differences in therapies offered children with similar behavioral problems among developed countries or among different professionals within the same country or center. These differences depend on multiple factors, such as training, theoretical orientation, personal style, and experience, as well as cultural background and social context. The training of child psychiatrists is a very long process. Compared with most other medical disciplines, the life of the practicing child psychiatry therapist is short. Further they may practice in the isolation of their offices, trying to help children without ever knowing for certain if their work is effective. Since many biological, psychological, and social factors are involved, therapy may be done poorly. Treatment-resistant children are often referred from one therapist to another. Conversely, many children are treated by the same therapist, or by the same method, for long periods of time with no attempt to modify the treatment strategy or to quantify any clinical changes. Therefore, it is important that child therapists become more open to different approaches to practice and learn to evaluate treatment effects on an ongoing basis.

Discussions on effectiveness and cost-benefit analysis of psychiatric interventions and child mental health programs often result in conflicting viewpoints as to whether the "best approach" is prevention, community-based treatment programs, or clinic-based interventions. Obviously, all of these approaches are important. The real challenge, however, lies in how to integrate them, so that they complement each other rather than compete for resources. Most of the advances in child psychiatry have benefited the individual patient, while progress on a broader level depends on prevention, which in turn depends on a range of social and political factors. The focus of child psychiatry training and responsibility remains the treatment of individual children and families. While there is now widespread interest in more global prevention programs, the present state of our knowledge is not adequate to implement such programs effectively. While child psychiatrists have an important role to play in these developments, at this time we believe it would be inappropriate for the discipline to shift its main focus away from treatment.

Prior to any therapeutic intervention, it is essential to undertake a comprehensive diagnostic evaluation. Any therapy where the diagnostic process is viewed as unnecessary, or as "labeling possibly harmful to the child," is doomed to failure. Diagnostic evaluation represents much more than the assignment of a classification. It is the process by which all the child's deficits, symptoms, and disorders are described and assessed, and other disorders are ruled out. The diagnostic process lays the foundation for the treatment, and the evaluation of its efficacy. Therapists must also learn to use recently developed rating scales and diagnostic interview techniques. In most cases, it is important to obtain careful information from several sources since the child's problems may manifest in several contexts. Improvements in therapeutic interventions on a more global scale depend on the evolution of valid diagnostic entities for which effective treatments can be developed. For this reason, the broad acceptance of clearly operationalized diagnostic criteria (e.g., DSM-III-R, ICD-10) represents an essential first step; these classification systems must be reviewed and refined on the basis of further research findings. Through the use of such systems, compilation of a body of knowledge regarding treatment outcome could be a very useful tool in deciding the optimal therapy for specific children. To achieve these goals, communication on an international level is urgently needed.

This book is based on an international conference on treatment in child psychiatry that took place in Vienna, Austria, March 1988. We have attempted to present therapeutic viewpoints from a variety of specialties or "schools" as they are practiced in different countries. It is addressed to all professionals who treat children. It emphasizes documented advances in therapy with children and families, and the need to continuously evaluate our therapeutic endeavors. This volume is not a comprehensive text on therapies in child psychiatry but covers selected topics representing the views of experienced therapists. Treating psychopathology in children usually requires simultaneous therapeutic efforts in several modalities (e.g., in cases of attention deficit disorders, one could combine parent management training with medication and cognitive training for the child). In most cases this requires a knowledge of available approaches and the coordination of a multidisciplinary group of professionals. The art of therapy is never "learned" but must be exercised as a never-ceasing challenge to one's skills. However, the development of better systems of multimodal and integrated approaches to therapy seem essential. Since we view such integration of therapeutic approaches as essential, the book is organized primarily around groups of disorders. However, since there have been significant developments within specific therapeutic areas (e.g., pharmacotherapy, family therapy), these have been presented as separate chapters.

It is hoped that this volume will promote communication among professionals dealing with disturbed children and adolescents across different centers and countries. Perhaps the sharing of these different perspectives will help advance our understanding of disorders and the art of therapy. Through a greater ability to understand children and treat their problems, child therapists may assume leadership roles in society.

# Contents

**1. Diagnosis and Treatment of Attention Deficit and Conduct Disorders in Children and Adolescents** .................... 1
*Walid O. Shekim*

Attention Deficit Hyperactivity Disorder .......................... 2
   Associated Features of ADHD ................................. 3
   Problems With the Diagnosis of ADHD ........................ 3
   Differential Diagnosis ......................................... 4
   Prevalence .................................................... 4
   Course ....................................................... 5
   Family History ................................................ 5
   Etiologies .................................................... 5
   Treatment .................................................... 6
Conduct and Oppositional Disorders .............................. 9
   Terminology .................................................. 10
   Associated Features .......................................... 10
   Prognosis .................................................... 10
   Prevalence and Sex Ratio ..................................... 11
   Treatment .................................................... 11
Summary ....................................................... 14
References ..................................................... 15

**2. Adolescent Depression: A Treatment Review** ................. 19
*S. P. Kutcher and P. Marton*

Psychological Therapies ......................................... 20
   Cognitive–Behavioral Approaches to Therapy ................... 21
   Psychodynamic Psychotherapy ................................. 22
   Family Therapy ............................................... 23
Social Therapies ................................................ 23
Biological Therapies ............................................. 23
   Antidepressants .............................................. 23
   Lithium Carbonate ............................................ 25

*xiii*

| | |
|---|---|
| Antidepressant Guidelines | 25 |
| Other Biological Treatments | 25 |
| Combined Treatment | 26 |
| Conclusions | 26 |
| References | 26 |

### 3. Psychopharmacological Treatment of School Phobia ......... 31
*Barry D. Garfinkel*

| | |
|---|---|
| Introduction | 31 |
| The Diagnosis of School Phobia | 32 |
| Family Pedigrees | 34 |
| The Epidemiological Basis of Anxiety Symptoms | 35 |
| Evaluation Techniques | 36 |
| Family Dynamics | 37 |
| General Considerations of Treatment | 38 |
| Previous Studies | 39 |
| Clinical Trials Comparing Alprazolam and Imipramine | 41 |
| A School Reentry Program | 43 |
| Conclusions | 44 |
| References | 45 |

### 4. Treatment of Childhood Obsessive–Compulsive Disorder: A Review in the Light of Recent Findings ................... 49
*Martine F. Flament and Luis Vera*

| | |
|---|---|
| Psychoanalytic Treatment | 51 |
| Other Forms of Psychotherapy | 52 |
| Behavioral Treatment | 53 |
|    The Behavioral Models of OCD | 54 |
|    Behavioral Treatment of OCD | 56 |
| Pharmacological Treatment | 61 |
| Conclusion | 68 |
| References | 70 |

### 5. Autism and Aggression ....................................... 77
*Magda Campbell, Richard P. Malone, and Vivian Kafantaris*

| | |
|---|---|
| Introduction | 77 |
| Autism | 77 |
|    History | 77 |

|     |     |
| --- | --- |
| Advances in Assessment | 78 |
| Comprehensive and Individualized Treatment Programs | 79 |
| Pharmacotherapy: An Overview of the Literature | 79 |
| Aggression | 83 |
| Assessment of Aggressive Behavior and SIB | 85 |
| Pharmacotherapy: An Overview of the Literature | 85 |
| Summary and Conclusions | 90 |
| References | 92 |

### 6. *Treatment of Children and Adolescents with Substance Abuse Disorders* ......... 99
*Nicholas L. Rock*

|     |     |
| --- | --- |
| Introduction | 99 |
| Treatment Program | 100 |
| Attitude | 101 |
| Knowledge and Skills | 101 |
| Diagnosis | 102 |
| Treatment | 103 |
| Detoxification | 104 |
| Rehabilitation | 106 |
| Summary | 107 |
| Appendix 1 | |
| A Model Alcohol Withdrawal Procedure | 107 |
| Appendix 2 | |
| Specific Sedative/Hypnotic Withdrawal | 110 |
| Appendix 3 | |
| Narcotic Withdrawal Procedures | 111 |
| References | 112 |

### 7. *Treatment of Anorexia Nervosa: Current Status* ......... 115
*Kai Tolstrup*

|     |     |
| --- | --- |
| Introduction | 115 |
| The Treatment of Anorexia Nervosa | 116 |
| A Model for Integrated Treatment | 117 |
| Core Therapy | 121 |
| Family Contact | 121 |
| Group Therapy | 122 |
| Patient Groups | 122 |
| Parent Groups | 122 |

Art Therapy ................................................. 123
Motoric Training ............................................ 123
Pharmacological Treatment ..................................... 124
Pharmacotherapy ............................................ 124
Hospitalization ............................................. 124
Discharge .................................................. 125
Treatment Outcome ......................................... 127
Indications for and Need of Treatment—Resources .............. 128
Who Should Treat AN? ...................................... 129
What About Prevention? ....................................... 130
Conclusion .................................................... 130
References .................................................... 131

## 8. Child Adolescent Psychopharmacology .................... 133
*Jovan G. Simeon*

Introduction .................................................. 133
General Guidelines of Prescribing ............................... 134
Stimulants .................................................... 135
Antidepressants ................................................ 137
Enuresis ................................................... 138
Attention Deficit and Conduct Disorders ...................... 138
Separation Anxiety and School Phobia ........................ 139
Depression ................................................. 139
Obsessive–Compulsive Disorder .............................. 140
Eating Disorders ............................................ 140
Antipsychotics ................................................. 141
Infantile Autism ............................................ 142
Tourette's Syndrome ........................................ 142
Anxiolytics .................................................... 143
Antiaggressive Drugs .......................................... 144
Conclusion .................................................... 144
References .................................................... 145

## 9. Recent Developments in Diet Therapy .................... 151
*H. Bruce Ferguson*

Food Allergies and Behavior .................................... 152
Food Colors and Preservatives—The Feingold Hypothesis ........... 154
Sugar and Children's Behavior .................................. 155
Study 1 .................................................... 156
Study 2 .................................................... 158

General Conclusions ... 160
References ... 161

## 10. Treatment of Developmental Language Disorders ... 163
*Michel Dugas and Christophe Gérard*

Introduction ... 163
Motivations for Treatment ... 164
Conceptualization of Treatment ... 165
A Neuropsychological Model ... 166
Therapeutic Strategies ... 168
Academic Acquisitions ... 170
Organization of Treatment ... 170
A Medical Model ... 173
Prospects ... 174
References ... 175

## 11. Child Psychotherapy ... 177
*Denis M. Donovan and Deborah McIntyre*

Introduction ... 177
  Persistence of an Adult Model ... 177
A Developmental-Contextual Approach ... 178
  How Children Think, Interact, Communicate, and Change ... 179
  The Interactive Style of Children ... 181
  Communication and Speech ... 183
The Real Worlds of Children ... 184
The Therapeutic Process ... 186
  Therapeutic Space ... 187
The Evaluation of Therapeutic Aptness ... 189
  An Operational Assessment of "Play" ... 189
The "Ecology" of Child Psychotherapy ... 192
  Parents and Teachers as Allies or Saboteurs of the Therapeutic Process ... 193
Psychotherapy as a Problem-Solving Process ... 194
References ... 195

## 12. Family Therapy: A Context for Child Psychiatry ... 199
*Vincenzo F. DiNicola*

Mapping the Family Field ... 200
  The Family ... 200

| | |
|---|---|
| Family Therapy | 200 |
| A Relational Context | 201 |
| Family Therapy Models of Mental Disorders | 202 |
|     Relational Disorders | 202 |
|     Triggering Events | 202 |
|     Maladaptive Responses | 203 |
| Tools of the Trade | 204 |
| Major Family Therapy Approaches | 205 |
|     The Structural School | 205 |
|     The Strategic Approach | 207 |
|     The Systemic Model | 208 |
| How Family Therapy Functions | 210 |
| Maturity of Family Therapy | 211 |
| Controversies | 214 |
| Conclusion | 215 |
| References | 216 |
| | |
| *Index* | 221 |
| | |
| *About the Editors* | 233 |

# Diagnosis and Treatment of Attention Deficit and Conduct Disorders in Children and Adolescents

## Walid O. Shekim

The three diagnostic categories in DSM-III of attention deficit disorders (ADD), oppositional disorder, and conduct disorders (CD) were grouped together in DSM-III-R into a subclass, disruptive behavior disorders. These disorders are characterized by disruptive behavior distressing to others and not to the person with the disorder. Research has demonstrated that the symptoms of these disorders covary to a high degree. For example, Cantwell (1977), Connors (1969), and Quay (1979) have demonstrated strong relationships between aggressive and hyperactive behavior. The dimension of aggressivity has been added to hyperactivity and inattention to differentiate children with ADD and to predict long-term outcome (Langhorne & Loney, 1979; Loney, Langhorne & Paternite, 1978; Milich, Loney, & Landau, 1982). Werry, Reeves, and Elkind (1987) have reviewed the literature comparing attention deficit hyperactivity disorder (ADHD) and conduct disorder. They conclude that there are remarkable similarities across diagnostic groups. They further suggest that ADHD is primarily a disorder of cognitive impairment, more impulsive responding, and poorer achievement in school, and that it is associated with increased motor activity and neurodevelopmental abnormalities. Conduct disorder, on the other hand, is characterized by egocentricity and higher degrees of hostility. Association between ADHD and CD increases the severity of the handicap. Reeves, Werry, Elkind, and Zametkin (1987) found, in a clinic sam-

---

*Walid O. Shekim*  Department of Psychiatry and Biobehavioral Sciences, UCLA Neuropsychiatric Institute and Hospital, Los Angeles, California 90024.

ple, that conduct and oppositional disorders resembled each other and rarely occurred in the absence of ADHD.

The relationship between ADHD and conduct disorder is a debated issue. The diagnosis of ADHD is rarely made in the U.K., probably because of the lack of differentiation between ADHD and CD in the U.K., where the diagnosis of CD is more likely to be applied. In the United States the existence of pure and mixed forms of ADHD, oppositional defiant disorder (ODD), and CD is suggested, but further research is needed to document the validity of these diagnostic categories. There are several studies (cited in Reeves et al., 1987) that demonstrate the existence of pure ADHD, and that ADHD and CD resemble ADHD with greater social handicaps and more adverse family environments coupled with alcoholic antisocial fathers. More research is needed to elucidate whether ADHD is distinct from ADHD with CD or whether psychosocial environmental factors interacting with the cause of ADHD produce ADHD + CD (Reeves et al., 1987). Edelbrock, Costello, and Kessler (1984) found that ADHD boys are more aggressive than other clinically referred boys, while boys diagnosed as ADD without hyperactivity (DSM-III) are less aggressive and in fact are more socially withdrawn. Hyperactivity was present in the past history of many antisocial persons, and it has been suggested that it may be a precursor of antisocial behavior (Kazdin, 1985). Many children with hyperactivity exhibit symptoms of conduct disorder and vice versa. DSM-III and DSM-III-R permit both diagnostic categories to be given to the same child or adolescent.

Prior to DSM-III, much of the research on children with ADHD and children with CD dealt with children who had both disorders. It is only recently that researchers have started analyzing the relationship between antisocial behavior and symptoms of attention deficit hyperactivity disorder. Important questions as to prognosis, treatment, and outcome are facilitated by such an approach (Kazdin, 1985).

Though there is plenty of research on the existence and validity of ADHD and CD, the existence of ODD is disputed, and there are no data on its validity (Werry, Reeves, & Elkind, 1987). The distinction between ODD and CD is also controversial. Research has failed to show differences on several variables (Reeves et al., 1987; Werry et al., 1987). There is agreement that the distinction is more quantitative than qualitative.

## Attention Deficit Hyperactivity Disorder

In DSM-III, the diagnosis of ADHD was determined by a minimum number of symptoms in each of three separate categories: inattention, impulsivity, and hyperactivity. A problem with this approach was that no matter how numerous the symptoms in two categories, the diagnosis could not be determined without the minimum number of symptoms in the third category. There was no empirical evidence to suggest that the symptoms from the three categories are necessary for the diagnosis. Therefore, DSM-III-R attempted to remedy this problem by merging all three categories. The items were selected to better discriminate the disorder from conduct and oppositional defiant disorders. The list of symptoms and the threshold for determining the diagnosis were based on the results of a field trial of several hundred children.

In DSM-III, ADD included two types: ADD with hyperactivity and ADD without hyperactivity. In ADD without hyperactivity, symptoms of inattention and impulsivity were present and symptoms of hyperactivity were absent. In DSM-III-R, the diagnosis of ADD without hyperactivity was deleted, and disturbances involving attentional difficulties that do not meet the criteria for ADHD are diagnosed in DSM-III-R as undifferentiated ADD. Further research is needed to define and validate undifferentiated ADD.

## Associated Features of ADHD

Many children with ADHD present no additional complications. The clinical impression is that this is usually more likely to be the case in the brighter child who has both a stable family and a warm home environment (American Psychiatric Association, 1987; Gittelman, 1980).

A large proportion of children with ADHD present with a specific developmental disorder, such as reading and arithmetic difficulties. Some ADHD children may have fine and gross motor coordination problems. They may present with nonlocalizing soft neurologic signs and motor-perceptual dysfunctions. Electroencephalographic abnormalities also may be present. In only 5% of the cases, however, is attention deficit disorder associated with a diagnosable neurologic disorder. Because of their impulsivity, these children may be reactively aggressive, excitable, and easily frustrated. Such behavior may lead to poor peer relations. Often they may be described as socially immature and emotionally labile.

## Problems with the Diagnosis of ADHD

One of the major problems in making the diagnosis of ADHD is the variability of the presenting symptomology coupled with the inconsistency of the reports from professionals, parents, and teachers (Gittelman, 1980; Palfrey, Levine, Oberklaid, Levaer, and Aufseeser, 1981). Variability is in fact a typical pattern of this disorder. The clinical phenomena will vary according to motivation, day-to-day fluctuation in focus, rapport with the examiner, level of anxiety, and preoccupying concerns. Furthermore, situational variability often leads to variability in clinical picture; for example, the presenting behaviors often worsen in group situations but improve in one-to-one or structured settings. The nature of the demand of the task is a major determinant of attention deficits (Palfrey et al., 1981). Children seem to have fewer attentional difficulties during active physical and motor engagement than during more passive efforts demanding sustained listening, sequential processing, and the retention of verbally presented input. The latter circumstances may approximate much of the experience in a regular classroom. Children with this disorder show little difficulty with attention during the physical examination; this finding is consistent with the observation that such deficits are less likely to manifest themselves during a traditional office visit. In new situations, which are often intimidating, the behavior of these children on a one-to-one basis is often unremarkable, especially in the older children. The problem of situational variability is confounded by the inconsistencies of the reports of parents and teachers. The use of parent and teacher questionnaires is advocated, but these may be subject to strong observer biases and may generate conflicting results.

## *Differential Diagnosis*

In the differential diagnosis of ADD, it is important to be aware that age-appropriate overactivity is different from the haphazard and poorly organized overactivity of ADD children. Children in an inadequate, disorganized, or chaotic environment may have difficulty in sustaining attention and goal-oriented behavior. Neglected children may present with the same symptom pattern as ADHD children. In such cases, it helps to compare the child with his or her siblings (Gittelman, 1980). In severe and profound mental retardation, the additional diagnosis of ADD should not be made; it would make sense only if the retardation were mild or moderate.

Many cases of CD and/or ODD present with symptoms of ADHD. Here the additional diagnosis of ADHD is acceptable. Symptoms of ADHD may also be present in schizophrenia and affective disorders with manic features; the presence of these diagnoses preempts the diagnosis of ADHD.

## *Prevalence*

Earlier estimates that between 5 and 15% of all schoolchildren have some form of hyperactivity, minimal brain dysfunction, or learning disabilities depended on differing definitions and diagnostic criteria. DSM-III-R lists the prevalence as up to 3% of prepubertal children.

Almost all of the studies that examined the sex ratio in hyperactivity revealed that the disorder is more common in boys than in girls. Ratios of 4 boys to 1 girl and of 10 boys to 1 girl were found in the majority of clinical studies. In community samples, the ratio of boys to girls is less than 3:1

(Shekim et al., 1985). DSM-III-R states that ADHD is ten times more common in boys than in girls. On the other hand, in adulthood the disorder is equally common in women and in men (Wender, Reimher, and Wood, 1981; Shekim, Masterson, Cantwell, Hanna, & McCracken, 1989).

## Course

Onset is around the age of 3, though sometimes it may occur as early as infancy. Some mothers may report that the child was overactive in utero. Frequently the disorder does not come to clinical attention until some time during the first 4 years of grade school.

The course is variable. In the past we often thought the disorder to be self-limited, with all of the symptoms disappearing during puberty. We now know that this may be true in some cases; in others, however, the disorder with all its ymptoms persists into adult life. In a third group, hyperactivity may disappear, but impulsivity and attentional problems may persist into adult life.

## Family History

There is enough evidence to suggest that the disorder is more common in family members than in the general population (APA, 1987). Earlier family studies have suggested that alcoholism in the biologic parents, antisocial personality in the biologic fathers, and hysterical personality in the biologic mothers are more prevalent among adult family members of hyperactive children, when compared with adopting parents of hyperactive children and biologic parents of nonhyperactive children (Wender et al., 1981). However, these earlier studies were not done blind, did not define rigorous criteria of hyperactivity, and used normal children as controls. Therefore, the specificity of the association between alcoholism, antisocial personality, and hysterical personality with hyperactivity was in doubt (Stewart, Cummings, Singers, and Debois, 1979). More recent studies on controls with psychiatric diagnoses based on structured interviews failed to demonstrate such a relationship. Antisocial personality and alcoholism were more common in natural fathers of aggressive antisocial boys than in fathers of the other boys, but the prevalence of these disorders did not distinguish fathers of hyperactive boys from father of boys who were not hyperactive (Stewart et al., 1979).

## Etiologies

It is generally accepted that the diagnostic category of ADHD consists of heterogeneous groups with different etiologies. Etiologies that are often considered include maturational lag, brain damage at birth or in early infancy, a disorder of the inhibitory arousal nervous system, food additives, and a disorder in the metabolism and/or the interaction between the catecholamines norepinephrine and dopamine (Shekim et al., 1982a; Zametkin & Rapoport, 1987). It has been suggested that some of these disorders may result from a familial-genetic predisposition and that genetic components of the disorder may be different in different groups (Cantwell, 1975). Most of the earlier works described the families of children with ADHD + CD. More recent work on ADHD children without CD could not find any association with parental psychopathology (Biederman, Munir, & Knee, 1987; Lahey, 1988).

## Treatment

Several modalities are used in the treatment of children, adolescents, and adults with ADHD. The treatment of choice is pharmacotherapy, and stimulants are the most effective. However, other treatment approaches are advocated, and several modalities are used in the single child depending on his or her and family needs. Behavior therapies, including classroom behavior modification, parent training, and cognitive behavioral training, are often used and found effective. Remedial education, environmental (classroom and home) manipulation, individual, family, and group therapies are all modalities used with some success depending on the individual child and family. There is some evidence that ADHD children who receive multimodality treatment with medications are further ahead educationally, demonstrate less antisocial behavior, are more attentive, and are better adjusted at home and at school than ADHD children receiving less treatment (Satterfield, Satterfield, & Cantwell, 1981).

### Psychotropic Drugs

*Psychostimulants.* These include dextroamphetamine, which has been in use longer than any other drug in this group, and methylphenidate, which has been in use for more than 20 years. There is controversy about their use because of their potential for abuse in adolescents and adults. However, most of the evidence seems to show that their use in ADHD children and adolescents decreases chances for alcohol and drug abuse later in life (Cantwell & Hanna, 1989; Loney, Kramer, & Milich, 1981). The two drugs are equally effective in therapeutic doses on hyperactive children. It is also though that dextroamphetamine may have more side effects than methylphenidate. Milligram for milligram, d-amphetamine is twice as potent as methylphenidate. Methylphenidate is used for preschoolers with beneficial results and is also used with success in adolescents and adults with ADHD (Varley, 1983; Wender, Reimherr, Wood, and Ward, 1985). Both medications are short-acting (from 2 to 6 hours, usually 4 hours). Because of this, it has been the practice to prescribe twice-a-day administration. However, several studies have reported good results using a single morning dose. The pattern of clinical use suggests that the milder the symptomatology, the more often the medicines are given once daily.

Magnesium pemoline is a more recently introduced slow-acting psychostimulant. It is not as effective as the other two stimulants; it takes from 2 to 4 weeks before beneficial effects start to show (Conners & Taylor, 1980).

It is customary to start treatment with methylphenidate given once or twice daily (morning and noon). Doses often found effective are 0.3 mg/kg to 0.6 mg/kg of methylphenidate/dose with a maximum of 1 mg/kg/dose and 2 mg/kg/day, not to exceed 60 mg/day except in cases where there are no side effects and the child is showing partial response to the medication. Methylphenidate and d-amphetamine have relatively similar pharmacological mechanisms of action and are expected to be effective in the same child. However, there is evidence now that some children may respond to one and not to the other. Therefore, if methylphenidate is found ineffective, the clinician may want to prescribe dextroamphetamine; d-amphetamine is given in doses half those of methylphenidate, not to exceed 40 mg/day. There is some evidence that d-amphetamine effects may last an extra hour or so; therefore, the clinician may want to use d-amphetamine when therapeutic effect is short-lived.

When there is evidence of drug dependence or when methylphenidate and d-amphetamine are ineffective, the patient should be given magnesium pemoline. The dose given is around 3 mg/kg/day. It has a long half-life and can be given once daily. Occasionally it may be given in the morning and in the afternoon. Insomnia and anorexia, which are more common with methylphenidate and d-amphetamine, do not occur as often with pemoline.

The stimulants are best used for the ADHD child with or without ODD or CD symptoms when symptoms of Tourette's disorder are absent. In the author's experience, stimulants are not very effective when there is a family history of schizophrenia or a schizotypal disorder. Furthermore, when there is a family history of depression and when there are symptoms suggestive of an affective disorder, stimulants may not be the best medication.

It is recommended that the patient's height, weight, pulse, and blood pressure be taken once a month or at least several times a year. It is also suggested that a complete blood count with differential and liver function test be done annually. Furthermore, it is suggested that the need for continued treatment with medication be ascertained by taking the child off medication periodically, perhaps during summer vacation.

*Tricyclic Antidepressants (TCAs).* Antidepressants such as imipramine and desipramine may be used with some beneficial results in children with ADHD. But antidepressants are not as effective as stimulants, and children often become tolerant to these medications (Pliszka, 1987). The general clinical impression is that the tricyclics may be more useful in an ADHD child who also has affective symptoms. Furthermore, a few ADHD children who do not respond to stimulants may respond to tricyclics in doses similar to antidepressant doses (5 mg/kg/day) after 2 to 4 weeks of treatment (Biederman, Gastfriend, & Jellinek, 1986). Moreover, TCAs may be used when the response of the ADHD child to stimulants is very short (less than 2 hours) and when the child rebounds from stimulant effect in the afternoon. TCAs in ADHD treatment are used in 2.5- to 3-mg/kg body weight/day doses. The response to tricyclic antidepressants in ADHD occurs within the first 3 days. One thing that needs to be kept in mind is that in treating ADHD, TCAs should be prescribed in the morning and at noon and not at bedtime, as is customarily done in the treatment of adult depression. This is because of a shorter half-life for imipramine and desipramine in children and because the inhibition of neurotransmitter reuptake, thought to be the mechanism of action in ADHD, is more immediate, while down regulation of the receptor, thought to be the mechanism of action in depression, depends on a steady-state plasma level and is more delayed.

Clonidine, an alpha$_2$ adrenergic receptor agonist, has been shown to be effective in the treatment of ADHD especially in those who have symptoms of anxiety, impulsivity, and aggression. Furthermore, it is also used when symptoms of tics are present (Hunt et al., 1985).

*Antipsychotic Drugs*

The phenothiazines, thioridazine and chlorpromazine, are occasionally used when the stimulants fail to improve the symptoms of ADHD. One must remember, however, that antipsychotics, especially in larger doses, may lead to a decrease in cognitive functioning and impair learning. Antipsychotics may also cause bothersome symptoms of tardive dyskinesia, which now are observed more frequently in children.

L-dopa, lithium, lead chelating agents, and special diets (free from salicylates, additives, preservatives, and food colors) have been used in the treatment of ADD children. More research is needed to establish the true efficacy of such methods. Diet studies are reviewed in another chapter in this volume.

*Behavior Therapy*

Several reports on the effects of behavior therapy in hyperactive children have been published (Barkley, 1981; Cayton & Russo, 1985; Gittelman, 1980; Pelham, 1986). In these reports, a few investigators have concluded that behavior modification may be as effective as the stimulants are. So far, the majority of the evidence suggests that behavior therapy leads to improvement that is perceptible to teachers and parents (Gittelman, 1980). Furthermore, the combination of behavior therapy with psychostimulants produces greater amelioration of symptoms (Barkley, 1981; Gittelman, 1980).

Several methods of behavior modification that can be used to manage the disruptive behavior of children with ADHD have been described (Barkley, 1981; O'Leary & O'Leary, 1976; Pelham, 1986). In addition, some of these methods have been found to improve academic functioning. As with other behavior therapy, it has been found that combining classroom behavior modification with pharmacotherapy proved to be more efficacious than either alone (Barkley, 1981; Pelham, 1986).

Parent training is another method of behavior therapy that is used effectively in the management of disruptive ADHD children. It is suggested that maladaptive behavior results from, and is perpetrated by, faulty interaction between parents and child. Therefore, parents are trained in several procedures that they can utilize to eliminate the undesirable behavior of their child. Several programs have been described (Barkley, 1981; Kazdin, 1985; Patterson, Reid, Jones, & Conger, 1975).

Cognitive behavioral therapies utilize several techniques that use thought processes, self-instruction, and problem-solving skills (Kazdin, 1985; Kendall & Braswell, 1984; Kendall & Hollon, 1979; Meichenbaum & Goodman, 1971). Children are trained to make self-statements; i.e., impulsive children are trained to make statements of becoming more deliberate and more reflective or are taught specific problem-solving skills that help them to come up with more appropriate alternative solutions to interpersonal problems.

*Psychotherapy*

No data are available on the effect of psychotherapy in hyperactive children. Several modalities are used, however, depending on the needs and strengths of the child and the family. For the child, these include individual and group psychotherapy, instruction in socialization skills, activity groups, and educational therapy; for the parents, individual and group psychotherapy.

## Conduct and Oppositional Disorders

Factor-analytic studies have resulted in two factors relating to childhood aggression: overt oppositional or coercive behavior directed toward another person, usually an adult (yelling, screaming, whining, crying), and conduct problems usually involving covert behavior (lying, stealing, firesetting) against property. Antisocial aggressive children function at a normal level when contingencies for performance involve instrumental rewards or punishment. Their common characteristics include short-term gratification of gain and lower levels of competency in academic achievement, sports, job skills, and peer relationships. Finally, there is an apparent decreased sensitivity to both social approval and disapproval compared with normal children.

*Terminology*

DSM-III-R defines conduct disorders as a persistent pattern of behavior that violates the rights of others and deviates from age-appropriate norms set by society. One of the difficulties in making the diagnosis is that many conduct symptoms develop and disappear during formative years. Several factors have been identified that place a child at risk for developing conduct disorders. Difficult and unmanageable behavior in early childhood are significant predictors. Family characteristics such as parents' criminality, antisocial behavior, alcoholism, marital difficulties, inconsistent discipline, and harsh punishment are important risk factors (Kazdin, 1985).

DSM-III classified conduct disorders according to two dimensions of aggression and socialization. Classifications of conduct problems according to these two dimensions resulted in four subgroups: aggressive socialized, nonagressive socialized, aggressive unsocialized, and nonaggressive unsocialized. Since there was little empirical evidence for this subgrouping, DSM-III-R abandoned the two-dimensional approach in favor of the unidimensional socialized–nonsocialized dichotomy. DSM-III-R diagnostic subtyping is more similar to the DSM-II CD categories of unsocialized aggressive reaction and group delinquent reaction, which were based on some empirical work done earlier by Jenkins and Glickman (1946).

*Associated Features*

Symptoms of attentional difficulties, hyperactivity, and impulsivity may be present and may meet the criteria for ADHD. Occasionally, anxiety, depression, low self-esteem, low frustration tolerance, and irritability may be severe enough to warrant an associated diagnosis. Within DSM-III-R, an axis II diagnosis of specific developmental disabilities may often be present.

*Prognosis*

Aggressive symptoms can start early in life, with earlier onset having poorer prognosis. Different types tend to appear at different ages; for example, solitary aggressive type tends to appear before the group type, while in females it usually appears in adolescence.

Many of the symptoms may disappear with time especially in milder forms. Fifty percent of all cases may continue to exhibit antisocial disorder in

## Attention Deficit and Conduct Disorders

adulthood, especially the severer forms. The disorder may be more severe if family background includes parental psychopathology, parental criminality, inconsistent discipline, harsh punishment, comorbidity with ADHD, and/or learning disabilities.

### Prevalence and Sex Ratio

Many children manifest antisocial behaviors at one time or another in their development; symptoms remit and others appear. Some behaviors are more common in boys; other are more common in girls. Boys are more likely to be referred for aggressive behavior, stealing, and lying. There is also evidence that there are gender differences related to the age of onset of the disorder. For example, age of onset for the majority of boys, was around 8 to 10 years, while in the majority of girls age of onset was around 14 to 16 years (Kazdin, 1985). Generally, as many as 15% of children may demonstrate some antisocial behavior at one point or another in their lives; however, it is not known how many of these children can be given the diagnosis of conduct disorder according to DSM-III or DSM-III-R criteria (Cantwell, 1989).

### Treatment

There is a large body of literature on a variety of treatment modalities used in children with conduct disorder. However, most of these studies are plagued with methodological problems that do not allow for clear conclusions on treatment effectiveness. The traditional methods of treatment in psychiatry, such as individual and group psychotherapies and especially the insight-oriented therapies, have not proven to be effective. There is some evidence that behavior therapy, parent training techniques, and pharmacotherapy may be more effective.

### Behavior Therapy

*General Approach.* (For a more detailed description of the different approaches, see Barkley, 1981). Parents and therapist select and define a target behavior as the focus of behavioral intervention. Parents are then instructed to "tally" the target behavior as to its frequency, the time of day it occurs, what cues precipitate it, and what consequences the parents provide. Records are reviewed with the parents, and an attempt is made to alter the controlling cues for the target behavior, the consequences, and their timing. The therapist needs to evaluate the changes continuously. Finally, the program is reviewed on the basis of success or failure.

*Positive Reinforcement Method.* With an ODD or CD child it is better to begin any behavior modification program with positive reinforcements for desirable alternatives to the targeted inappropriate behaviors. Numerous studies have shown that positive reinforcers after a child's display of appropriate behavior frequently increases the occurrence of that behavior. Praise and social attention upon occurrence of positive behavior are the most common reinforcements used. Food, recreational pursuits, games, or outings are frequently used reinforcers. Tokens, points, or stars can be exchanged with established reinforcers. A reinforcement menu can be designed for 10 to 15 activities or items with a corresponding point value for each (Barkley, 1981).

The type of reinforcers that are chosen for any particular program will have some influence on the effectiveness of the program. Reinforcement given continuously is more likely to increase the desired behavior than are reinforcers given intermittently. However, the desired behavior is more likely to disappear faster when reinforced continuously. A solution to this problem is to start a program with continuous reinforcement and then switch to an intermittent schedule.

*Punishment Methods.* Punishment methods include one of two procedures: the use of an aversive or unpleasant event following an undesirable behavior, or the removal of a positive reinforcer. Most commonly used is the withdrawal of attention from the child; this may temporarily increase the behavior, but with time the behavior will decrease gradually.

Another approach is the "response cost." The occurrence of undesirable target behavior results in the child's giving back tokens or points. This may be more effective than the use of positive reinforcers.

Another method of punishment procedure is the "time-out" from reinforcement. Duration of the time-out may vary with the age of the child and the severity of the misbehavior. The location of the time-out is extremely important.

Disapproval or reprimand also can be considered as forms of punishment.

*Self-Control.* Deficiencies in self control in children are thought to be either the result of poor training or the result of a dysfunction of neuronal circuits involved in the development of self-control skills, especially in the prefrontal cortical region.

Research has focused on the use of language in the training of self-control. Fantasies and mental images also can play a role in teaching self-control. One of the shortcomings of self-control training is that behavior changes do not persist after treatment termination and do not generalize outside the situation in which the procedure has been taught (Barkley, 1981).

*Parent Training*

Parent training techniques have been shown to be an effective modality of treatment. Parent training is done within the home and uses parents as therapists. Improvement has been demonstrated in the home and school settings and was shown to last for a year or more (Cantwell, 1989). Parent training requires high motivation and commitment from parents. Many families are not good candidates for such training, and a selection is always attempted initially.

*Pharmacotherapy*

The primary treatment approach for conduct disorders is a combination of psychosocial and behavioral approaches. A trial of psychotropic medications may facilitate other types of therapy. When other psychiatric conditions are present (e.g., ADHD, depression) medications also may be used.

*Lithium.* There is evidence that lithium carbonate is useful in the treatment of children with severe aggressive behavior disorders, with bipolar disorder, or with unsocialized aggressive conduct disorder (Campbell, Perry, & Green, 1984a; Campbell, Small, et al., 1984; Platt, Campbell, Green, & Grega, 1984). Lithium has been found to help children and adolescents characterized by explosive anger, hostility, and irritability, many of who met criteria of conduct disorder and in the absence of affective disorder. When used judiciously, lithium is relatively safe and is well tolerated.

*Stimulants.* Aggression appears to respond to stimulant treatment when conduct disorder is present in association with ADHD. Several studies demonstrated a decrease of hyperactivity and conduct problems in ADHD children treated with stimulants (Shekim, Dekimenjan, Chapel, Javaid, & Davis, 1979; Shekim et al., 1982; Zametkin et al., 1985). Clinical experience also suggests that ADHD children's disruptive behaviors decrease when treated with stimulants. However, there is no evidence that stimulants have any beneficial effects in "pure" conduct or oppositional defiant disorders.

*Antidepressants.* The presence of depressive illness in association with conduct disorder has been documented (Carlson & Cantwell, 1980; Puig-Antich, 1982). Depressive symptoms may precede the onset of conduct problems. When the depressive symptoms respond to antidepressants, conduct problems improved and often reappeared when the children relapsed into a depressive illness (Puig-Antich, 1982). There are no studies examining the effects of antidepressants, either tricyclics or monoamine oxidase inhibitors, in CD. However, there is evidence that symptoms of disruptive behavior and impulsivity in children with ADHD respond to treatment with tricyclic antidepressants (Pliszka, 1987). More research on the effect of antidepressants in pure and mixed conduct disorder is needed.

*Neuroleptics.* Neuroleptics are commonly used in the treatment of aggressive children (Campbell et al., 1984b; Platt et al., 1984). In one well-designed placebo-controlled study in a carefully diagnosed large sample of hospitalized children with undersocialized aggressive type conduct disorder, haloperidol was found to be better than placebo in controlling aggressive symptoms (Campbell et al., 1984b). These children had failed to respond to previous treatment attempts. Neuroleptics have short- and long-term adverse effects, and they should be used only when other treatments have failed.

Clonidine has also been shown to reduce impulsive and disruptive behavior in children with ADHD, ODD, and/or CD (Hunt, Minderra, & Cohen, 1985). There is no evidence that clonidine is beneficial in pure CD or ODD. Clonidine has been found to be effective in the treatment of mania in adults (Hardy, Leerubier, & Widlocker, 1986) and has been used in the treatment of children and adolescents with manic symptoms. More research is needed in this area.

*Anticonvulsants.* If CD is present in association with epilepsy, carbamazepine (Tegretol) and valproic acid (Depakene) may be helpful in decreasing aggressive conduct problems, especially if there are EEG abnormalities (McElroy, Keck, & Pope, 1987; O'Donnell, 1985). Carbamazepine and valproic acid have been shown to be effective in the treatment of aggressive and hypomanic symptoms in the presence of a mildly abnormal or borderline EEG findings not diagnostic of a seizure disorder.

*Propranolol.* There is some evidence that propranolol, a beta-adrenergic blocker, may effectively control aggressive outbursts and violent behavior (Mattes, 1986). Propranolol may be tried when everything else has failed.

### Summary

Diagnostic issues, boundaries, and phenomenology of disruptive behavior disorders are being clarified and delineated. Improved and more specific assessment methods have enabled researchers and clinicians to communicate their findings more clearly. Improved diagnostic work-up (see Table 1) has resulted in a proliferation of more scientific work with different treatment modalities. Effectiveness and limitations of each treatment modality may now be substantiated. There is evidence that pharmacotherapy and behavior therapies are two effective treatments of disruptive behavior disorders; their combination in the same child may have additive effects.

Several issues in the diagnosis and treatment of disruptive behavior disorders still remain controversial. The relationship between ADHD and CD needs

## Table 1
### Diagnostic Work-Up for Disruptive Behavior Disorders

1. Diagnostic interview with the parent and child: pregnancy, birth, and infancy, developmental history, family history, emotional, social interaction, school performance, mental status exam
2. Information from school: educational, psychoeducational
3. Parent and teacher rating scales—baseline and drug follow-up: Parent and teacher (Conners, 1970); Child Behavior Checklist—parent and teacher (Achenbach & Edelbrock, 1983); ACTeRS (Ullman, Sleater, & Sprague, 1986); Child Depression Inventory
4. Review of systems, medical history, physical and neurological exam: EEG, audiometry, visual screening, neurological consult if needed
5. Psychoeducational testing, psycholinguistic testing, neuropsychological testing, as needed
6. Optional: structured interview, Continuous Performance Test of attention and impulsivity, Matching Familiar Figure Test of impulsivity and reflectivity, Paired Associate Learning Test— in diagnostic challenges or in clinical/research program

to be further clarified. The effectiveness of pharmacotherapies in pure ADHD or pure CD also needs to be explored. Newer and possibly more effective treatments heed to be tried. In the opinion of the author, improved treatment depends on an increase in the understanding of the pathophysiological mechanisms of ADHD and CD.

## References

Achenbach, T. M., & Edelbrock, C. S. (1983). *Manual for the Child Behavior Checklist and Revised Child Behavior Profile.* Burlington, VT.

American Psychiatric Association. (1987) *Diagnostic and statistical manual of mental disorders* (3rd ed.-rev.) Washington, DC: Author.

Barkley, R. A. (1981). *Hyperactive children: A handbook for diagnosis and treatment* (pp. 237–270), New York: Guilford Press.

Biederman, J., Gastfriend, D. R., & Jellinek, M. S. (1986). Desipramine in the treatment of children with attention deficit disorder. *Journal of Clinical Psychopharmacology, 6*, 359–363.

Biederman, J., Munir K., & Knee, D. (1987). Conduct and oppositional disorder in clinically referred children with attention deficit disorder: A controlled family study. *Journal of the American Academy of Child and Adolescent Psychiatry, 26*, 724–727.

Campbell, M., Perry, R., & Green, W. H. (1984). Use of lithium in children and adolescents. *Psychosomatics, 25*, 95–106.

Campbell, M., Small, R. M., Green, W. H., Jennings, S. J., Perry, R., Bennett, W. G., & Anderson, L. (1984) Behavioral efficacy of haloperidol and lithium carbonate. *Archives of General Psychiatry, 41*, 650–656.

Cantwell, D. P. (1975). Genetics of hyperactivity. *Journal of Child Psychology and Psychiatry, 16*, 261–264.

Cantwell, D. P. (1977). Hyperkinetic syndrome. In M. Rutter & L. Hersov (Eds.), *Child psychiatry, modern approaches.* London: Blackwell Scientific.

Cantwell, D. P. (1989). Conduct disorder. In H. I. Kaplan & B. J. Sadock (Eds.), *Comprehensive textbook of psychiatry* (Vol. 5). Baltimore: Williams & Wilkins, pp. 1821–1828.

Cantwell, D. P., & Hanna, G. L. (1989). Attention deficit disorder. In A. Tasman, R. E. Hales, & A. J. Frances (Eds.), *Review of psychiatry,* (Vol. 8).

Carlson, G. A., Cantwell, D. P. (1980). Unmasking masked depression in children and adolescents. *American Journal of Psychiatry, 137,*455–459.

Cayton, T. G., & Russo, D. C. (1985). The behavior therapies. In D. Shaffer, A. A. Ehrhardt, & L. L. Greenhill (Eds.), *The clinical guide to child psychiatry* (pp. 519–538). New York: Tree Press.

Conners, C. K. (1969). A teacher rating scale for use in drug studies with children. *American Journal of Psychiatry, 126,*152–156.

Conners, C. K. (1970). Symptom patterns in hyperkinetic, neurotic, and normal children. *Child Development, 41,*667–682.

Conners, C. K., & Taylor, E. (1980). Pemoline, methylphenidate and placebo in children with minimal brain dysfunction. *Archives of General Psychiatry, 37,*922–930.

Edelbrock, C., Costello, A. J., & Kessler, M. D. (1984). Empirical corroboration of attention deficit disorder. *Journal of the American Academy of Child and Adolescent Psychiatry, 23,*285–290.

Gittelman, R. (1980). Diagnosis and drug treatment of childhood disorders. In D. F. Klein, R. Gittelman, F. Quitkin, *Diagnosis and treatment of psychiatric disorders* (pp. 590–775). Baltimore: Williams & Wilkins.

Hardy, M. C., Lecrubier, Y., & Widlocher, L. (1986). Efficacy of clonidine in 24 patients with acute mania. *American Journal of Psychiatry, 143,*1450–1453.

Hunt, R. D., Minderra, R., & Cohen, D. J. (1985). Clonidine benefits children with attention deficit disorder and hyperactivity: Report of a double-blind placebo crossover therapeutic trial. *Journal of the American Academy of Child and Adolescent Psychiatry, 24,*617–629.

Jenkins, R. L., & Glickman, S. (1946). Common syndromes in child psychiatry: I. Deviant behavior traits. II. The Schizoid child. American Journal of Orthopsychiatry, 16,244–261.

Kazdin, A. (1985). *Treatment of antisocial behavior in children and adolescents.* Homewood, IL: Dorsey Press.

Kendall, P. C., & Braswell, L. (1984). *Cognitive behavioral therapy for impulsive children.* New York: Guilford Press.

Kendall, P. C., & Hollon, S. D. (Eds.) (1979). *Cognitive-behavioral interventions: Theory, research, and procedures.* New York: Academic Press.

Lahey, B. B., Pianceutini, J. C., McBurnett, K., Stove, P., Martdagen, S., and Hynd, G. (1988). Psychopathology in the parents of children with conduct disorder and hyperactivity. *Journal of the American Academy of Child and Adolescent Psychiatry, 27,*163–170.

Langhorne, J. E., & Loney, J. (1979). A 4-fold model for subgrouping the hyperkinetic/MBD syndrome. *Child Psychiatry and Human Development, 9,*153–159.

Loney, J., Kramer, J., & Milich, R. (1981). The hyperkinetic child grows up: Predictors of symptoms, delinquency, and achievement at follow-up. In K. D. Gadow & J. Loney (Eds.), *Psychosocial aspects of drug treatment for hyperactivity.* Boulder, CO: Westview Press.

Loney, J., Langhorne, H. E., Jr., & Paternite, C. E. (1978). An empirical basis for subgrouping the hyperkinetic/minimal brain dysfunction syndrome. *Journal of Abnormal Psychology, 87,*431–441.

Mattes, J. A. (1986). Propranolol for adults with temper outbursts and residual attention deficit disorder. *Journal of Clinical Psychopharmacology, 6,*299–302.

McElroy, S. L., Keck, P. E., & Pope, H. G. (1987). Sodium valproate: Its use in primary psychiatric disorders. *Journal of Clinical Psychopharmacology, 7,*16–24.

Meichenbaum, D. H., & Goodman, J. (1971). Training impulsive children to talk to themselves: A means of developing self-control. *Journal of Abnormal Psychology, 77,*115–126.

Milich, R., Loney, J., & Landau, S. (1982). Independent dimensions of hyperactivity and aggression: A validation with playroom observation data. *Journal of Abnormal Psychology, 91,*183–198.

O'Donnell, P. J. (1985). In J. M. Wiener (Ed.) Conduct disorders in diagnosis and psychopharmacology of childhood and adolescent disorders (pp. 250–287). New York: Wiley.
O'Leary, K. D., & O'Leary, S. G. (1976). Behavior modification in the school. In *Handbook of behavior modification and behavior therapy.* New York: Appleton-Century-Crofts.
Palfrey, S. J., Levine, M. D., Oberklaid, F., Lerner, M., and Anfseeser, C.L. (1981). An analysis of observed attention and activity patterns in preschool children. *Journal of Pediatrics, 98,*1006–1011.
Patterson, G. R., Reid, J. B., Jones, R. R., & Conger, R. E. (1975). *A social learning approach to family intervention.* Eugene, OR: Castalia.
Pelham, W. E. (1986). Behavior therapy. In *Attention Deficit Disorder.* E. K. Sleator & W. E. Pelham (Eds.), (pp. 127–161). Norwalk, CT: Appleton-Century-Crofts.
Platt, J. E., Campbell, M., Green, W. H., & Grega, D. M. (1984). Cognitive effects of lithium carbonate and haloperidol in treatment-resistant aggressive children. *Archives of General Psychiatry, 41,*657–662.
Pliszka, S. R. (1987). Tricyclic antidepressants in the treatment of children with attention deficit disorder. *Journal of the Academy of Child and Adolescent Psychiatry, 26,*127–132.
Puig-Antich, J. (1982). Major depression and conduct disorder in prepuberty. *Journal of the American Academy of Child Psychiatry, 21,*118–128.
Quay, H. C. (1979). Classification. In H. C. Quay & J. S. Werry (Eds.), *Psychopathological disorders of childhood* (2nd ed., pp. 1–42). New York: Wiley.
Reeves, J. C., Werry, J. S., Elkind, G. S., & Zametkin, A. *(1987). Attention deficit, conduct, oppositional, and anxiety disorders in children: II. Clinical characteristics. Journal of the American Academy of Child and Adolescent Psychiatry, 26,*144–155.
Satterfield, J. H., Satterfield, B. T., & Cantwell, D. P. (1981). Three-year multimodality treatment study of 100 hyperactive boys. *Journal of Pediatrics, 98,*650–655.
Shekim, W. O., Dekirmenjian, H., Chapel, J. L., Javaid, J., & Davis, J. M. (1979). Norepinephrine metabolism and clinical response to dextroamphetamine in hyperactive boys. *Journal of Pediatrics, 95,*389–394.
Shekim, W. O., Dekirmenjian, H., Javaid, J., Bylund, D. B., & Davis, J. M. (1982a). Dopamine-norepinephrine interaction in hyperactive boys treated with d-amphetamine. *Journal of Pediatrics, 100,*830–834.
Shekim, W. O., Javaid, J., Dekirmenjian, D., Chapel, J. L., & Davis, J. M. (1982b). Effects of d-amphetamine on urinary metabolites of dopamine and norepinephrine in hyperactive boys. *American Journal of Psychiatry, 139,*485–488.
Shekim, W. O., Masterson, A., Cantwell, D. P., Hanna, G. L., & McCracken, J. T. (in press). Nomifensine maleate in adult ADD. *Journal of Nervous and Mental Disease.*
Shekim, W. O., Kashani, J., Beck, N., Cantwell, D. P., Martin, J., Rosenberg, J., & Costello, A. J. (1985). The prevalence of attention deficit disorder in a rural sample of nine-year-old children. *Journal of the American Academy of Child and Adolescent Psychiatry, 24,* 765–770.
Stewart, M. A., Cummings, C., Singer, S. (1981). The overlap between hyperactive and unsocialized aggressive children. *Journal of Child Psychology and Psychiatry, 22,*35–45.
Ullmann, R. K., Sleator, E. K., & Sprague, R. L. (1986). Introduction to the use of ACTeRS. *Psychopharmacology Bulletin, 21,*915–920.
Varley, C. (1983). Effects of methylphenidate in adolescents with attention deficit disorder. *Journal of the American Academy of Child Psychiatry, 22,*351–354.
Wender, P. H., Reimheer, F. W., & Wood, D. R. (1981). Attention deficit disorder (minimal brain dysfunction) in adults: A replication study of diagnosis and drug treatment. *Archives of General Psychiatry, 38,*449–456.
Wender, P. H., Reimheer, F. W., Wood, D. R., & Ward, M. (1985). A controlled study of methylphenidate in the treatment of attention deficit disorder, residual type (ADD, RT or "minimal brain dysfunction" in adults). *American Journal of Psychiatry, 142,*547–552.

Werry, S. J., Reeves, J. D., & Elkind, G. S. (1987). Attention deficit, conduct, oppositional, and anxiety disorders in children: I. A review of research on differentiating characteristics. *Journal of the American Academy of Child and Adolescent Psychiatry, 26*,133–143.

Zametkin, A. J., Karoum, F., Linnoila, M., Rapoport, J. L., Brown, G. L., Chang, L. W., & Wyatt, R. J. (1985). Stimulants, urinary catecholamines and indoleamines in hyperactivity: A comparison of methylphenidate and dextroamphetamine. *Archives of General Psychiatry, 42*,251–255.

Zametkin, A. J., & Rapoport, J. L. (1987). Neurobiology of attention deficit disorder with hyperactivity: Where have we come in 50 years. *Journal of the American Academy of Child and Adolescent Psychiatry, 26*,676–686.

# 2

# Adolescent Depression
# A Treatment Review

## S. P. Kutcher and P. Marton

Major depression in adolescents has recently been well characterized, and its phenomenological, epidemiological, interpersonal, social, and biologic aspects are now subjected to serious empirical study (Carlson & Strober, 1979; Kutcher & Marton, 1989; Rutter, Izard, & Read, 1986; Ryan & Puig-Antich, 1986). Previously advocated theories of the "normality" or "inevitability" of depression in adolescents (Baker, 1978; Blos, 1967; Freud, 1958) have given way to an understanding of adolescent depression as a serious psychiatric disorder with significant short- and long-term sequelae (Kutcher & Marton, 1989; Rutter et al., 1986; Ryan & Puig-Antich, 1986; Weller, Weller, & Herjanic, 1983). For example, declining academic performance, disturbed interpersonal and family relationships, substance abuse, disordered eating, and suicide are all associated with depression in adolescents. Long-term sequelae include recurrent depressive illnesses, academic and vocational difficulties, problems with intimate relationships, and use of mental health services. Given the seriousness of the effects of depressive illness on a wide variety of social, interpersonal, and vocational areas, demonstrated effective treatment of acute depressive episodes and the prevention of relapses is vital.

Although a variety of psychological and biological therapies have been shown to be effective in the treatment of adult depression (Baldessarini, 1983; Klerman, DiMasco, and Weissman, 1974), the extrapolation of the "adult" treatments to adolescents is fraught with difficulties. Psychologically, adolescents demonstrate different cognitive and emotional sets than do adults (Keating, 1980). The social milieu and support systems of the adolescent differ significantly from those of the adult (Coleman, 1980). Thus, psychological therapies designed for adults may not be applicable in the adolescent age group.

---

*S. P. Kutcher and P. Marton*   Department of Psychiatry and Department of Psychology, Sunnybrook Medical Centre, University of Toronto, Toronto, Ontario M4N 3M5, Canada.

Similarly, the biologic milieu of the adolescent is rapidly changing over the entire pubertal period (Johnson & Singer, 1982; Nottelman et al., 1987; Seifert, Foxx, & Butler, 1980). The neuroendocrine and central nervous system responses to biologic manipulations often differ between adults and adolescents (Popper, 1987). Further, early pubertal teens may differ significantly from late pubertal teens, both psychologically and biologically, possibly necessitating different therapeutic approaches even within the adolescent age group. Therefore, specific therapies must be developed, and their efficacy must be demonstrated in adolescents as a group and not simply transferred to teens on the basis of previous success in adult populations. Different stages of adolescence may also require different therapeutic approaches; thus, treatments may need to be shown to be subspecific. Treatments for adolescent depression must therefore arise out of carefully implemented studies of specific modalities in which the variables of age, pubertal stage, cognitive level, and social capabilities are considered.

As with any treatment for a psychiatric disorder, treatment for adolescent depression must meet specific criteria prior to general acceptance (Kazdin, 1986a). First, it must be shown to be effective through the use of carefully constructed and empirically validated studies, preferably using untreated control groups. Presumed psychological, social, or biologic etiological constructs may be useful in the development of treatment methods, but they should never be advocated as a priori validation of any treatment. Second, specific treatment factors that ameliorate the disorder must be identified and separated from more general or nonspecific treatment effects. Third, treatments must be shown not to be harmful, or at least they should do less harm than good. Not only must this be shown for every specific modality but the use of one modality to the exclusion of another must be shown to be more beneficial, so that the patient will not be denied a potentially more effective treatment. Fourth, predictors of treatment outcome must be identified. An extension of this principle is the identification of relapse predictors.

This chapter will review the different psychological, social, and biological treatments advocated for adolescent depression. They will be described and evaluated using the four criteria noted above. It is hoped that the issues raised in this review for adolescent depression will stimulate thoughtful consideration of current treatment modalities, an awareness of their strengths and limitations, and a critical approach to one's own clinical strategies.

## *Psychological Therapies*

Psychotherapy for the depressed adolescent is commonly given during the acute episode. However, as the work of DiNicola and Simeon (1988), Garber,

Kriss, Koch, & Lindholm (1988), and McCauley et al. (1988) suggests, depressed adolescents treated during the acute phase often are functioning poorly at follow-up. Further, a substantial number develop recurrent depressive episodes.

Studies of psychotherapeutic approaches in adult depression have mostly evaluated cognitive, behavioral, and interpersonal methods, both with and without concurrent pharmacologic interventions (Shea, Elkin, & Hirschfeld, 1988). In general, no one treatment approach has been shown to be superior to the others. A clear understanding of why psychotherapy is effective is not yet available. These three psychotherapeutic approaches share a number of common features that may account—at least in part—for their effects: They are structured, they advocate a goal-oriented approach arising from collaboration between an active therapist and an active patient, and they all emphasize current issues. Insight-oriented long-term psychotherapy has not been shown to be effective in treating adult depression.

A number of authors have adapted treatments for depressed adolescents that have initially been shown to be effective for depressed adults (Molick & Pinkston, 1982; Schloss, Schloss, & Harris, 1984; Trautman & Rotheram-Borus, 1988; Wilkes & Rush, 1988). These have included cognitive techniques and behavioral interventions. However, in spite of the variety of possible approaches, only two studies of psychotherapy in depressed teens meet the treatment criteria outlined above.

## Cognitive–Behavioral Approaches to Therapy

Reynolds and Coates (1986) compared a cognitive behavior therapy program with both a progressive muscle relaxation approach and a waiting list control group. Thirty adolescent high school students not identified as clinically depressed were randomly assigned to one of the above groups on the basis of self-reported depression scores in the clinical range on one of the following instruments: Beck Depression Inventory (BDI, cutoff score of 11); Reynolds Adolescent Depression Scale (RADS, cutoff score of 71); and the Bellevue Index of Depression (BID, cutoff score of 19). Both treatment groups underwent structured, goal-oriented interventions involving "homework" and face-to-face contract with an experienced school psychologist for 10 one-hour sessions.

Six subjects dropped out of the active treatment groups (3 in each), leaving 14 treatment completers. Ten subjects remained as waiting list controls during the study. Both treatments resulted in statistically significant within-group improvement on all depression ratings; no differences were found between the two treatments. At 1-month follow-up, improvement was maintained across both modalities.

Although the authors argue that these results show that cognitive behavior treatment may be an effective intervention in adolescent depression, great care must be taken in generalizing from the study. The subjects were not clinically depressed, and the same measures used to select subjects were used to evaluate outcome—introducing the possibility of response bias. The two treatment modalities were equally effective, showing no superiority for the cognitive-behavioral approach; however, the study sample was too small to evaluate possible between-treatment differences. Finally, while the authors claim a 79% treatment response; when dropouts are counted, the improvement rates drops to 55%—basically identical to the 44% improvement found in the untreated waiting list group.

Lewinsohn, Clarke, Hops, Andrews, & Osteen (1987) assessed the efficacy of a 7-week course of cognitive-behavioral therapy in adolescent depression diagnosed by DSM-III criteria using the K-SADS. Sixty-one depressed teens were randomly assigned to three treatment conditions: a cognitive behavioral psychoeducation group, cognitive-behavioral therapy plus parental involvement in a separate but complementary group, and a wait list condition. Forty-six percent of treated adolescents were rated as improved, with no significant difference between types of treatment noted. Treatment gains were found to be maintained up to 2 years at follow-up. Of interest is that parental involvement was not found to significantly improve treatment response.

Methodological difficulties make interpretation of some of the above findings difficult, and although treatment outcome was not exceedingly robust in either the Lewinsohn et al. (1987) or the Reynolds and Coates (1986) studies, these results suggest that cognitive therapies may be useful in the treatment of adolescent depression. Much further research remains to be done in this area before efficacy is clearly established.

Future studies should demonstrate more clearly how treatment influences the natural course of the depression by tracking the time of onset, duration, and offset of the depressive episode. Furthermore, in addition to addressing symptom change, the treatment effect on the features thought to be antecedents, correlates, or consequences of depression—such as cognitive and attitudinal distortions, impaired social skills, disturbed self-concept, and personality problems—should be assessed. In addition, the specificity of particular therapeutic techniques needs to be determined and isolated from general therapeutic effects that can be demonstrated across a wide variety of psychotherapies.

## Psychodynamic Psychotherapy

The literature on psychodynamic psychotherapy of adolescent depression usually describes presumed dynamic models of depression and defines treatment from these assumptions (Anthony, 1970; Bemporad, 1988). The state of the art in evaluating this form of adolescent psychotherapy has recently been reviewed and lamented by Kazdin (1986a, b) and Shaffer (1984). No evidence exists as to the effectiveness, positive cost-benefit, or specific indications for psychodynamic treatment in adolescents.

To date, no attempts have been made to adopt and evaluate in adolescents the Interpersonal Psychotherapy model developed by Klerman, Weissman, Rounsaville, and Chevon (1984). This particular psychotherapy model holds promise because it operationally addresses prominent areas of dysfunction and has clearly specified treatment procedures.

## Family Therapy

There is little if any literature on the effectiveness of family therapy in treating adolescent depression, probably owing to the lack of attention given by family therapists to diagnostic issues and the underdeveloped state of family therapy evaluation. Nevertheless, this is an important research area. Family therapists emphasize clear and operationally defined techniques, such as family sculpting, the use of genograms, and paradoxical interventions, which are amenable to outcome evaluation (Coyne, Kahn, & Gotlib, 1987; Rutter, 1982). Further, good studies of specific models of family intervention in adult schizophrenia (Kuipers & Babbington, 1988) may suggest possible treatment approaches that could be modified for use in adolescent depression. To date, however, the value of any kind of family therapy in treating depressed adolescents remains intuitively appealing but essentially unproven.

## Social Therapies

The literature on social difficulties associated with adolescent depression has noted that many problems in social and interpersonal functioning persist beyond remission of the depressive disorder (Korenblum et al., 1988; Puig-Antich, Lukens, Doris, Goetz, Brennan-Quattrock, & Todak, 1985). Whether these impairments in interpersonal functioning actually constitute risk factors for future episodes is yet unclear. However, although social treatments have been described for depressed adults, no such approaches seem to be currently under study in teens. The development of such treatments may significantly contribute to the improvement of specific deficits associated with depression and to the prevention of recurrences.

## Biological Therapies

### Antidepressants

Studies of tricyclic antidepressant (TCA) treatment in depressed adolescents have been few, and no clear directions for the use of these medications have yet been determined (Kramer & Feiguine, 1981; Ryan & Puig-Antich, 1986; Ryan et al., 1986). Kramer and Feiguine (1981) treated 10 depressed teens with a fixed dose (200 mg/day) of amitriptyline (AMI) and compared them with an equal number of controls. They were unable to demonstrate a positive drug effect. However, their study exhibited serious deficiencies, including no placebo washout, lack of standardized diagnostic and evaluative tools, and no monitoring of plasma levels. These deficiencies, when compounded by the very small sample size, make *any* conclusions drawn from this study tenuous at best.

Ryan et al. (1986) reported an open 6-week trial of imipramine (IMI) in 34 depressed younger adolescents. Although only 44% were clinically judged as improved, the lack of both a placebo washout and a double-blind placebo design makes interpretation difficult. In a companion report on 29 depressed adolescents, Ryan et al. (1987) noted that single daily IMI dosage did not significantly alter cardiac parameters over three times per day dosage—suggesting that a single dose of IMI may be the preferred dosage schedule. Ryan et al. (1986) further reported a ninefold range in plasma levels of IMI and its major metabolites, suggesting great variability in achievable plasma levels at a fixed dose of IMI in teens. These findings support the monitoring of plasma drug levels to determine dosage requirements in clinical practice.

Extein, Pottash, Gold, Goggans, & Lydiard (1986) have reported a 75% response rate in an open trial of nortriptyline (NPT) in depressed hospitalized adolescents. Drug treatment was directed at maintaining a plasma level of 50 ng/ml to 140 ng/ml for at least 21 consecutive days. They reported no significant side effects and suggested that adolescents require lower doses than adults. Kutcher and Marton (1989) have noted that an open trial of 200 mg/day of desipramine (DMI) in older hospitalized depressed teens resulted in a 60% improvement rate. Currently, the efficacy of DMI in this population is being evaluated in proper placebo washout, double-blind controlled trials.

Although suggestive of a positive therapeutic effect in adolescents, TCAs have not been adequately evaluated in this age group. No studies to date have met the four treatment evaluation criteria outlined above. Further, TCA treatment is not without its risks—particularly in higher dosages or overdose (Biggs, Spiker, Petit, & Ziegler, 1977). Thus, although the treatment literature suggests a useful role for TCA treatment in adolescent depression, such a conclusion must be qualified by the verdict of "not proven."

Studies of monoamine oxidase inhibitors (MAOIs) as a first-line treatment of adolescent depression have not to our knowledge been reported. Ryan et al. (1988a) reviewed the charts of 23 depressed adolescents, of whom 21 had been previously refractory to TCA treatment. These patients were then treated either with MAOI alone or in combination with a TCA, and 74% were rated as clinically improved. Side effects and dietary problems were infrequently noted. Although these findings are encouraging, MAOI use in adolescents awaits a proper treatment study. The issue of dietary restrictions in this age group do not make MAOIs at this time the initial drugs of choice, except in teens who can be trusted with dietary compliance.

## Lithium Carbonate

Lithium carbonate augmentation of TCA nonresponse has been described in adult depressives (De Montigny, Mayer, & Deschines, 1981; De Montigny, Cournoyer, Morisette, Langlois, & Caville, 1983). Ryan, Meyer, Dachille, Mazzie, & Puig-Antich (1988b) have recently reported that a similar regime was effective in 43% of depressed adolescents previously refractory to a TCA alone. Lithium augmentation did not appear to significantly increase side effects, but the time period needed for lithium therapy to be clinically effective was longer than that reported in adults. Although this was an open clinical trial, the data suggest that further studies of lithium in depressed adolescents are indicated—both as a primary and a secondary treatment.

## Antidepressant Guidelines

The lack of sufficient outcome studies of antidepressant use in teenage depressives make clinical guidelines for their use difficult. Effective doses have not been firmly established, nor have "adult" serum levels been shown to correlate with clinical response. The dangers of their use in a potentially suicidal population are well known. Using the general guideline of the least "toxic" approach, antidepressants should probably be introduced only after an initial trial of individual, family, or social treatment lasting at least 3 to 4 weeks has proven ineffective. Antidepressants, particularly those with the best-tolerated side effect profiles (NTP, DMI), should be added only after a full medical workup. Weekly cardiac function monitoring and steady-state serum drug levels should be used to titrate dosage requirements.

Careful medication monitoring is essential, and pharmacotherapy should not be prescribed outside of a comprehensive treatment plan that includes individual, family, and social interventions. Drug education must precede drug prescription, and weekly reviews of medication efficacy and side effects should be part of the treatment routine. If no significant clinical improvement is noted following an adequate trial (6 weeks at "adult" steady-state levels), a course of lithium augmentation following the same strict guidelines is a reasonable approach. Continued nonresponsiveness should lead to an inpatient evaluation or consultation with a specialized pharmacological treatment unit.

## Other Biological Treatments

A number of other somatic treatments have been described as successful in treating adult depressions, including thyroid hormone (Whybrow & Prange,

1981), sleep deprivation (Roy-Byrne, Uhde, & Post, 1984), methylphenidate (Janowsky, El-Yousef, Dorris, & Sekerke, 1973), electroconvulsive therapy (Fink, 1979), and phototherapy (Issacs, Stainer, Sensky, Moor, & Thompson, 1988). No properly conducted evaluative studies of these treatment modalities have, to our knowledge, been reported in adolescents. Their effectiveness in the depressed adolescent remains speculative to date, and they should not be undertaken outside of a specialized treatment research center well versed in their use, and then only with full informed consent in ethically approved research protocols or in exceptional clinical circumstances.

## Combined Treatment

No studies to date have evaluated the effectiveness of combining various forms of psychotherapies with biological treatments. However, given the multiplicity of interpersonal and biological disturbances found in adolescent depression, multimodal treatment approaches may hold greater promise than single treatments used alone. Although this approach is logical, it too awaits proper evaluation.

## Conclusions

Although adolescent depression is a relatively common psychiatric illness with a serious clinical course, its treatment to date is often based on practitioner preference, unproven etiologic hypotheses, or uncritical applications of methods designed for adult patients. Well-conducted research studies of *all* types of treatment modalities in adolescent depression are urgently needed, and they should be a priority in the development of research programs in this age group.

## References

Anthony, E. (1970). Two contrasting types of adolescent depression and their treatment. *Journal of the American Psychoanalytic Association, 18*, 841–859.

Baker, R. (1978). Adolescent depression illness or developmental task? *Journal of Adolescence, 1*, 309–317.

Baldessarini, R. (1983). *Biomedical aspects of depression and its treatment*. Washington, DC: American Psychiatric Press.

Bemporad, J. (1988). Psychodynamic treatment of depressed adolescents. *Journal of Clinical Psychiatry, 49*, 26–31.

Biggs, J., Spiker, D., Petit, M., & Ziegler, V. (1977). Tricyclic antidepressant overdose. *Journal of the American Medical Association, 238*, 135–138.

Blos, P. (1967). The second individuation process of adolescence. *Psychoanalytic Study of the Child, 24*, 162–186.

Carlson, G., & Strober, M. (1979). Affective disorders in adolescence. *Psychiatric Clinics of North America, 2,* 511–526.
Coleman, J. (1980). Friendship and the peer group in adolescence. In J. Adelson (Ed.), *Handbook of adolescent psychology.* New York: Wiley.
Coyne, J., Kahn, J., & Gotlib, I. (1987). Depression. In T. Jacob (Ed.), *Family interaction and psychopathology.* New York: Plenum.
De Montigny, C., Cournoyer, G., Morissette, R., Langlois, R., & Caille, G. (1983). Lithium carbonate addition in tricyclic antidepressant resistant unipolar depression. *Archives of General Psychiatry, 40,* 1327–1334.
De Montigny, C., Mayer, A., & Deschines, J. (1981). Lithium induces rapid relief of depression in tricyclic antidepressant drug non-responders. *British Journal of Psychiatry, 138,* 252–256.
DiNicola, V., & Simeon, J. (1988, October). *Managing adolescent depression: A follow-through study.* Poster presentation at the Annual Meeting of the American Academy of Child and Adolescent Psychiatry, Seattle.
Extein, I., Pottash, A., Gold, M., Goggans, F., & Lydiard, B. (1986). Antidepressants: Predictory response/maximizing efficacy. In M. Gold, R. Lydiard, & J. Carmen (Eds.), *Advances in psychopharmacology: Predicting and improving treatment response.* Boca Raton, FL: CRC Press.
Fink, M. (1979). *Convulsive therapy: Theory and practice.* New York: Raven Press.
Freud, A. (1958). Adolescence. *Psychoanalytic Study of the Child, 13,* 255–278.
Garber, J., Kriss, M., Koch, M., & Lindholm, L. (1988). Recurrent depression in adolescents: A followup study. *Journal of the American Academy of Child and Adolescent Psychiatry, 27,* 49–54.
Issacs, C., Stainer, D., Sensky, T., Moor, S., & Thompson, C. (1988). Phototherapy and its mechanisms of action in seasonal affective disorder. *Journal of Affective Disorders, 14,* 13–19.
Janowsky, D., El-Yousef, M., Davis, J., & Sekerke, J. (1973). Antagonistic effects of physostigmine and methylphenidate in man. *American Journal of Psychiatry, 130,* 1370–1376.
Johnson, M., & Singer, H. (1982). Brain neurotransmitters and neuro regulators in pediatrics. *Pediatrics, 70,* 57–68.
Kazdin, A. (1986a). The evaluation of psychotherapy: Research design and methodology. In S. Garfield & A. Bergin (Eds.), *Handbook of psychotherapy and behavior change: An empirical analysis.* New York: Wiley.
Kazdin, A. (1986b). Treatment of antisocial behavior in children: Current status and future directions. *Psychological Bulletin, 102,* 187–203.
Keating, D. (1980). Thinking processes in adolescence. In J. Alderson (Ed.), *Handbook of adolescent psychology.* New York: Wiley.
Klerman, G., DiMascio, A., Weissman, M., Prusoff, B., & Paykel, E. (1974). Treatment of depression by drugs and psychotherapy. *American Journal of Psychiatry, 131,* 186–191.
Klerman, G., Weissman, M., Rounsaville, B., & Chevon, E. (1984). *Interpersonal psychotherapy of depression.* New York: Wiley.
Korenblum, M., Marton, P., Kutcher, S., Stein, B., Kennedy, B., & Pakes, J. (1988, October). *Personality dysfunction in depressed adolescents: State or trait?* Poster presentation at the annual meeting of the American Academy of Child and Adolescent Psychology, Seattle.
Kramer, A., & Feiguine, R. (1981). Clinical effects of amitriptyline in adolescent depression. *Journal of the American Academy of Child and Adolescent Psychiatry, 20,* 636–644.
Kuipers, L., & Babbington, P. (1988). Expressed emotion research in schizophrenia: Theoretical and clinical implications. *Psychological Medicine, 18,* 893–910.
Kutcher, S. P., & Marton, P. (1989). Parameters of adolescent depression. *Psychiatric Clinics of North America, 4,* 896–918.
Lewinsohn, P., Clarke, G., Hops, H., Andrews, J., & Osteen, V. (1987, November). *Treatment of depression in adolescents.* Paper presented at the annual meeting of the Association for the Advancement of Behavior Therapy, Boston.

McCauley, E., Mitchell, J., Burke, P., Myers, K., Calderon, R., & Schloredt, B. (1988, October). *Clinical course of depression in young people: A three year prospective study.* Poster presentation at the Annual Meeting of the American Academy of Child and Adolescent Psychiatry, Seattle.

Molick, R., & Pinkston, E. (1982). Using behavioral analyses to develop adaptive social behavior in a depressed adolescent girl. In E. Pinkston, J. Levitt, G. Green, et al. (Eds.), *Effective social work practice.* San Francisco: Jossey-Bass.

Nottelmann, E. D., Susman, E. J., Dorn, L., Ineff-Germain, G., Lorianx, D., Cutler, G., & Chromos, G. (1987). Developmental processes in early adolescence. *Journal of Adolescent Health Care, 8,* 246–260.

Popper, C. (Ed.). (1987). *Psychiatric pharmacosciences of children and adolescents.* Washington, DC: American Psychiatric Association Press.

Puig-Antich, J., & Gittelman, R. (1982). Depression in childhood and adolescence. In E. Paykel (Ed.), *Handbook of affective disorders.* New York: Basic Books.

Puig-Antich, J., Lukens, E., Davis, M., Goetz, D., Brennan-Quattrock, J., & Todak, G. (1985). Psychological functioning in prepubertal major depressive disorders: Interpersonal relationships after sustained recovery from affective episode. *Archives of General Psychology, 42,* 511–517.

Reynolds, W., & Coates, K. (1986). A comparison of cognitive-behavioral therapy and relaxation training for the treatment of depression in adolescents. *Journal of Consulting and Clinical Psychology, 54,* 653–660.

Roy-Byrne, P., Uhde, T., & Post, R. (1984). Antidepressant effects of one night's sleep deprivation: Clinical and theoretical implications. In R. Post & J. Ballander (Eds.), *Neurobiology of mood disorders,* Baltimore: Williams and Wilkins.

Rutter, M. (1982). Family and school influences: Meanings, mechanisms and implications. In A. Nichol (Ed.), *Practical lessons from longitudinal studies.* Chichester: Wiley.

Rutter, M., Izard, C., & Read, P. (Eds.). (1986). *Depression in young people.* New York: Guilford Press.

Ryan, N., Meyer, V., Dachille, S., Mazzie, D., & Puig-Antich, J. (1988). Lithium augmentation in TCA-refractory depression in adolescents. *Journal of the American Academy of Child and Adolescent Psychiatry, 27,* 371–376.

Ryan, N., & Puig-Antich, J. (1986). Affective illness in adolescence. In A. J. Francis & R. E. Hales (Ed.), *American Psychiatric Association annual review* (Vol. 5). Washington, DC: American Psychiatric Press.

Ryan, N., Puig-Antich, J., Cooper, T., Pabinovich, H., Ambrosini, P., Davies, M., King, J., Torres, D., & Fried, J. (1986). Imipramine in adolescent major depression. *Acta Psychiatrica Scandinavica, 73,* 275–288.

Ryan, N., Puig-Antich, J., Cooper, T., Rabinovich, H., Ambrosini, P., Fried, J., Davies, M., Torres, D., & Suckow, R. (1988). Relative safety of single versus divided dose imipramine in adolescent major depression. *Journal of the American Academy of Child and Adolescent Psychiatry, 26,* 400–406.

Ryan, N., Puig-Antich, J., Rabinovich, H., Fried, J., Ambrosini, P., Meyer, V., Torres, D., Dachille, S., & Mazzie, D. (1988). MAOIs in adolescent major depression unresponsive to tricyclic antidepressants. *Journal of the American Academy of Child and Adolescent Psychiatry, 27,* 755–758.

Schloss, P., Schloss, C., & Harris, L. (1984). A multiple baseline analysis of an interpersonal skills training program for depressed youth. *Behavioural Disorders, 9,* 182–188.

Seifert, W., Foxx, J., & Butler, I. (1980) Age effect on dopamine and serotonin metabolite levels in CSF. *Annals of Neurology, 8,* 38–42.

Schaffer, D. (1984). Notes on psychotherapy research among children and adolescents. *Journal of the American Academy of Child Psychiatry, 23,* 552–561.

Shea, M., Elkin, I., & Hirschfeld, R. (1988). Psychotherapeutic treatment of depression. In A. Francis & R. Hales (Eds.), *Review of psychiatry* (Vol. 7). Washington, DC: American Psychiatric Press.

Trautmann, P., & Rotheram-Borus, M. J. (1988). Cognitive therapy with children and adolescents. In A. Frances & R. Hales (Eds.), *Review of psychiatry* (Vol. 7). Washington, DC: American Psychiatric Press.

Weller, R., Weller, E., & Herjanic, B. (1983). Adult psychiatric disorders in psychiatrically ill young adolescents. *American Journal of Psychiatry, 140,* 11585–1588.

Whybrow, P., & Prange, A. (1981). Perspectives: A hypothesis of thyroid-atecholamine receptor interaction. *Archives of General Psychiatry, 38,* 106–113.

Wilkes, T., & Rush, J. (1988). Adaptations of cognitive therapy for depressed adolescents. *Journal of the American Academy of Child and Adolescent Psychiatry, 27,* 381–386.

# 3

# Psychopharmacological Treatment of School Phobia

## Barry D. Garfinkel

### Introduction

In order to review the pharmacological treatment of school phobia, a number of clinical and behavioral issues should be examined. The purpose of studying school phobia is to establish a model from which anxiety disorders can be better understood. The scientific study of school phobia allows for a better conceptualization of the underlying diagnostic problems, classification issues, severity ratings, family functioning, behavioral genetics, outcome, and eventually treatment. Historically the assumption has been that school phobia was synonymous with separation anxiety disorder (Kolvin, Berney, & Bhatz, 1984). It is likely that this assumption will have to be reexamined and possibly discarded.

Recently, school phobia has been replaced by the term *school refusal*. This less specific term reflects the changing empirical evidence that suggests that the inability of a child or adolescent to attend school may reflect fearfulness as well as periods of worry and sadness. Originally symptoms of fear, worry, and dysphoria were associated with separation anxiety disorder alone. More recently, Bernstein and Garfinkel (1986) and Tisher (1983) demonstrated that the majority of school-phobic youngsters met diagnostic criteria for depressive disorders. These findings suggest that treatment should be directed more to an affective disorder rather than to a phobia or panic attack.

The reexamination of school phobia requires that clinicians understand the context in which treatment is provided. The home environment creates a situation whereby the psychodynamics within the family take on even greater significance. Because of an exceedingly high placebo response rate and a high

---

*Barry D. Garfinkel*   Division of Child and Adolescent Psychiatry, University of Minnesota Medical School, Minneapolis, Minnesota 55455.

noncompliance rate associated with psychopharmacological treatments of childhood disorders, it is necessary to have as complete an understanding as possible of the underlying clinical interpersonal issues. Psychodynamic theorists have repeatedly emphasized the hostile dependent nature of the mother in association with oppositional, defiant, and conduct symptoms primarily arising from the child and having an impact on the child–mother relationship. If this hostile dependency were empirically established, one would predict that psychiatric management of this disorder would be hampered since refusal to take the medicine would be one more battleground for this oppositional defiant relationship to be acted out. This chapter will specifically describe, using empirical studies, the family context and interpersonal relationships that influence the overall management and treatment of this disorder.

## *The Diagnosis of School Phobia*

The first issue in utilizing pharmacological treatment is to establish a specific diagnosis for which appropriate medications are available. It is important to emphasize that medications are not helpful for treating specific or general behavioral or emotional problems. Medicine is least effective when it is used to manage problematic behaviors instead of treating syndromes and disorders. The first task, therefore, is to establish the underlying diagnostic and syndromatic entities determining children's refusal to attend school. Obviously, school nonattendance can reflect many factors, including social, economic, geographic, and familial, as well as psychiatric diagnostic issues. In 1986 Bernstein and Garfinkel, using structured interview techniques and depression and anxiety rating scales, identified that in a group of 26 school-phobic youngsters (with a mean age of 13 years 7 months) 69% met DSM-III criteria for depression. Baker and Wills (1978) demonstrated that 24% of their sample were given the diagnosis of depression, and Davidson (1961) indicated that 76% of school phobics that they studied were depressed. Tisher (1983) evaluated a sample of school refusers who were remarkably similar in family and socioeconomic characteristics to those studied in the Bernstein and Garfinkel sample. Compared with students who were regularly attending school, the school-phobic sample scored in the 85th percentile on the Children's Depression Scale.

This is not to say, however, that the samples studied did not meet criteria for anxiety disorders. In fact, 62% of the same sample met anxiety disorder criteria. Therefore, there was a large and significant comorbidity in these patients for these two diagnoses. Of all the school-phobic patients, 50% fulfilled the criteria for anxiety and depressive diagnoses (Bernstein & Garfinkel, 1986). The clinicians studying these youngsters could not distinguish which diagnosis was primary and which was secondary. All that could be concluded was that the two diagnoses coexisted to this extent and that the temporal sequencing of the diagnoses was impossible to establish.

Within the total sample of school-phobic children there were two other groupings that are noteworthy. The first was that there was a subsample of children that met the diagnostic criteria for either oppositional defiant disorder or conduct disorder. A number of these children also met criteria for affective and anxiety disorders; the primary diagnosis in these cases was that of a disruptive behavioral disorder of childhood. This suggests, however, that the negative, disruptive, and defiant behaviors predominate in some children who refuse to go to school. There was an even smaller group of youngsters in which no diagnostic entity could be established. This suggests that school refusal or phobia can also be a behavioral set of symptoms that does not represent an underlying disorder. This finding in particular has important ramifications related to treatment.

The severity rating of the underlying disorders is also noteworthy. Severity was measured using depression rating scales, including the Children's Depression Rating Scale (CDRS; Poznanski, Cook, & Carroll, 1979), a Children's Depression Index (CDI; Kovacs & Beck, 1977), and the Children's Depression Scale (CDS; Lang & Tisher, 1978). Anxiety was measured using the Anxiety Rating Scale for Children (ARC; Erbaugh, 1984, personal communication), the Children's Manifest Anxiety Scale (CMAS; Reynolds & Richman, 1978), and a Visual Analogue Scale for anxiety (Garfinkel, Bernstein, & Erbaugh, 1984, personal communication). The severity ratings indicated that those school-phobic children who met criteria for both disorders were most highly symptomatic as rated on these scales. The group that had the combination of the disorders (i.e., both anxiety and depressive disorders) were indistinguishable from the affective disorder group alone. The group that had only anxiety disorders was rated as being least symptomatic on both of these general scales. These severity ratings raise a number of questions. The first question that needs to be addressed is whether or not severe anxiety disorder merges into an affective disorder and becomes indistinguishable from it. This suggests that severe anxiety disorder may be misdiagnosed as an affective disorder. The second problem is whether or not severe anxiety disorder is indeed separate from an affective disorder and that the symptoms of worry and fearfulness may possibly reflect affective disorder more than an anxiety disorder. What this suggests is that anxious children may simply endorse multiple symptoms of depression (Hershberg, Carlson, Cantwell, & Strober, 1982). It was also encouraging to note that there was a pure group of anxiety-disordered youngsters who were mildly symptomatic and had very few symptoms of depression. It is likely that this overlap of the two diagnoses partially reflects a severity dimension of the existing disorder.

The diagnostic issues from these studies leads one to conclude that there may be a group of symptomatic youngsters who have two disorders coexisting simultaneously. This finding of the comorbidity of affective and anxiety disorders led to a series of studies examining the family pedigrees of school-phobic youngsters who meet criteria for both disorders. The purpose of the investigations was to determine whether a specific familial pattern could be established that would indicate that the adult relatives had also an overrepresentation of these two disorders. If this were the case, it would suggest that these comorbid individuals would have a lifetime risk for these two disorders and that school phobia may be a behavioral marker for these diagnoses.

## Family Pedigrees

Leckman, Merikangas, Parls, & Prusoff (1983) and Weissman, Leckman, Merikangas, & Gammer (1984) demonstrated that there was a group of adult patients who possessed both major depression and various anxiety disorders. The former study demonstrated that first-degree relatives of adults with both major depression and panic disorder have significantly higher rates of major depression, phobias, and panic disorder, as well as alcoholism. This was demonstrated in comparison with normal individuals as well as patients with pure depression (i.e., no evidence of anxiety disorder). The latter study demonstrated that the combination of depression plus panic disorder or agoraphobia in the parent created additional risk for these combination disorders in the children. There was a threefold increased risk for separation anxiety disorder in children of parents who had panic disorder. Furthermore, Livingston, Nugent, Rader, & Smith (1985) demonstrated that family studies of children with severe anxiety disorders and those with family histories with major depression equally demonstrated a high rate of affective disorder and alcoholism, and that there were no discernible differences between the two groups of families.

Bernstein and Garfinkel (1988) studied six families of children with anxiety and depressive disorders manifesting as school phobia. Three generations of relatives were studied. A total of 82 first- and second-degree relatives were evaluated, and they were compared with a psychiatric control group of children (mainly ADHD and conduct disorder) along with their first- and second-degree relatives. Most of the parents of the school-phobic children met criteria for either anxiety, depressive disorders, or alcoholism. The anxiety disorder group of parents was represented by two who had agoraphobia with panic attacks, one who had agoraphobia, three who had generalized anxiety disorder and one who had social phobia. Two-thirds of the parents of children with school phobia who had depressive and/or anxiety disorders also had a substance abuse disorder in contrast to only one parent in the comparison psychiatric control group. These different studies support the diagnostic findings suggesting that the families of school-phobic individuals have higher rates of pure anxiety disorder, pure depressive disorder, combinations of both anxiety and depressive disorders, and alcoholism and substance abuse. The findings suggest that these three groups of disorders may be frequently observed within specific children and within their family environment. Treatment for the children, as well as other family members, may be directed at specific disorders—namely, depression and/or anxiety. These findings may also suggest that children with school phobia, which is a behavioral manifestation of an underlying set of disorders, are more vulnerable to the adult variants of these disorders in their adult years if untreated. Similarly, there may be a greater probability that these individuals will turn to self-medication to ameliorate the symptoms of depression and anxiety in the adolescent and young adult years. School phobia, untreated, then may be a risk factor for future substance abuse. The need for effective treatments is therefore emphasized from these family studies.

## The Epidemiological Basis of Anxiety Symptoms

The study of the anxiety disorders from adult population studies shows that there is a relatively high prevalence rate. Three percent of the population had a lifetime prevalence of panic disorder, 6% for agoraphobia, 3% for generalized anxiety, 2% for simple phobia, and 1.5% for social phobia (Reich, 1986). The estimated prevalence rate for the United States is somewhere between 8 and 15%, with a disproportionate number of women affected compared with men (2 to 1 ratio). Anxiety symptoms therefore have a high rate of endorsement in community studies (Orvaschel & Weissman, 1986). Orvaschel and Weissman (1986) demonstrated that girls were affected more often than boys and that race and lower socioeconomic class predicted anxiety symptoms.

A study completed by Bernstein, Garfinkel, and Hoberman (1989) of over 1,000 high school students showed that 6% reported a severe level of anxiety symptoms, confirming the previously determined prevalence of anxiety symptoms in adults. The anxious adolescents were more likely to have a history of multiple somatic complaints, physical and sexual abuse, recent suicide attempts, street drug usage, poor academic performance, and prior treatment with antidepressant medication. The family histories also were significant for depression and suicide attempts. In this community sample, when both a Beck Depression Inventory and the Revised Children's Manifest Anxiety Scales were used simultaneously, a marked comorbidity for anxiety and depressive symptoms was found. The correlation coefficient in this sample of adolescents was $r = .59$. This finding suggests that anxiety and depression coexist and possibly overlap much in the same manner that these diagnoses do in clinical samples of school-phobic individuals. This epidemiological survey also supports the family and outcome studies previously mentioned—namely, emphasizing the familial linkage with depression, anxiety, and substance abuse. The finding that highly anxious symptomatic high school students are already involved in a higher rate of street drug usage suggests that self-medication and self-treatment become an issue well before the adult years.

The population studies highlight another vexing problem in the area of anxiety symptoms and school phobia in particular. This problem relates to the evaluation, assessment, and recognition of such symptoms. Because anxiety symptoms are not disruptive but are internalized, does an adequate evaluation schedule exist that reflects our ability to elicit these symptoms from the children using current psychometric techniques? Assessment questions and psychological tests may not be tapping the correct underlying symptom complex. Symptoms that are commonly associated with anxiety may also reflect an underlying depression. The best example of this is where anxiety scales ask for the endorsement of multiple somatic, nonspecific physical complaints. These symptoms, along with sleep and appetite changes, may be more accurately associated with depression. The same may be true for the nonspecific questions concerning "worry." Worry as a term may be more commonly observed in depressed youngsters than in anxious individuals. Symptom endorsement studies may therefore reflect equally the evaluation of both conditions and the circumstance that both disorders overlap and resemble each other clinically.

## *Evaluation Techniques*

Because of the overlap of affective and anxiety disorders in school-phobic individuals, the clinician must be able to complete a thorough and broad-ranging psychiatric clinical evaluation. Structured psychiatric interviews, especially the DICA and DICA-P (Herjanic & Campbell, 1977), have been particularly useful in enumerating the broad range of diagnoses affecting these youngsters. Evaluation should also include semistructured interview techniques that address the specific disorders—namely, the Children's Depression Rating Scale (CDRS; Poznanski, 1979); a scale derived from the Hamilton Anxiety Scale for adults was modified for children and is entitled the Anxiety Rating Scale for Children (ARC; Erbaugh, 1984, personal communication).

There are a number of other psychometric measures that provide severity ratings as well as providing a basis for establishing a categorical diagnosis. These scales should be used in evaluating symptom amelioration and response to treatment. The most specific and reliable scales include the following: the Children's Manifest Anxiety Scale-Revised (RCMAS; Reynolds & Richman, 1978), the State-Trait Anxiety Inventory for Children (STAIC; Spielberger, Edwards, Lushene, Montuori, & Platzek, 1973), a visual analogue scale for anxiety (Garfinkel et al., 1984, personal communication). These three scales are all paper-and-pencil self-report measures. They primarily establish a severity rating for symptoms associated with fearfulness, worry, and nonspecific somatic symptoms. As one would imagine, there can be a substantial overlap with measures of depression. One must be cautious in concluding that treatment is specifically ameliorating and directed to anxiety symptoms when using these scales to judge clinical response. In truth, treatment may be more directed to the symptoms of depression. At the present time, it appears that these scales evaluate for anxiety not as a totally independent construct, and as such are only approximate instruments.

## Family Dynamics

Psychoanalytic theory postulated that separation anxiety/school phobia occurred within the context of a mutually hostile dependent relationship between the patient and his/her mother (Johnson et al., 1941). Whereas mothers were viewed as being dominant and overbearing, fathers were seen as absent, weak, or ineffective (Takagi, 1972). The families of school-phobic children were viewed as having difficulty in tolerating autonomy and separation and that the parents fostered dependency (Waldron, Shirier, Stone, & Tobin, 1975). Previously, these dynamic issues were never systematically investigated. Current thinking is that the anger, dependency, and confrontation are not clearly established as causative but may likely be a consequence of school phobia or a result of the family adapting to a highly symptomatic child. Earlier research has not empirically identified marked evidence of family dysfunction in a hospitalized sample of school-phobic youngsters (Berg, Butler, Fairbairn, & McGuire, 1981). Bernstein, Svingen, and Garfinkel (1990) studied more than 75 families of school-phobic children. Using a structured measure of family functioning (FAM; Skinner, Steinhauer, & Santa-Barbara, 1983) they were able to demonstrate specific areas of problematic functioning in the parent–child relationship. There were two main areas of family dysfunction—namely, in role performance and in establishing the values and norms of the general community within the family. The role performance problems in the school-phobic families showed that the parents and the children were vying for identical roles within the context of family life. Role definition was poor. The parents were not authoritarian and were not successful in directing their children back to school. In turn, the school-phobic child was described as becoming hostile and controlling within that dysfunctional system. The difficulties associated with values and norms in the school-phobic families were contradictory communications between the parents and the children negatively regarding independence, autonomy, and school attendance.

What was most surprising was that these areas of family dysfunction as measured by this empirical evaluation scale were described only by the parents. The children minimized the problems in the family and did not identify the severity of problems identified by the parents. The other very striking finding was that family dysfunction as measured by the FAM was not observed in the group that had anxiety disorders alone. The families of children in other diagnostic groups—especially conduct disorder, depression, and the mixed depression and anxiety disorders group—had the most severe family dysfunction. Elevation of specific FAM subscales appeared only in these other diagnostic subgroups. A child refusing to attend school frustrates the parents and reinforces the parents belief that the child is noncompliant and is in a power struggle with them. This situation may reflect the fact that these other groups had a more severely symptomatic child and therefore these families had a more difficult time responding to the more disturbed children. Like the Berg et al. (1981) findings, it may also indicate that youngsters with school refusal that arose out of separation anxiety do not have marked family dysfunction. Therefore, family dysfunction may not be causative of the school refusal. While these data support the contention that families of school-phobic children are dysfunctional, the critical variable is **not** the school refusal but likely the severity and category of the present underlying child's diagnosis. These data suggest that highly symptomatic children have a very disruptive influence on parents' carrying out their assigned roles and prevent them from establishing a value system within the family that is consistent within their community. This inability to provide effective parenting may also have a marked influence on their ability to have the children comply with their treatment program, especially taking their medication and attending regular therapy sessions.

### *General Considerations of Treatment*

The preceding discussion modifies the clinicians' view of intervention for school-phobic children and adolescents. Initially, most clinicians viewed school phobia as an extreme form of separation anxiety disorder. Subsequently, the clinical opinion that has emerged is that one may be managing separation anxiety disorder but what is more likely is that one will be dealing with a combination of anxiety and depressive disorders or pure depression alone. Clinicians have also been impressed with the fact that there is a high rate of psychopathology in other family members and that the family pathology clusters around three chief disorders (depression, anxiety, and substance abuse). Whether as a result of these adult disorders or as a consequence of living with a highly symptomatic youngster, family communication and roles are distorted. All these factors affect how one would intervene in working with a school-phobic youngster and his or her family. These considerations suggest that individual psychotherapy, family therapy, therapy for the adult family members, and medication directed to both anxiety and depressive disorders in various individuals must be considered.

Depending on the severity of the symptoms, one might consider using medication. If it were pure separation anxiety disorder of a mild to moderate type, one would likely choose a cognitive behavioral therapeutic program as well as a school reintegration program without medication to treat that situation. The reason for withholding medication only for those who have severe disorders is that treatment studies suggest that school phobia is highly responsive to psychotherapy. Studies in general have shown that there is an exceedingly large placebo response rate associated with this clinical entity. Whereas in the treatment of attention deficit hyperactivity disorder the placebo response may be somewhere between 30 and 50%, for this disorder it is between 50 and 70% (Garfinkel, 1986). The other consideration for using medication is to be aware of the side effects associated with the use of benzodiazepines and tricyclic antidepressant medications, the two most commonly used medicines in the treatment of school phobia. Various studies have shown that there is a high dropout rate while taking these drugs because of the emergence of intolerable side effects. In general, the conclusion is that clinicians must reserve the use of medication only for the severely disordered youngsters. One would also rely on existing rating scales that could provide a severity score above which one would prescribe medicine.

## Previous Studies

Since the early 1960s antidepressant medication and anxiolytics have been used in the treatment of child and adolescent anxiety disorders and school-phobic individuals in particular. During this same time period there were hundreds of pharmacological studies on adults with anxiety disorders. The first documented report on children was by D'Amato (1962), who used chlordiazepoxide in treating elementary school-aged school-phobic youngsters, in doses ranging from 10 to 30 mg daily. Within 14 days, eight out of the nine children were attending school regularly. Kraft, Ardali, Duffy, Hart, and Pearce (1965) used the same medication but in much higher doses in a group of children with various psychiatric conditions. Chlordiazepoxide was most effective in the subgroup of youngsters with school phobia. While on the anxiolytic, over two-thirds of the school-phobic sample received a clinical rating of between good and excellent. Frommer (1967) employing a double-blind design compared phenelzine, an MAO inhibitor with chlordiazepoxide to a barbiturate, phenobarbital, in 15 school-phobic individuals. The combination of the

MAO inhibitor and the benzodiazepine was far superior to phenobarbital and suggests that the MAO inhibitor in combination with the benzodiazepine is a highly effective treatment of school phobia. Furthermore, these drugs may work well individually in ameliorating the symptoms of school phobia, and the combination of these two drugs may only obscure the conclusion. Unfortunately, no objective ratings of improvement were used to assess drug response, so it is difficult to determine the magnitude of the drugs' effect. It is not known whether the positive therapeutic response is secondary to the anxiolytic effect or the antidepressant effect of this drug combination. This study, as well as the earlier reports, corroborates the use of MAOI's and benzodiazepines in the treatment of adult, adolescent, and childhood anxiety disorders (Quitkin, Rifkin, & Klein, 1979). What these studies do not address is the finding from adult studies demonstrating the superiority of tricyclic antidepressants over benzodiazepines in the treatment of adult anxiety disorders. The conclusions drawn from the study of this limited literature suggests that antidepressants (TCAs and MAOI's) may be better antianxiety drugs than existing anxiolytics. Abe (1975) in Japan studied the use of sulpiride in 21 school-phobic youngsters. This study found 13 who responded to the medication within the first week and successfully returned to school. Not only did they return to school but they also had a marked decrease in symptoms of anxiety and affective disorders. In the nonresponding group a number were subsequently placed on imipramine, with 2 of them showing a very positive response.

Gittelman-Klein and Klein (1973) conducted a double-blind placebo-controlled study of imipramine in 35 elementary school-aged children who had all demonstrated a partial or no response to psychotherapy. The children were all in the early elementary school years. They received high doses of imipramine, receiving approximately 100–200 mg per day. The placebo response rate in this group was 47%, whereas the imipramine response rate was approximately 80%. Although these findings are very encouraging, this study has never been replicated. A number of methodological problems affect this study. Foremost among them are the observations that these children were part of a young group of school-phobic children (aged 7–10 years) and almost all had the diagnosis of separation anxiety disorder alone. Of particular concern was the procedure to administer extremely high doses of medication, frequently exceeding 3.5 mg per kg per day. Other investigators studying this disorder tend to work with the early adolescent junior high school population, where there is a greater occurrence of comorbidity with depression.

Berney et al. (1981) studied 51 school-phobic children and adolescents following a double-blind placebo-controlled procedure. Clomipramine was administered in doses ranging from 40 to 75 mg. This study was unable to distinguish clomipramine from placebo. The Berney study differed from the Gittelman-Klein study on a number of characteristics, including (1) older age group, (2) comorbidity for depression, (3) dosage of tricyclic antidepressant, and (4) different medications; (5) both studies employed different types of concurrent psychotherapy (behavioral vs. insight-oriented). By reviewing both of these studies it can be concluded that tricyclic antidepressant medication may be one of the promising forms of treatment for this disorder. Relying on this medication, however, as the sole form of treatment without either individual or family-based psychotherapy would be premature at this time.

Alprazolam, has been investigated as a treatment of anxiety symptoms in children and adolescents. In adults alprazolam has been shown to decrease anticipatory anxiety and panic attacks and in specific individuals to ameliorate symptoms of depression (Chouinard, Annabler, Fountaine, & Solyom, 1982). There are only two studies examining this medication in the pediatric population. Pfefferbaum et al. (1987) demonstrated that alprazolam was effective in treating anticipatory and situational anxiety in youngsters having bone marrow aspiration as part of their treatment for a malignancy. This study simply documented symptom relief at the time of the procedure. Two-thirds of the youngsters benefited from this medication. Although it appears that alprazolam was effective, no placebo response was studied. Simeon and Ferguson (1987) administered alprazolam to 12 youngsters with overanxious/avoidant disorders. Seven of the 12 youngsters responded in a moderate to marked manner, whereas 5 of them showed only a minimal to absent response. Because neither of these alprazolam trials was blinded or placebo-controlled, it is difficult to speculate about the medication's efficacy. One can only conclude that these results are promising and should be studied further under controlled conditions.

### Clinical Trials Comparing Alprazolam and Imipramine

There were two types of studies conducted—namely, an open trial and a double-blind placebo-controlled trial. A number of important background characteristics must be defined before the procedures concerning the drug administration are reviewed. Critical variables that have been found to determine treatment response include age (i.e., younger children responding more favorably to medications than older children) and diagnosis (separation anxiety disorder responding better than depression). Other variables include severity of illness, chronicity of illness (responding less well to treatment), and failure to respond to outpatient psychotherapies. All of these variables can have a significant effect either by enhancing the probability of drug response or decreasing its effect. Similarly, the placebo effect, the spontaneous remission rate, and observer bias in the evaluation of drug response will also determine treatment outcome. The systems' issues indicate that medication studies evaluating treatment effects for anxiety disorders are much more difficult to complete compared with treatment studies of ADHD or depression. Methods of improving the probability of observing a treatment response include (1) using only treatment failures, (2) having a "placebo washout" entry phase, (3) crossover design, (4) large sample size ($N = 60$ or greater), (5) random assignment to study groups, and (6) independent concurrent psychotherapy group.

In the research by Bernstein, Garfinkel, and Borchardt (1990), 17 chronic (two-thirds of the subjects having a length of illness of approximately 1.5 years), older (mean age of approximately 14 years), primarily severely depressed (some had both depression and anxiety) school-phobic youngsters were openly assigned to either an alprazolam or imipramine treatment. Those who were treated with alprazolam received 1.4 mg daily on the average, and those who received imipramine received a mean dose of 135 mg daily. Of the 9 patients who received alprazolam, 6 showed a marked to moderate improvement on anxiety and depressive symptoms. Five of the 9 subjects returned to school. Four of the 6 in the imipramine group showed a moderate to marked improvement. Three of the 6 on imipramine returned to school on a regular basis. The alprazolam produced only mild sedation, whereas imipramine produced constipation, orthostatic hypotension, dry mouth, and sedation.

Because of the generally positive response, 25 additional youngsters were enrolled in a double-blind placebo-controlled study of these two active pharmacological agents. Each of the three groups of youngsters was treated identically. Medication was gradually raised to 3 mg per kg per day for imipramine and .03 mg per kg per day for alprazolam. Children were extensively evaluated at baseline and weeks 4 and 8 utilizing anxiety and depression ratings. All the youngsters received individual psychotherapy and a school reentry program along with the medication.

On the clinician rating scale for anxiety the medication groups showed statistically significant improvement compared with the placebo group (Bernstein et al., 1990). It is unclear whether the group differences were because of initial baseline differences on rating scales or actual drug effects. The overall functional response to the medication has been reported elsewhere (Bernstein et al., 1990). There were, however, specific areas in which the symptoms were ameliorated (Bernstein, Garfinkel, & Borchardt, 1987). Responses based on items from the Children's Manifest Anxiety Scale for children who were receiving imipramine showed a significant decrease in the area of depression. From individual items on rating scales, imipramine was observed to decrease/improve the somatic anxiety, energy level, and mood, and to enhance socialization. Alprazolam showed specific areas in which improved response was observed—namely, sleep and the ability to concentrate on schoolwork. The placebo group, which actually appears as a group receiving psychotherapy alone, improved in areas of perfectionism and being less pessimistic. In general, one can conclude that there are specific areas that show a positive therapeutic response to these active agents. Given these findings and the earlier Gittelman-Klein and Klein (1973) report, one would cautiously recommend imipramine in the dose used in the Bernstein et al. studies over the dosage of alprazolam used. The positive response observed in these two double-blind studies and the lack of tolerance or dependence at this dose and duration supports its use. The conclusion, however, that alprazolam is also a very effective treatment is justified, and because it was associated with a limited range of side effects, it should be readily considered in treating these youngsters. There were, however, fewer side effects with the alprazolam, and because of the relative safety one would think that alprazolam in doses up to 4 mg per day could be used in this particular group of youngsters for up to 12–15 weeks of treatment. This would be followed by a gradual tapering off period lasting up to 4 weeks. If the school-phobic youngster had multiple physical complaints and tended to have frequent somatization and vegetative symptoms, alprazolam would be the drug of first choice. Medication without psychotherapy would not be recommended.

## A School Reentry Program

Medication certainly has a role to play in the overall management program of school-phobic children and adolescents. Because of the large placebo response rate and the high spontaneous remission rate, it must be emphasized that rather than simply relying on medication, a complete multimodality therapeutic program would be in order. The first component of treatment is a systematic desensitization to the school environment based on a school reentry program spanning a 4-week period. The program is designed on the basis of clinical observation of the diurnal fluctuation in mood. Because the youngsters are low in energy, tired, and most irritable in the morning, the first 2 weeks of the program emphasize activities and exposure to school in the afternoons. The first week requires that the youngster attend school for 1 to 2 hours approximately two to three times per week. During these school visits the youngster does not join the class but visits with guidance counselors and other school personnel. It is best that a nonfamily member or school person accompany the youngster to the school. This could be a social worker or other mental health professional.

The second week increases school attendance to daily attendance for up to 2 hours per day, all within the afternoon. The youngster meets a designated staff member of the school's faculty, who welcomes the youngster and makes certain that the youngster attends the classes contained within that time period. In the third week the youngster starts school somewhere between 10:00 and 11:00 in the morning and attends school 5 days a week. By the fourth week, the youngster attends school all day each day of the week. The youngster is allowed to ventilate his or her feelings with a guidance counselor or social worker at school at least twice each week and with a therapist on an outpatient basis. The overarching concept of this program is that the youngster is being exposed in vivo to the dreaded and feared situations. The youngster is not maintained at home and is not encouraged to remain at home when the peer group is at school.

Along with the reentry schedule, youngsters are encouraged to engage in individual cognitive behavioral psychotherapy. The principles underlying the psychotherapy include the ability to model after a therapist, to engage in role-playing with the therapist, and to self-monitor and self-instruct oneself to do things that one fears. While working with the therapist the patient, ideally, incorporates strategies by which self-instruction, self-direction, and self-reward can occur.

In conjunction with individual cognitive behavioral therapy, family therapy following a systems model has also been shown to be effective. Family therapy can be effective especially when it addresses the specific problems around role definition, limit setting, parental direction, and discipline. Communication concerning the incorporation of the communities' values and norms must be addressed since these youngsters tend to develop clinical characteristics suggesting oppositionality and defiance. Parents often benefit from having some parent management educational programs. These parent management technique classes can be done independently of any other psychotherapy provided.

## Conclusions

Initially, when embarking on the systematic study of school phobia, a number of the surprising findings from this empirical research could not have been predicted. The most surprising finding of all has been the high rate of affective disorder in this population of youngsters. This has been corroborated by the remarkable predisposition of the school-phobic families to have the triad of disorders including affective disorder, anxiety disorders, and substance abuse. The family dynamic issues were only partly in agreement with the theoretical psychoanalytic models proposed a number of years ago. What was demonstrated, however, was that family dysfunction could be identified by the parents, but it was most often associated with the severity of symptoms and the appearance of depression and conduct disorders. School phobia alone was not associated with a particular pattern of abnormal family functioning. As one would predict, living with a chronic dysfunctional oppositional youngster, parents were seen who were not able to effectively direct their children and to convey their values to them. In general, this older group of chronic school refusers was not particularly responsive to medication treatment. Medication, however, in combination with family and individual therapy and a school reentry program resulted in improvement in school attendance and symptomatic relief in approximately two-thirds of the individuals treated.

Medication trials for school-phobic individuals should compare benzodiazepines, monoamine oxidase inhibitors, and tricyclic antidepressants. Their therapeutic efficacy must also be compared with a placebo treatment as well as psychotherapeutic interventions. At this time one must assume that treatment may be directed to the diagnostic clinical disorders (affective and anxiety) as much as it is to the symptom of school refusal.

## References

Abe, K. (1975). Sulpiride in school phobia. *Psychiatric Clinics, 8,* 95–98.
Baker, H., & Wills, V. (1978). School phobia: classification and treatment. *British Journal of Psychiatry, 132,* 492–499.
Berg, I., Butler, A., Fairbairn, I., & McGuire, R. (1981). The parents of school phobic adolescents—A preliminary investigation of family life variables. *Psychological Medicine, 11,* 79–83.
Berney, T., Kolvin, I., Bhate, S. R., Garside, R. F., Jeans, J., Kay, B., & Scarth, L. (1981). School phobia: A therapeutic trial with clomipramine and short-term outcome. *British Journal of Psychiatry, 138,* 110–118.
Bernstein, G. A., & Garfinkel, B. D. (1986). School phobia: The overlap of affective and anxiety disorders. *Journal of the American Academy of Child Psychiatry, 25,* 235–241.
Bernstein, G. A., & Garfinkel, B. D. (1988). Pedigrees, functioning, and psychopathology in families of school phobic children. *American Journal of Psychiatry, 145,* 70–74.
Bernstein, G. A., Garfinkel, B. D., & Borchardt, C. (1987). *Imipramine versus alprazolam for school phobia.* Paper presented at the Annual Meeting of the American Academy of Child and Adolescent Psychiatry, Washington, D.C.
Bernstein, G. A., Garfinkel, B. D., & Borchardt, C. (1990). Comparative studies of pharmacotherapy for school refusal. *Journal of the American Academy of Child and Adolescent Psychiatry.*
Bernstein, G. A., Garfinkel, B. D., & Hoberman, H. M. (1989). Self-reported anxiety in adolescents. *American Journal of Psychiatry, 146,* 384–386.
Bernstein, G. A., Svingen, P. H., & Garfinkel, B. D. (1990). School phobia: Patterns of family functioning. *Journal of the American Academy of Child and Adolescent Psychiatry, 29,* 24–30.
Chouinard, G., Annabler, L., Fountaine, R., & Solyom, L. (1982). Alprazolam in the treatment of generalized anxiety and panic disorders: A double-blind placebo-controlled study. *Psychopharmacology, 77,* 229–233.
D'Amato, G. (1962). Chlordiazepoxide in management of school phobia. *Diseases of the Nervous System, 5,* 292–295.
Davidson, S. (1961). School phobia as a manifestation of family disturbance: its structure and treatment. *Journal of Child Psychology and Psychiatry, 1,* 270–287.
Frommer, E. A. (1967). Treatment of childhood depression with antidepressant drugs. *British Medical Journal, 1,* 729–732.
Garfinkel, B. D. (1986). Recent developments in attention deficit disorder. *Psychiatric Annals, 16*(1), 11–15.

Gittelman-Klein, R., & Klein, D. F. (1973). School phobia: Diagnostic considerations in the light of imipramine effects. *Journal of Nervous and Mental Disease, 156,* 199–215.

Herjanic, B., Campbell, W. (1977). Differentiating psychiatrically disturbed children on the basis of a structured interview. *Journal of Abnormal Child Psychology, 5,* 127–134.

Hershberg, S. G., Carlson, G. A., Cantwell, D. P., & Strober, M. (1982). Anxiety and depressive disorders in psychiatrically disturbed children. *Journal of Clinical Psychiatry, 43,* 358–361.

Johnson, A. M., Falstein, E. I., Szurek, S. A., & Svendsen, M. (1941). School phobia. *American Journal of Orthopsychiatry, 11,* 702–711.

Kolvin, I., Berney, T. P., & Bhate, S. R. (1984). Classification and diagnosis of depression in school phobia. *British Journal of Psychiatry, 145,* 347–357.

Kovacs, M., & Beck, A. (1977). An empirical-clinical approach toward a definition of childhood depression. In J. G. Schulterbrandt & A. Raskin (Eds.), *Depression in childhood* (pp. 1–25). New York: Raven Press.

Kraft, I. A., Ardali, C., Duffy, J. H., Hart, J. T., & Pearce, P. (1965). A clinical study of chlordiazepoxide used in psychiatric disorders of children. *International Journal of Neuropsychiatry, 9,* 433–437.

Lang, M., & Tisher, M. (1978). *Children's Depression Scale.* Melbourne: Australian Council for Educational Research.

Leckman, J. F., Merikangas, K. R., Pauls, D. L., & Prusoff, B. A. (1983). Anxiety disorders and depression: Contradictions between family study data and DSM-III conventions. *American Journal of Psychiatry, 140,* 880–882.

Leckman, J. F., Weissman, M. M., Merikangas, K. R., Prusoff, B. A., & Pauls, D. L. (1983). Panic disorder and major depression: Increased risk of depression, alcoholism, panic, and phobic disorders in families of depressed probands with panic disorder. *Archives of General Psychiatry, 40,* 1055–1060.

Livingston, R., Nugent, H., Rader, L., & Smith, G. R. (1985). Family histories of depressed and severely anxious children. *American Journal of Psychiatry, 142,* 1497–1499.

Orvaschel, H., & Weissman, M. M. (1986). Epidemiology of anxiety disorders in children: A review. In R. Gittelman (Ed.), *Anxiety disorders of childhood* (pp. 58–72). New York: Guilford Press.

Pfefferbaum, B., Overall, J. E., Boren, R. N., Frankel, L. S., Sullivan, M. P., & Johson, K. (1987). Alprazolam in the treatment of anticipatory and acute situational anxiety in children with cancer. *Journal of the American Academy of Child and Adolescent Psychiatry, 26,* 532–535.

Poznanski, E. O., Cook, S. C., & Carroll, B. J. (1979). A depression rating scale for children. *Pediatrics, 4,* 442–450.

Quitkin, F., Rifkin, A., & Klein, D. F. (1979). Monoamine oxidase inhibitors. A review of antidepressant effectiveness. *Archives of General Psychiatry, 36,* 749–760.

Reich, J. (1986). The epidemiology of anxiety. *Journal of Nervous and Mental Disease, 174,* 129–136.

Reynolds, C. R., & Richman, B. O. (1978). What I think and feel: A revised measure of children's manifest anxiety. *Journal of Abnormal Child Psychology, 6,* 271–280.

Simeon, J. G., & Ferguson, H. B. (1987). Alprazolam effects in children with anxiety disorders. *Canadian Journal of Psychiatry, 32*(7), 570–574.

Skinner, H. A., Steinhauer, P. D., & Santa-Barbara, J. (1983). The Family Assessment Measure. *Canadian Journal of Community Mental Health, 2,* 91–105.

Spielberger, C. D., Edwards, C. D., Lushene, R. E., Montuori, J., & Platzek, D. (1973). *STAIC preliminary manual.* Palo Alto, CA: Consulting Psychologists Press.

Takagi, R: (1972). The family structure of school phobics. *Acta Paedopsychiatrica, 39–40;* 131–146.

Tisher, M. (1983). School refusal: A depressive equivalent. In D. P. Cantwell & G. A. Carlson (Eds.), *Affective disorders in childhood and adolescence: An update* (pp. 29–144). New York: Spectrum.

Waldron, S., Shirier, D. K., Stone, B., & Tobin, S. (1975) School phobia and other childhood neuroses: A systematic study of the children and their families. *American Journal of Psychiatry, 132,* 802–808.

Weissman, M. M., Leckman, J. F., Merikangas, K. R., & Gammon, G. D. (1984). Depression and anxiety disorders in parents and children: Results from the Yale family study. *Archives of General Psychiatry, 41,* 845–852.

Weissman, M. M., Prusoff, B. A., Gammon, G. D., Leckman, J. F., Merikangas, K. R., & Kidd, K. K. (1984). Psychopathology in the children (ages 6–18) of depressed and normal parents. *Journal of the American Academy of Child Psychiatry, 23,* 78–84.

# 4

# Treatment of Childhood Obsessive–Compulsive Disorder
# A Review in the Light of Recent Findings

## Martine F. Flament and Luis Vera

Obsessive–compulsive disorder (OCD) can develop early in life. The classical psychiatric and psychoanalytic literature contains detailed clinical descriptions of the disorder in young children. Janet reported a case of obsessional neurosis in a 5-year-old boy (Janet, 1903), and Freud's famous patient, the Rat Man, had his first symptoms around age 6 (Freud, 1909).

However until recently, OCD was thought to be rare in children, at least from estimates of its incidence in child psychiatric populations. Berman (1942) found 6 cases of obsessive compulsive neurosis out of almost 3000 pediatric cases admitted to the Bellevue Hospital between 1935 and 1942, an incidence of 0.2% of the child psychiatric population. In 1965, Judd's retrospective chart examination of 405 children seen at UCLA Neuropsychiatric Institute yielded 5 cases meeting strict diagnostic criteria for obsessive compulsive neurosis, which made up 1.2% of the children's psychiatric cases (Judd, 1965). More recently in the same center, Hollingsworth, Tanguay, Grossman, and Pabst (1980) found only 17 cases in a retrospective examination of more than 8000 in- and outpatient clinical records, again an incidence of 0.2% of the child psychiatric cases.

If children with OCD are relatively rare in child psychiatry clinics, adult obsessive–compulsive patients often trace the origin of their symptoms back into childhood. In a cumulative review of eight different retrospective studies on the age of onset of obsessive–compulsive symptoms, Black (1974) has shown that the highest incidence of first obsessive–compulsive symptoms

---

Martine F. Flament     International Hospital of the University of Paris, 75014 Paris, France.    Luis Vera    Robert Debre Hospital, 75019 Paris, France.

49

occurred between the ages of 10 and 15, by which age the disorder had started in nearly one-third of the cases.

Moreover, a recent epidemiological study (Flament, Whitaker, Rapoport, et al., 1989) revealed that OCD in adolescence was much more frequent than previously thought. In an unselected adolescent population of about 5600 subjects, the point-prevalence rate of the disorder was estimated to be 1% of the general population, and its lifetime prevalence rate, 1.9%. Most of the OCD subjects identified in the study had never been under psychiatric care, and the study showed that OCD was clearly underdiagnosed and undertreated during adolescence.

Recent data from a prospective follow-up study of children with OCD (Flament, Koby, Rapoport, et al., 1990) suggest that the disorder is likely to become chronic: In early adulthood, 68% of the subjects still suffered from OCD, and 48% presented another complicating psychiatric disorder, most commonly a depressive and/or an anxiety disorder.

These recent findings call for greater sensitivity to the diagnosis of OCD during childhood or adolescence, and for its early treatment before chronicity and complications occur.

Childhood OCD, unlike most other childhood disorders, presents in a form virtually identical to the full adult syndrome (Flament & Rapoport, 1984). The same diagnostic criteria apply to both adults and children, the clinical phenomenology is strikingly similar (Swedo, Rapoport, Leonard, Lenane, & Cheslow, 1989), and the disorder when it arises early in life is remarkably continuous from childhood to adulthood (Flament, Koby, Rapoport, et al., 1990).

The diagnosis of OCD in children is usually straightforward once it is considered. As in adults, it manifests itself through obsessions (recurrent, persistent ideas, thoughts, or impulses that are experienced, at least initially, as intrusive and senseless) and/or compulsions (repetitive, purposeful behaviors, perceived as unwanted and unnecessary, that are performed in response to an obsession, according to certain rules, or in a stereotyped fashion). OCD children are acutely aware that their rituals or repetitive thoughts are irrational. They accurately describe how the symptoms interfere with their lives, and how they fight against the thoughts and impulses.

Presenting symptoms for children with OCD closely resemble adult symptomatology. In the National Institute of Mental Health (NIMH) series of 70 consecutive children and adolescents with OCD (Swedo et al., 1989), the most common obsessions concerned fear of contamination with dirt, germs, or toxins (40%); fear of something terrible happening (24%); need for symmetry or exactness (17%); and scrupulosity or religious obsessions (13%). Compulsions most often consisted of excessive or ritualized handwashing, showering, or grooming (85%); repeating rituals (51%); checking (51%); rituals to remove contact from contaminants (23%); touching (20%); counting (18%); ordering or arranging (17%); and measures to prevent harm to self or others (16%).

Measurement of the severity of the obsessive–compulsive symptoms is an important part of both inital diagnostic evaluation and assessment of treatment results. Observer's rating scales used for adult patients, such as the Comprehensive Psychiatric Rating Scale-Obsessive Compulsive Subscale (CPRS-OC; Thorén, Asberg, Cronholm, et al., 1980) or the NIMH-OC Scale (Insel, Murphy, Cohen, et al., 1983), apply very well to children. On the same model, an Obsessive Compulsive Rating Scale (OCR) has been designed for a treatment study with children (Rapoport, Elkins, & Mikkelson, 1980). Among the self-rated scales for obsessive–compulsive symptoms, one has been specifically adapted for children—that is the Leyton Obsessional Inventory-Child Version (LOI-CV; Berg, Rapoport, & Flament, 1986), which gives three scores: one for the number of symptoms present, one for the resistance of the subject to his or her obsessive–compulsive thoughts or behaviors, and one for their interference in the subject's life.

## Psychoanalytic Treatment

The treatment literature on childhood OCD includes fascinating and detailed case studies by psychoanalytic and psychodynamic therapists. These reports provide invaluable material for conceptualization of the psychopathology of childhood OCD.

Psychoanalysis tells us about the internal and external clinical picture of the disorder, giving a sense to symptoms. For Anna Freud (1966), the ego devices used for the purpose of warding of the *id* content from consciousness are, in varying combinations, denial, repression, regression, reaction formation, isolation, undoing, magical thinking, doubting, indecision, intellectualization, rationalization—all of them, with the exception of regression, operating strictly within the area of the thought processes. In the external clinical picture, the prominence of the reaction formations provides the impression of stability and immutability, the intensity of the countercathexes provides the mental strain, and the profusion of intellectualizations is an attempt to bind *id* energies through secondary process thinking. About etiology, Anna Freud proposes that "obsessional outcomes are promoted by a constitutional increase in the intensity of the anal-sadistic tendencies...probably as the result of inheritance combined with parental handling."

However, despite the "classical" nature of the obsessional neurosis, so illustrative of unconscious thought processes, and despite the well-understood dynamics of obsessional symptoms, few successful treatment cases involving children have been reported in the literature.

Muriel Barton Hall (1935) wrote very enthusiastic reports on psychodynamic treatment of children with obsessive–compulsive neurosis; Ramzy (1967) and Silverman (1972) reported the stories and analyses of little boys aged 5 and 3, respectively.

Morton Chethik (1969), in an interesting report on the 3-year psychoanalysis of an 11-year-old boy with rituals, obsessions, fears, and anxiety, comments on the specifics of analytic processes for childhood OCD. He says that his young patient could maintain a treatment alliance with him that was motivated by suffering: "He seemed to have an early awareness that in the rituals and obsessions he had to establish, he was at the mercy of the unknown and compelling forces that made him act in senseless ways." Chethik emphasizes the enormous treatment advantages when analysis begins early in the patient's life, before this fast-developing neurosis becomes consolidated with entrenched defense mechanisms, and while the prominent original sources of conflicts (father and mother) continue to play a direct and immediate part in his affective life. Chethik also stresses the concept of mixed pathology, or "mixed neurosis," saying that, although the boy had developed a highly organized and structured obsessional neurosis, other forms of pathology were also present, and this concept provided for flexibility throughout the treatment.

However, most psychoanalysts recognize with Fenichel (1945) that the analytic process with compulsive neurotic patients is often arduous and sometimes interminable. Fenichel notes the difficulty these patients have with free association, and how their discussions turn to intellectualized brooding. He describes how magical thinking interferes with the patient's ego observations, how intense ambivalence produces continuous road blocks in the treatment relationship, and how affects and emotions are tenaciously warded off, though memories are available. Anna Freud (1966) says that obsessional neurosis is hard to unravel not in spite of the pathology but because the pathology is located in the thought processes themselves, thereby attacking the patient's very means of communicating with us, as well as our ability to identify with them and with the aberrations of their logic and reasoning.

## Other Forms of Psychotherapy

There have been few published reports on the efficacy of other forms of psychotherapy for treatment of childhood OCD. Most are anecdotal case reports. We still lack real efficacy studies.

A few individual cases of successful outcome with *strategic, problem-focused therapy* have been reported: Weiner (1967) successfully treated a 15-year-old boy with pervasive compulsive rituals using directive psychotherapy, with behavioral prescriptions providing alternate socially acceptable and relatively economic rituals. O'Connor (1983) describes the five-session therapy of a 10-year-old boy using the Palo Alto theory of problem development and change, with behavioral and family prescriptions.

*Family therapy* has also been used for childhood OCD, on the assumption that families, and interpersonal relationships in general, are crucial to the creation and maintenance of obsessive symptoms in children. Bolton, Collins, and Steinberg (1983) state that family involvement is able to maintain both the anxiety of the child and his conviction in his obsessional coping strategies; they included family sessions in the multimodal treatment of 15 obsessive–compulsive adolescents. Other reports of successful treatment of obsessive–compulsive symptoms in children with family therapy include one case by Hafner, Gilchrist, Bowling, and Kalucy (1981) where a definite family conflict and a familial precipitating event were identified at the onset of the patient's illness, and a report by Fine (1973) on two young compulsive boys for whom the development of motor rituals and ruminative thoughts was thought to be related to the family members' inability to verbalize their feelings, particularly angry feelings.

*Milieu therapy* has proven useful, often in synergy with individual treatment approaches, especially for adolescents (Apter, Bernhout, & Tyano, 1984; Bolton et al., 1983; Friedmann & Silvers, 1977). The weird and time-consuming nature of the symptoms, the considerable isolation that the illness has sometimes created, and the lack of social skills associated with the personality style of some patients create additional distress. Milieu therapy represents a valuable support; it can bring stable behavioral changes and provide social skills training. It is a useful adjunct to any form of inpatient therapy.

*Supportive psychotherapy* is always necessary, if only to relieve the guilt and isolation generated by the disorder. As with other rare conditions, it is of considerable support to these patients just to meet with therapists who have had contact with others with the same disorder. Parents tend to form mutual support groups with an intensity that testifies to their need for such support. Some of the children appear to benefit at least from the supportive and reassuring features of therapy. Associated problems, such as depression and family conflict, may be helped, perhaps indirectly lightening the severity of the burden of the disorder. In addition, therapy may, in a preliminary way, serve as a kind of baseline record-keeping function, which may in itself prove helpful in attenuating the frequency of some of the symptoms.

## Behavioral Treatment

For OCD, as for other anxiety disorders, behavioral theories and behavioral treatment have greatly enlightened both the understanding of the symptoms and the prognosis of the disorder.

## The Behavioral Models of OCD

Behavioral treatment is based on the analysis of the components and determinants of each behavior, and on the capacity of the human subject to learn alternate behaviors. Four behavioral models have been proposed to account for development and maintenance of obsessive–compulsive symptoms. These models combine biological and learning theories.

From a behavioral point of view, obsessive–compulsive symptoms are classified according to their function. Thoughts, images, and impulses that elicit anxiety are denoted as obsessions. Overt behaviors and other conditions that are anxiety-reducing are termed compulsions: washing (or cleaning) rituals, checking rituals, repetition rituals (counting, repeating actions), but also behaviors consisting of active or passive avoidance, which are close to phobic avoidance behaviors.

### The First Behavioral Model: Mowrer's Two-Factor Learning Theory

First, Mowrer (1960) adapted the concept of *avoidance conditioning,* usually cited to explain phobic behaviors, for obsessive–compulsive patients: the avoidance behavior prevents the aversive stimulus from appearing; avoiding the object avoids anxiety. One difference between phobic patients and OCD patients with avoiding rituals (for example, from fear of contamination) is that, for the obsessionals, the fear concerns less the situation in itself (being in contact with a dirty object) than the consequences of the encounter with the situation (having to wash or to check). OCD patients can accept confrontation with the situation but then rush to perform rituals. In contrast, phobic patients strongly resist encountering the feared situation. Another difference between obsessive–compulsive and phobic patients concerns the larger role of cognitive factors in OCD: The obsessional patient who *knows* he can wash can more easily face dirt.

Then Mowrer (1960) developed a specific model for obsessive–compulsive behaviors, the *two-factor learning theory.* The first process is a *classical conditioning process:* The obsessive thought provokes anxiety because, for reasons known or unknown, this thought has been associated for the subject with a past traumatic experience. Intrusion of the obsessive thought (a word, number, sentence, image, or memory, even neutral in appearance) induces a conditioned anxiety response.

The second process is an *instrumental conditioning:* the subsequent behavior (checking, washing, or magical counter-behavior) is reinforced and maintained because it decreases anxiety by eliminating its source; the subject learns to use a ritual to decrease anxiety created by the obsessive thought.

### The Second Behavioral Model: Hernstein's Model

Despite its success, Mowrer's model has been contested because, in some cases, an increase, not a decrease, in anxiety occurs after the ritual is performed. For Hernstein (1969), if rituals are reinforced and maintained, it is because they induce a relative decrease in anxiety, compared with what would have been had the ritual not been performed.

According to this model, the obsessional idea induces an anxiety response that can be arbitrarily rated 60 on a 100-point scale and provokes an urge to ritualize. Then there are two alternatives: (1) The ritual is performed, but the ritual itself creates its own anxiety response (due to the guilt of having "given up," the uncertainty about having done it "right"); this anxiety response can be rated 80. (2) The ritual is impeded, and anxiety increases from 60 to 100. Thus, performing the ritual has produced only a relative decrease in anxiety: 80 instead of 100.

### The Third Behavioral Model: The Rachman and Hodgson Model

For Rachman and Hodgson (1980), there are four determinants of the obsessive–compulsive behavior: a genetic component of hyperarousability, mood disturbances, a particular social learning, and specific learning exposures. Thus, there are multiple determinants for each obsessive–compulsive behavior, and the authors propose that it makes little sense to ask what is the cause of the behavior. Rather, they sense that the actual conditions that currently promote the excessive compulsive behavior should be the focus of treatment, through exposure techniques.

### The Fourth Behavioral Model: The Activation Theory of Beech and Perrigault

Beech and Perrigault (1974) also focus on the notion of hyperarousability. For them, the concept of *activation,* or arousal, replaces the concept of avoidance.

Beech and Perrigault affirm the OCD patients are predisposed to pathological states of arousal and that, by a mechanism not yet fully understood, this activation produces morbid thoughts and aberrant behaviors. The state of emotional activation induces a mood disturbance, and when it reaches a critical level, associative processes occur where an event becomes randomly linked to an internal state. This model is based on the concepts of pseudoconditioning and habituation: (1) OCD subjects are prone to pseudoconditioning—that is, a tendency to respond to a stimulus in the absence of an actual contingency; (2) they have difficulty developing habituation in response to repeated stimulation.

It is interesting that the activation theory is a model that can now be supported by recent biological findings in OCD. Electrophysiological studies have actually shown, notably in children (Rapoport, Elkins, Langer, et al., 1981), differences in electrodermal response, an index of habituation, between OCD patients and matched normal controls. Current research with brain-imaging techniques have found increased metabolic rates (that is, hyperactivity) in certain areas of the brain of obsessive–compulsive subjects compared with depressed and normal controls (Baxter, Phelps, Maziotta, et al., 1987).

## Behavioral Treatment of OCD

Two main therapeutic strategies can be used for treatment of obsessive–compulsive symptoms (see Table 1): one intends to modify the anxiety associated with obsessions and compulsions; the other is directed to changing the obsessive or compulsive behavior itself. If the target symptom is anxiety, there are two types of behavioral techniques: in imagination or in vivo.

### Techniques Addressing Anxiety

*Systematic Desensitization in Imagination.* The evoking stimulus is a situation (dirt, untidiness) that induces an evoked response, the obsessive thought (feeling dirty, fear of contamination). The evoked response (the obsession) can in turn become an evoking stimulus and induce another evoked response (the ritual), such as running away from the situation, washing hands, or arranging rituals.

*Cognitive Flooding.* Cognitive flooding is a prolonged and repeated exposure to obsessive thoughts to decrease the evoked anxiety. For instance, the

*Table 1*
Behavior Therapy of OCD

| Target symptom | Behavioral treatment |
| --- | --- |
| Anxiety response | In imagination |
|  |    Systematic desensitization |
|  |    Cognitive flooding |
|  |    Aversive conditioning |
|  | In vivo |
|  |    Systematic desensitization |
|  |    Exposure |
|  |       Immersion |
|  |       Implosive exposure |
| Obsessional idea | Thought stopping |
| Compulsive ritual | Response prevention |

patient can be asked to repeatedly watch himself discussing the sources of his anxiety on a videotape (Milby, Meredith, & Rice, 1981).

*Aversive Conditioning.* This method, used by Lazarus (1958) for treatment of diverse checking rituals, consists of having the patient imagine the evoking stimuli or the rituals themselves, and associate them to unpleasant experiences (such as nausea, vomiting) also presented in imagination.

*In Vivo Systematic Desensitization.* Systematic desensitization is often used in vivo. It has been used for checkers (Worsley, 1968), washers (Walton, 1960), and even ruminators (Bevan, 1960).

*Exposure.* Exposure can use immersion: sudden and prolonged exposure to the situation (as opposed to the brief, gradual exposure of systematic desensitization). With immersion, the subject manifests intense emotional reactions. Immersion is the treatment of choice for compulsive ritualizers (Marks, 1981).

Rachman, De Silva, and Roper (1976) provided a detailed view of how discomfort and the urge to ritualize decrease with continued exposure: in an experiment with 11 compulsive ritualizers, a brief contact with the evoking stimulus led to immediate feelings of being contaminated, with resultant discomfort and the urge to ritualize. Both discomfort and the urge to ritualize dropped sharply when patients were allowed to carry out the usual rituals (e.g., washing). Next, patients were again exposed to similar stimuli, but this time they were asked to refrain from ritualizing (washing), thus prolonging contact with the symbolic evoking stimulus of feeling contaminated. Contact with the evoking stimulus was rapidly followed by urges to ritualize and by discomfort, but once the patients no longer immediately escaped from these reactions by washing, the discomfort and the urge to ritualize gradually subsided over the next 3 hours.

Implosive exposure is a prolonged exposure to stimuli that are still more anxiety-provoking than those reported by the patient (Lamontagne, 1977).

### Techniques Addressing the Obsessions or Compulsions

*Thought Stopping.* In this procedure (Cautela, 1969; Marks, 1981), the patient is relaxed and is asked to think of the obsessive thought. The therapist shouts "stop," and makes a sudden noise at the same time. The patient is then told to shout "stop" himself to dispel the thought and then to whisper and eventually to employ a subvocal command (e.g., snap an elastic band worn on his wrist).

Thought stopping can be viewed in different ways: as an exercise in self-regulation or coping (whereby patients learn to control their own thoughts), as a form of short-lasting exposure to the obsessional thought, or as an aversive conditioning.

Thought stopping is useful because it is one of the very few techniques that can be used for pure obsessional patients—those who do not have rituals.

*Response Prevention.* Response prevention allows the anticipation of change, by experiencing that the expected dreaded consequences of not performing the rituals actually do not occur (Meyer, 1966). Treatment combines two elements: in vivo exposure to the evoking stimulus, and interruption or prevention of the evoked ritualistic behavior.

## Group Studies of Behavioral Treatment of OCD

Numerous studies (see Table 2) have found that various forms of exposure in vivo effectively reduce compulsive rituals up to several years' follow-up (Marks, 1981). These studies were done with samples of adult OCD patients.

The studies by Marks, Rachman, and Hodgson (1975), and Marks, Stern, Mawson, Cobb, & McDonald (1980), and Roper, Rachman, and Marks (1975) were controlled with relaxation as the nonexposure condition. All showed that

*Table 2*
Behavioral Treatment of OCD Group Studies of Ritualizers[a]

| Study | Number of subjects | Results |
|---|---|---|
| Marks et al., 1975 | 20 | Exposure + response prevention better than relaxation |
| Roper et al., 1975 | 10 | |
| Marks et al., 1980 | 40 | |
| Robertson, 1975 | 13 | 24-hour = 1-hour response prevention |
| Meyer et al., 1974 | 10 | Lasting improvement after exposure in vivo |
| Marks et al., 1978 | 28 | |
| Boulougouris, 1977 | 15 | |
| Foa & Goldstein, 1978 | 21 | |
| Foa et al., 1980 | 8 | Exposure + response prevention better than either alone |
| Emmelkamp & Kraanen, 1977 | 13 | Therapist-controlled = self-controlled exposure |
| Steketee et al., 1982 | 49 | In vivo + imaginal exposure better than in vivo exposure alone at follow-up |

[a]Adapted from Marks (1981).

exposure associated with self-imposed response prevention for about 3 weeks of daily sessions was significantly more effective than relaxation for treatment of compulsive rituals. The overall level of moderate depression and anxiety reported by the patients at the beginning of therapy was unchanged by improvement of rituals. Amelioration in compulsive behaviors was maintained at 1- to 2-year follow-up.

Robertson's study (1975, unpublished) compared the results of 24-hour versus 1-hour daily response prevention treatment and found no advantage for continuous supervision.

Several uncontrolled studies have found lasting improvement in compulsive rituals after treatment by exposure in vivo (Boulougouris, 1977; Foa & Goldstein, 1978; Marks, Bird, & Lindley, 1978; Meyer, Levy, & Schnurer, 1974). In general, improvement in ritualistic behavior seemed greater than that in obsessive ideation, and patients' depression, if any, did not improve. Foa, Steketee, and Milby (1980) showed that the combination of exposure with response prevention was more effective than either technique alone.

Emmelkamp and Kraanen (1977) contrasted therapist-controlled exposure in vivo in the client's home with self-controlled exposure in vivo in the hospital and found little difference between the two approaches, although the former treatment was twice as long as the latter.

Steketee, Foa, and Grayson (1982) compared the effects of daily sessions of exposure in vivo to those of daily imaginal exposure followed by in vivo exposure. The addition of imaginal exposure to in vivo exposure did not affect short-term treatment gains but did increase the maintenance of such gains.

## Behavioral Treatment of Children with OCD

There have been no systematic studies on the effects of behavior therapy for children with OCD. The only published data consist of individual case reports of successful treatment of children with obsessions or compulsions using some of the behavior modification techniques described above (often associated with other treatment modalities).

Mills, Agras, Barlow, and Mills (1973) successfully treated a 15-year-old boy with morning and bedtime rituals using response prevention. Yamagami (1978) reports the successful treatment of a 15-year-old boy with fear of contamination and compulsive handwashing, using a variant of the response prevention technique. After nine repeats of a series of sessions, a marked decrease in fear and handwashing time was obtained, as well as change in the thoughts concerning the symptoms.

Ong and Leng (1979) treated a 13-year-old Malaysian Chinese girl obsessed with cleanliness. Behavior treatment included exposure in vivo with participant modeling, response prevention, and operant conditioning. Treatment was effective; a mild relapse at 2 years responded to a second course of treatment.

As with adults, treatment of "ruminators" (pure compulsives) is more difficult, but Campbell (1973) utilized a variation of the thought-stopping technique to treat a 12-year-old boy who had distressing and persistent posttraumatic obsessive thoughts related to the actual violent death of his sister, which he had witnessed. Four sessions of thought stopping, using counting loudly backwards, eliminated ruminations. At a 3-year follow-up, there had been no return of the symptoms.

Friedmann and Silvers (1977) describe the synergistic effects of combined standard psychotherapy, behavioral techniques, family therapy, and milieu therapy for an 18-year-old obsessive–compulsive young man. De Seixas Queiroz, Motta, Modi, Sossai, & Boren (1981) treated two children with behavioral procedures designed to counteract the specific variables that they had identified as maintaining the obsessive–compulsive behaviors (e.g., environmental, familial, and social variables; subject's own behavioral deficits)

More recently, Bolton et al. (1983) reported on 15 adolescents with OCD treated with behavior therapy, using response prevention and family sessions (some of the subjects simultaneously received other treatments). The outcome was generally good, and treatment gains were maintained at follow-up in most cases.

So, except for Bolton's study, concerning a pretty large series of adolescents (but in that study several types of treatment were used simultaneously, confounding results), most of the reports cited above are just anecdotal. The overall efficacy of behavior therapy for OCD children remains to be explored further (Wolff & Rapoport, 1988).

However, existing reports are interesting at least for two reasons. First, they show that techniques that have proven effective in controlled studies with adults appear to be applicable—and to produce the same results—with obsessive–compulsive children. Second, they show the advantages, while using sound techniques, of individualizing the global treatment strategy for each child and for each case. Standard methods should be adapted to the specific needs of each individual; different treatment approaches can be combined.

Besides formal behavior therapies, more casual behavioral strategies can be used as adjunctions to other types of treatment. For inpatients, an operant conditioning program may tie ward privileges to attainment of progressively more difficult goals, such as tolerating disorder, or reducing tardiness due to the rituals. Specific limits can be set to handle washing or other rituals (e.g., limited allocation of soap or bedclothes) and help the children to adhere to some daily routine in the hospital as well as at home or at school.

## Pharmacological Treatment

Besides behavior therapy, the other major breakthrough of the last decades in the treatment of OCD has come from psychopharmacology. Nearly every category of psychotropic drugs has been investigated for treatment of OCD, but only few have been recognized as effective by several independent groups of investigators, first, the antidepressant clomipramine, then more recently, new drugs with similar pharmacological properties, fluoxetine and fluvoxamine.

Most of the drug treatment studies of OCD have been done with adult patients. Although we will focus on the few pharmacological studies that have specifically concerned children or adolescents, we will also briefly review the adult studies since there is no evidence of a different responsivity of children to pharmacological treatment of the disorder.

### Clomipramine

There have been eight main controlled double-blind studies on the effects of treatment with clomipramine for OCD patients, six of them with adults and two with children. These studies are summarized in Table 3.

For adult patients, clomipramine, administered at doses from 75 to 300 mg/day for 4 to 6 weeks was superior to placebo in the studies by Insel et al. (1983), Marks et al. (1980), Montgomery (1980), Thorén, Asberg, Cronholm, Jörnestedt, & Träskman (1980). Clomipramine was found significantly more

Table 3
Clomipramine Treatment of OCD. Main Controlled Studies

| Study | Number of subjects | Results[a] |
|---|---|---|
| Thorén, Asberg, Cronholm, et al., 1980 | 24 | CMI > Plac, not NOR (5 weeks) |
| Montgomery, 1980 | 14 | CMI > Plac (4 weeks) |
| Marks et al., 1980 | 40 | CMI > Plac (4 weeks), depressed subgroup only |
| Ananth et al., 1981 | 20 | CMI improved from baseline, not AMI |
| Insel et al., 1983 | 13 | CMI > CLG and Plac (4 + 6 weeks) |
| Flament et al., 1985 | 19[b] | CMI > Plac (3 + 5 weeks) |
| Volavka et al., 1985 | 23 | CMI > IMI (6 weeks) |
| Leonard et al., 1988 | 21[b] | CMI > DMI (5 weeks) |

[a] CMI = clomipramine, Plac = placebo, NOR = nortriptyline, AMI = amitriptyline, CLG = clorgyline, DMI = desipramine.
[b] Subjects are children.

effective than clorgyline (Insel et al., 1983) and imipramine (Volavka, Nezirogu, & Yaryura-Tobias, 1985), while nortriptyline (Thorén et al., 1980) and amitriptyline were ineffective (Ananth, Pecknold, Van Der Steen, Engelsmann, 1981).

The first controlled pharmacological study done with OCD children is the study by Flament, Rapoport, Berg, et al., (1985), where clomipramine was compared with placebo in a double-blind randomized crossover design, with 5 weeks on each treatment condition. Nineteen subjects were included in the trial. Obsessive–compulsive, depressive, and anxiety symptoms were measured weekly on standard scales.

Compared with placebo, clomipramine produced significant improvement on all scales (observer's and self-rated scales) measuring obsessive–compulsive symptoms at week 3, week 4, and week 5 of treatment. On scales measuring depression and anxiety, scores were generally low at baseline and unchanged under any treatment condition.

Clomipramine was given at the mean daily dose of 134 mg, and plasma levels of clomipramine and its metabolites were in the range generally considered therapeutic for depression. Except for moderate anticholinergic side-effects often encountered with tricyclic antidepressants, the medication was well tolerated.

Unfortunately, not all patients improved to the same extent. At the end of 5 weeks, two subjects (10%) were entirely symptom-free, six (32%) were much improved, and another six (32%) only moderately improved; two patients (10%) were just slightly improved, and three (16%) were unchanged.

The second pharmacological study done with OCD children compared clomipramine with desipramine in a double-blind randomized crossover trial (Leonard, Swedo, Rapoport, et al., 1989). The study confirmed the efficacy of clomipramine in this age group and showed the specificity of its effect: there was a significant superiority of clomipramine over desipramine, with little difference between desipramine and an initial placebo phase. Significant differences between the two active treatments were seen by the third week of treatment. Relapse on desipramine was prompt, usually after 2 weeks, when this drug was given following clomipramine.

In addition to these large studies on the therapeutic effects of clomipramine on series of OCD patients, and although this is not the usual route of administration for this disorder, there had been early reports (Marshall, 1975; Walter, 1973) on the efficacy of IV clomipramine for treatment of anxious obsessional patients. Similar results have been reported more recently: Five adult patients (Warneke, 1984) and one 15-year-old adolescent girl with OCD (Warneke, 1985), all of whom had failed to respond to oral clomipramine, showed dramatic improvement of obsessive compulsive symptoms and mood, following six to eight infusions of clomipramine; the drug was much better tolerated in IV than during the previous oral course, and improvement was maintained with subsequent administration of the oral treatment.

## Other Tricyclic Antidepressants

The other tricyclic antidepressants do not seem to share clomipramine's efficacy for OCD.

Imipramine (Freed, Kerr, & Roth, 1972; Mavissakalian & Michelson, 1983), amitriptyline (Snyder, 1980), trimipramine (Bartucci, Stewart, & Kemph, 1987), and doxepin (Ananth et al., 1975) have been found beneficial for individual patients. However, imipramine was not better than placebo (Foa, Steketee, Kozak, & Dugger, 1987), and less effective than clomipramine (Volavka et al., 1985) in two controlled studies; desipramine (Leonard et al., 1989; Zohar & Insel, 1987) and amitriptyline (Ananth et al., 1981) were also negatively compared with clomipramine in controlled studies.

## Monoamine Oxidase Inhibitors (MAOI)

Phenelzine (Isberg, 1981; Jenike, Surman, Cassem, Zusky, & Anderson, 1983), tranylcypromine (Jenike, 1981; Jenike et al., 1983), and nialamide (Rihmer, Szántó, Arató, Szabó, & Bagdy, 1982) have been found to improve both obsessive–compulsive and anxiety symptoms in a few patients with OCD associated with panic or phobic disorder. However, clorgyline was less effective than clomipramine and not different from placebo in Insel's controlled study (Insel et al., 1983).

## Neuroleptics

Trifluperazine (Altschuler, 1962), haloperidol (O'Regan, 1970), chloroprothixene (Hussain & Ahad, 1970), and loxapine (Rivers-Bulkely & Hollender, 1982) were reported useful for some patients unresponsive to other treatment regimens. The only placebo-controlled double-blind study has concerned chlorpromazine (Trethowan & Scott, 1955), which was ineffective in a mixed diagnostic cohort of 59 patients with obsessions and compulsions.

## Benzodiazepines

Only anecdotal reports suggest that these agents can be useful in some cases. Oxazepam and chlordiazepoxide were reported better than placebo in a group of patients "with obsessive compulsive symptoms" (but various diagnoses) in one controlled study (Orvin, 1967). In another study, diazepam was not statistically different from placebo (Venkoba-Rao, 1964).

More recent reports of a few cases of OCD treated with alprazolam (Ketter, Chun, & Lu, 1986; Tesar & Jenike, 1984; Tollefson, 1985) showed some diminution of obsessive compulsive symptoms under this treatment.

## Lithium

A few reports (but not all) document success with lithium carbonate for OCD patients (Stern & Jenike, 1983). Of interest are two cases of improvement with lithium augmentation of clomipramine (Rasmussen, 1984) and desipramine (Eisenberg & Asnis, 1985) treatment.

## L-Tryptophan

There has been one open study, by Yaryura-Tobias (1977), concerning seven patients, all improved by L-tryptophan treatment; unfortunately, this study was never replicated.

Cases of improvement by L-tryptophan augmentation of clomipramine treatment have been reported (Rasmussen, 1984), but also a number of cases of toxic reactions following administration of L-tryptophan in association with fluoxetine or MAOIs (Steiner & Fontaine, 1986), toxic reactions resembling the "serotonin syndrome" described in animal studies.

## Other Classes of Pharmacological Agents

Among nontricyclic antidepressants, mianserin was found effective for 6 of 13 patients by one investigator (Jaskari, 1980).

There have been case reports of the successful treatment of OCD with clonidine (Knesevich, 1982). Practolol had some effect on the autonomic accompaniments of obsessive–compulsive symptoms but not on the symptoms themselves (Rabavilas, Boulougouris, Perissaki, & Stefanis, 1979). Antiandrogenic treatment has been reported to improve one male and four female OCD patients in Spain (Casas, Avarez, Duró, et al., 1986).

## Newer Drugs

Since clomipramine has been recognized effective for obsessive compulsive patients, four drugs from the newer generation of antidepressants have been studied, with partial success, for treatment of OCD.

*Zimelidine.* Zimelidine was first found beneficial in small groups of OCD patients in open studies (Fontaine, Chouinard, & Imy, 1985; Kahn, 1984). Zimelidine was better than imipramine in a very small study (3 patients in each group) by Prasad (1984) but less effective than clomipramine in a study by Insel, Mueller, Alterman, Linnoila, & Murphy (1985). Since zimelidine was subsequently declared unsafe for clinical use, there could be no further investigations.

*Trazodone.* Case reports of OCD patients successfully treated with trazodone have been published (Baxter, 1985; Lydiard, 1986; Won Kim, 1987). There have been two open group studies. One was positive: for Prasad (1986), 6 out of 8 patients improved; the other was negative: for Mattes (1986), 11 patients treated with an association of trazodone and L-tryptophan showed no significant clinical change.

*Fluoxetine.* One open study by Fontaine and Chouinard (1986) and one single-blind study by Turner, Jacob, Beidel, and Himmelhoch (1985) found significant group improvement in a small number of OCD patients, but, as mentioned earlier, five cases of toxic reactions to fluoxetine associated with L-tryptophan were also reported.

*Fluvoxamine.* Finally, the most recent pharmacological trials for OCD have concerned fluvoxamine, with significant group improvement first shown in one single-blind (Price, Goodman, Charney, Rasmussen, & Henninger, 1987) and one double-blind (Perse, Greist, Jefferson, Rosenfeld, & Dar, 1987) study. In a recent placebo-controlled trial with 42 OCD patients (Goodman, Price, & Rasmussen, 1989), fluvoxamine was found to be significantly better than placebo, although only about half of the patients responded to fluvoxamine.

## The Limits of Pharmacological Treatment

If clomipramine—and more recently fluoxetine and fluvoxamine—have shown, from all studies completed, the greatest promise for psychopharmacological treatment of OCD, there are several caveats to clomipramine treatment and, more generally, to pharmacotherapy of OCD.

First, medication generally induces an improvement but not a cure for obsessive–compulsive symptoms. Pooled data from the different clomipramine studies show a 40 to 60% reduction in symptoms at 4 to 6 weeks of treatment. Typically, most patients report that the symptoms persist, but they cause less interference and are resisted more successfully. As a result, patients are able to return to school or to work, and the increased activities successfully distract them from the remaining obsessions or rituals. Occasionally, the symptoms may ultimately disappear.

Not all patients are responsive to pharmacological treatment: of the studies in which individual responses to clomipramine were reported, 50 to 70% showed substantial improvement. In good responders, discontinuing the medication may precipitate a relapse, or a good response to treatment may fade after a few years.

Finally, because drug treatment is likely to be chronic, side-effects may pose a problem, although, in our experience, children and adolescents tolerated the drug relatively better than do adults.

A practical as well as theoretical question posed by the evidence of a therapeutic effect of clomipramine and newer antidepressant drugs for OCD is that of the specificity of this effect. Could the antiobsessional action observed be mediated by the drugs' antidepressant properties?

The question can be partly answered by the observation that many other antidepressant drugs that, as shown above, have also been tried for treatment of OCD did not prove effective. For clomipramine, the specificity of its antiobsessional effect of clomipramine has also been directly demonstrated in some of the studies cited above.

In our study with children (Flament et al., 1985), depression scores were generally low at baseline and were not affected by clomipramine treatment. Moreover, change scores in obsessive compulsive symptoms during active treatment were not related to pretreatment depression scores; that is, depressed and nondepressed children had similar improvement of their obsessive–compulsive symptoms with clomipramine.

Except for the Marks study (Marks et al., 1980), in which only the depressed subgroup of OCD patients improved significantly with clomipramine, the other adult studies have also shown the specificity of the antiobsessional effect of clomipramine: in the studies by Ananth, Pecknold, Van Der Steen, and Engelsmann (1981), Insel et al. (1983), and Thorén et al. (1980), clomipramine was effective in patients with and without depression, and improvement in obsessive–compulsive symptoms was not related to amelioration of secondary depressive symptoms.

*The Serotonin Hypothesis of Obsessive–Compulsive Disorder*

The recent advances in pharmacological treatment of OCD support what had been proposed in the 1970s as "the serotonin hypothesis of obsessive compulsive disorder." This hypothesis, that a dysfunction of the serotonin system in the brain might be involved in the pathogenesis of OCD, had come from the early report that L-tryptophan, a serotonin precursor, was effective in relieving obsessive–compulsive symptoms (Yaryura-Tobias, 1977). Clomipramine, a potent serotonin reuptake blocker, was consistently found to be effective for OCD, whereas less serotonergic tricyclics (nortriptyline, amitriptyline, imipramine, desipramine) did not appear useful. Moreover, other nontricyclic selective serotonin reuptake blockers, such as zimelidine, trazodone, fluoxetine, and fluvoxamine, have recently been reported to be effective in OCD.

Further support for a role of serotonin in OCD came from two studies of the biochemical effects of clomipramine treatment in obsessive–compulsive patients.

Thorén, Asberg, Bertilsson, et al. (1980) looked at the concentrations of monoamine metabolites in the cerebrospinal fluid of OCD patients, before and after treatment with clomipramine. Good responders had higher pretreatment concentrations of the serotonin metabolite 5-hydroxyindoleacetic acid (5-HIAA) than did the nonresponders, and during treatment, clinical improvement was strongly associated with the decrease in 5-HIAA concentration. These findings suggested that the antiobsessional effect of clomipramine was indeed related to the drug's ability to inhibit serotonin uptake, as reflected in the decreased amine turnover.

In Flament's study with obsessive–compulsive children (Flament, Rapaport, Murphy, Berg, & Lake, 1987), platelet serotonin concentrations were measured before and after treatment with clomipramine. There was a significant correlation between clinical improvement and the decrease in platelet serotonin concentration during treatment. This also indicated that clomipramine's pharmacological effect on serotonin uptake was essential to the drug's antiobsessional clinical effect.

Finally, the role of serotonin in OCD pathophysiology is supported by recent pharmacological challenge studies. Zohar & Insel (1987) found that single doses of a serotonin postsynaptic receptor agonist called metachlorophenylpiperazine (m-CPP) were able to produce acute modulation of obsessive–compulsive symptoms in OCD patients, without inducing them in normal controls. Still more recently, Benkelfat, Murphy, Zohar, et al., (1989) showed that administration of the serotonin receptor antagonist metergoline induced anxiety and obsessive–compulsive symptoms in OCD patients receiving clomipramine on a long-term basis (but not in untreated patients); this supported the hypothesis that clomipramine's therapeutic effects in OCD are mediated via serotonergic mechanisms.

Of course, current hypotheses on the role of the neurotransmitter serotonin in the pathophysiology and treatment of OCD remain speculative. There are contradictory findings and other neurotransmitter systems might be involved. Even if a neurochemical dysregulation has been partially demonstrated in OCD, its causal role in the disorder cannot be established.

It may seem contradictory to claim simultaneously that OCD has a neurochemical basis and that a psychological treatment such as behavior therapy is effective in reversing it. This is not contradictory. In primitive animals, cerebral amines have been shown to influence behavioral patterns and, in return, behavioral conditioning and repeated training have been demonstrated to modify neurobiochemical regulation (Marks, 1985). The human brain is both a biological organ and the recipient of sensory and psychological inputs, and it is only to be expected that strictly psychological causes do have biological effects.

## Conclusion

Obsessive–compulsive disorder was, until recently, considered to be a severe and chronic condition refractory to most treatment approaches. For many patients, the new developments in behavioral modification techniques and in pharmacological treatment with clomipramine or related drugs have completely changed the outcome of the disorder. Yet therapeutic results are still partial, and research on OCD pathogenesis and treatment is ongoing.

Behavior therapy is a safe and valuable tool for treating children and adolescents with OCD. In vivo exposure with response prevention is the treatment of choice for compulsive rituals. Other techniques should also be applied in number of cases. However, patients rarely find themselves entirely free of symptoms at the completion of treatment; maintenance of gains is problematic for about 20% of them, and brief booster treatment may at times be necessary.

Behavior therapy alone is effective for OCD. Yet severe symptoms of anxiety or depression can make patients unable to carry out the treatment. Anxiety prevents them from identifying the cognitive processes associated with their compulsive thoughts or behaviors. Depression hinders their participation in tasks required during (and between) the treatment sessions. In those two cases, the addition of drug treatment—particularly clomipramine—to behavioral modification techniques may facilitate patients' participation in behavior therapy as well as accelerating and consolidating their treatment gains.

Obsessive ruminators are less predictably responsive to the behavioral treatments used so far. Medication can decrease the anxiety associated with the obsessive thoughts, and if obsessions lead to avoidance behaviors, behavioral treatment can apply to these avoidance behaviors.

Obsessive–compulsive children generally respond to the same behavioral techniques as do adult patients. Emotional reactions to both symptoms and therapy are the same in all age groups. However, children—at least until 10 or 12 years of age—have more difficulties identifying and expressing the cognitive processes associated with their symptoms. Abstract thinking is less developed and "in imagination" techniques are more difficult. On the other hand, children have constructed less rationalization around their rituals, and this makes behavioral changes easier and treatment often faster. Although this is not emphasized in published studies, the role of modeling—the therapist's actually demonstrating the prescribed behaviors during therapy—is essential in children behavioral treatment.

There is now undisputed evidence that drug therapy with one of the serotonin uptake inhibitors—clomipramine, fluoxetine, or fluvoxamine—is a major treatment for childhood OCD. Clomipramine is still experimental in the United States, but it is available in Canada and in South American and European countries. Whenever possible, clomipramine should be the first medication to try for obsessive–compulsive children. Doses of 2.5 to 3 mg/kg/day are recommended and generally well tolerated, provided the posology is gradually attained over a few weeks (and gradually decreased at the end of treatment). Long-term treatment is often necessary, but discontinuation can be attempted approximately every 6 months. If symptoms return, treatment should be resumed.

If clomipramine is the one drug that has shown the best group efficacy for treatment of childhood OCD, not all children respond to this medication. For those who do not improve under clomipramine, fluoxetine, fluvoxamine, or one of the other medications that have proven effective in some cases of OCD should be tried. So far, this can be attempted only on an empirical basis since there is no evidence of differential clinical profiles or other predicting factors that can suggest treatment outcome with specific pharmacological agents.

Even if they are less efficacious alone, the other treatment modalities should not be neglected. Psychoanalytic or psychodynamic treatment remains indicated in some cases, especially children for whom personality problems, or suffering, extend beyond the area of their obsessive thoughts or behaviors. The relationship of obsessive children with their environment, their relations to peers and family, should be carefully evaluated. In many cases, group therapy, milieu therapy, and family therapy may help alleviate the isolation and incomprehension created by the disorder. In addition, obsessive–compulsive patients are likely to need long-term support and, at times, directive interventions. Encouraging patients and families to take risks and to push themselves into school or social activities may yield substantial improvements.

In conclusion, it needs to be emphasized that, for nearly all children and adolescents with obsessive–compulsive disorder, a multimodal approach to case conceptualization and treatment is necessary. Young people who suffer with obsessions and compulsions are usually guilt-ridden and feel very isolated. The psychological expressions, or consequences, of the disorder are profound. All efforts should be made, with drugs or with behavioral treatment, to alleviate what are very incapacitating symptoms. The context in which these symptoms have appeared, or persist, needs careful attention, and, in all cases, psychological treatment remains essential.

## References

Altschuler, M. (1962). Massive doses of trifluperazine in the treatment of compulsive rituals. *American Journal of Psychiatry, 119,* 367–368.
Ananth, J., Pecknold, J. C., Van Den Steen, N. & Engelsmann, F. (1981). Double-blind comparative study of clomipramine and amitriptyline in obsessive neurosis. *Progress in Neuropsychopharmacology, 5,* 257–262.
Ananth, J., Solyom, L., Solyom, C., et al. (1975). Doxepin in the treatment of obsessive-compulsive neurosis. *Psychosomatics, 16,* 185–187.
Apter, A., Bernhout, E., & Tyano, S. (1984). Severe obsessive compulsive disorder in adolescence: A report of eight cases. *Journal of Adolescence, 7,* 349–358.
Barton Hall, M. (1935). Obsessive-compulsive states in childhood and their treatment. *Archives of Disease in Childhood, 10,* 49–59.
Bartucci, R. J., Stewart, J. T., & Kemph, J. P. (1987). Trimipramine in the treatment of obsessive-compulsive disorder. *American Journal of Psychiatry, 144,* 964–965.
Baxter, L. R. (1985). Two cases of obsessive-compulsive disorder with depression responsive to trazodone. *Journal of Nervous and Mental Diseases, 173,* 432–433.
Baxter, L. R., Phelps, M. E., Maziotta, J. C., Guze, B. H., Schwertz, J. M., & Celin, C. E. (1987). Local cerebral rates in obsessive-compulsive disorder: A comparison with rates in unipolar depression and normal controls. *Archives of General Psychiatry, 44,* 211–218.
Beech, H. R., & Perigault, J. (1974). Toward a theory of obsessional disorder. In H. R. Beech (Ed.), *Obsessional states.* London: Methuen.
Benkelfat, C., Murphy, D. L., Zohar, J., Hill, J. L., Grover, G., & Insel, T. R. (1989). Clomipramine in obsessive-compulsive disorder: Further evidence for a serotonergic mechamism of action. *Archives of General Psychiatry, 1,* 23–28.
Berg, C. J., Rapoport, J. L. & Flament, M. F. (1986). The Leyton Obsessional Inventory-Child Version. *Journal of the American Academy of Child Psychiatry, 25,* 84–91.
Berman, L. (1942). The obsessive-compulsive neurosis in children. *Journal of Nervous and Mental Disease, 95,* 26–39.
Bevan, J. R. (1960). Learning theory applied to the treatment of a patient with obsessional ruminations. In H. J. Eysenck (Ed.), *Behavior therapy and the neurosis.* Oxford: Pergamon Press.
Black, A. (1974). The natural history of obsessional neurosis. In H. R. Beech (Ed.), *Obsessional states.* London: Methuen.
Bolton, D., Collins, S., & Steinberg, D. (1983). The treatment of obsessive-compulsive disorder in adolescence: A report of fifteen cases. *British Journal of Psychiatry, 142,* 456–464.
Boulougouris, J. C. (1977). Variables affecting the behaviour of obsessive-compulsive patients treated by flooding. In Boulougouris, Rabavilas, & Elmsford (Eds.), *Studies in phobic and obsessive-compulsive disorders.* New York: Pergammon Press.
Campbell, L. M. (1973). A variation of thought stopping in a twelve-year-old boy: A case report. *Journal of Behavior Therapy and Experimental Psychiatry, 4,* 69–70.
Casas, M., Alvarez, E., Duro, P., Garcia-Ribera, C., Udina, C., Velat, A., Abella, D., Rodrigues-Espinosa, A., Salva, P. & Jané, F. (1986). Antiandrogenic treatment of obsessive-compulsive neurosis. *Acta Psychiatrica Scandinavica, 73,* 221–222.
Cautela, J. R. (1969). Behavior therapy and self-control: Technique and implications. In C. M. Franks (Ed.), *Behavior therapy: Appraisal and status.* New York: McGraw-Hill.
Chethik, M. (1969). The therapy of an obsessive-compulsive boy. *Journal of the American Academy of Child Psychiatry, 8,* 465–484.
De Seixas Queiroz, L. O., Motta, M. A., Pinho Madi, M. B. B., et al. (1981). A functional analysis of obsessive-compulsive problems with related therapeutic procedures. *Behaviour Research Therapy, 19,* 377–388.

Eisenberg, J., & Asnis, G. (1985). Lithium as an adjunct treatment in obsessive-compulsive disorder. *American Journal of Psychiatry, 142,* 663.
Emmelkamp, P. M. G. & Kraanen, J. (1977). Therapist-controlled exposure in vivo versus self-controlled exposure in vivo: A comparison with obsessive-compulsive patients. *Behaviour Research Therapy, 15,* 491–495.
Fenichel, O. (1945). *The psychoanalytic theory of neurosis.* New York: Norton.
Fine, S. (1973). Family therapy and a behavioral approach to childhood obsessive-compulsive disorder. *Archives of General Psychiatry, 28,* 695–697.
Flament, M. F., Koby, E., Rapoport, J. L., Berg, C. J., Zahn, T., Cox, C., Denckla, M., & Lenane, M. (1990). Childhood obsessive compulsive disorder: A prospective follow-up study. *Journal of Child Psychology and Psychiatry, 31,* 363–380..
Flament, M., & Rapoport, J. L. (1984). Childhood obsessive-compulsive disorder. In T. R. Insel (Ed.), *New findings in obsessive-compulsive disorder.* Washington, D. C.: American Psychiatric Press.
Flament, M. F., Rapoport, J. L., Berg, C. J., Sceery, W., Kilts, C., Mellström, B., & Linnoila, M. (1985). Clomipramine treatment of childhood obsessive-compulsive disorder: A double-blind controlled study. *Archives of General Psychiatry, 42,* 977–983.
Flament, M. F., Rapoport, J. L., Murphy, D. L., Berg, C. J., & Lake, C. R. (1987). Biochemical changes during clomipramine treatment of childhood obsessive-compulsive disorder. *Archives of General Psychiatry, 44,* 219–225.
Flament, M. F., Whitaker, A., Rapoport, J. L., Davies, M., Berg, C. Z., Kalkow, K., Sceery, W., & Shaffer, D. (1989). Obsessive compulsive disorder in adolescence: An epidemiological study. *Journal of the American Academy of Child Psychiatry.*
Foa, E. B., & Goldstein, A. (1978). Continuous exposure and complete response prevention treatment of obsessive-compulsive neurosis. *Behavior Therapy, 9,* 821–829.
Foa, E. B., Steketee, G., Kozak, M. J., & Dugger, D. (1987). Effects of imipramine on depression and obsessive-compulsive symptoms. *Psychiatry Research, 21,* 123–136.
Foa, E. B., Steketee, G. S. & Milby, J. B. (1980). Differential effects of exposure and response prevention in obsessive-compulsive washers. *Journal of Consulting and Clinical Psychology, 48,* 71–79.
Fontaine, R., & Chouinard, G. (1986). An open clinical trial of fluoxetine in the treatment of obsessive-compulsive disorder. *Journal of Clinical Psychopharmacology, 6,* 98–101.
Fontaine, R., Chouinard, G., & Iny, L. (1985). An open trial of zimeldine in the treatment of obsessive compulsive disorder. *Current Therapeutic Research, 37,* 326–332.
Freed, A., Kerr, T. A., & Roth, M. (1972). The treatment of obsessional neurosis. *British Journal of Psychiatry, 120,* 590–591.
Freud, A. (1966). Obsessional neurosis: A summary of psycho-analytic views as presented at the congress. *International Journal of Psychoanalysis, 47,* 116–122.
Freud, S. (1959). Notes upon a case of obsessional neurosis. In *Collected Papers,* (Vol. 3). New York, Basic Books. (Original work published 1909)
Friedmann, C. T. H., & Silvers, F. M. (1977). A multimodal approach to inpatient treatment of obsessive-compulsive disorder. *American Journal of Psychotherapy 31,* 456–465.
Goodman, W. K., Price, L. H., Rasmussen, S. A., Delgado, P. L., Henninger, G. R., & Charney, D. S. (1989). Efficacy of fluvoxamine in obsessive-compulsive disorder: A double-blind comparison with placebo. *Archives of General Psychiatry, 46,* 36–44.
Hafner, R. J., Gilchrest, P., Bowling, J., & Kalucy, R. (1981). The treatment of obsessional neurosis in a family setting. *Australian and New Zealand Journal of Psychiatry, 15,* 145–151.
Hernstein, R. J. (1969) Method and theory in the study of avoidance. *Psychological Review, 76,* 49–69.
Hollingsworth, C. E., Tanguay, P. E., Grossman, L., & Pabst, P. (1980). Long-term outcome of obsessive-compulsive disorder in childhood. *Journal of the American Academy of Child Psychiatry, 19,* 134–144.

Hussain, M. Z., & Ahad, A. (1970). Treatment of obsessive-compulsive neurosis. *Canadian Medical Association Journal, 103,* 648.

Insel, T. R., Mueller, E. A., Alterman, I., Linnoila, M., & Murphy, D. L. (1985). Obsessive-compulsive disorder and serotonin: Is there a connection? *Biological Psychiatry, 20,*1174–1188.

Insel, T. R., Murphy, D. L., Cohen, R. M., Alterman, I., Kilts, C., & Linnoila, M. (1983). Obsessive-compulsive disorder: A double-blind trial of clomipramine and clorgyline. *Archives General Psychiatry, 40,* 605–612.

Isberg, R. S. (1981). A comparison of phenelzine and imipramine in an obsessive-compulsive patient. *American Journal of Psychiatry, 138,* 1250–1251.

Janet, P. (1903). *Les obsessions et la Psychasthénie* (2nd ed.) Paris: Bailliere.

Jaskari, M. O. (1980). Observations on mianserin in the treatment of obsessive neuroses. *Current Medical Research and Opinion, 6,* 128–131.

Jenike, M. A. (1981). Rapid response of severe obsessive-compulsive disorder to tranylcypromine. *American Journal of Psychiatry, 138,* 1249–1250.

Jenike, M. A., Surman, O. S., Cassem, N. H., Zusky, P., & Anderson, P. W. (1983). Monoamine oxidase inhibitors in obsessive-compulsive disorder. *Journal of Clinical Psychiatry, 44,* 131–132.

Judd, L. L. (1965). Obsessive compulsive neurosis in children. *Archives of General Psychiatry, 12,*136–143.

Kahn, R. S. (1984). Zimeldine treatment of obsessive-compulsive disorder. *Acta Psychiatrica Scandinavia, 69,* 259–261.

Ketter, T., Chun, D., & Lu, F. (1986). Alprazolam in the treatment of compulsive symptoms. *Journal of Psychopharmacology, 6,* 59–60.

Knesevich, J. W. (1982). Successful treatment of obsessive-compulsive disorder with clonidine hydrochloride. *American Journal of Psychiatry, 139,* 364–365.

Lamontagne, Y. (1977). Immersion et implosion. in R. Ladouceur, M. A. Bouchard, & L. Granges (Eds.), *Thérapies behaviorales.* Paris: Maloine.

Lazarus, A. A. (1958). New methods in psychotherapy: A case study. *South African Medical Journal, 33,* 660–663.

Leonard, H., Swedo, S., Rapoport, J. L., Koby, E. V., Lenane, M., Cheslow, D. L., & Hamburger, S. D. (1988). Treatment of obsessive-compulsive disorder with clomipramine and desmethylimipramine: A double-blind crossover comparison. *Psychopharmacological Bulletin, 24,* 93–95.

Lydiard, R. B. (1986). Obsessive-compulsive disorder successfully treated with trazodone. *Psychosomatics, 27,*858–859.

Marks, I. M. (1981). Review of behavioral therapy. I: Obsessive-compulsive disorders. *American Journal of Psychiatry, 138,* 584–592.

Marks, I. M. (1985). *Traitement et prise en charge des malades névrotiques.* Chicoutimi, Quebec, Canada: Gaetan Morin.

Marks, I. M., Bird, J., & Lindley, P. (1978). Psychiatric nurse therapy: Developments and implications. *Behavioural Psychotherapy, 6,*25–36.

Marks, I. M., Rachman, S., & Hodgson, R. (1975). Treatment of chronic obsessive-compulsive neurosis by in vivo exposure. *British Journal of Psychiatry, 127,* 263–267.

Marks, I. M., Stern, R. S. Mawson, D., Cobb, J., & McDonald, R. (1980). Clomipramine and exposure for obsessive-compulsive rituals: I and II. *British Journal of Psychiatry, 136,* 161–166.

Marshall, W. K. (1975). The role of intravenous clomipramine in the treatment of obsessional and phobic disorders. *Scottish Medical Journal, 20,* 49–53.

Mattes, J. A. (1986). A pilot study of combined trazodone and tryptophan treatment in obsessive-compulsive disorder. *International Clinical Psychopharmacology, 1,* 170–173.

Mavissakalian, M., & Michelson, L. (1983). Tricyclic antidepressants in obsessive-compulsive disorder: Antiobsessional or antidepressant agents? *Journal of Nervous and Mental Disease, 171,* 301–306.

Meyer, V. (1966). Modification of expectancies in cases with obsessional rituals. *Behaviour Research and Therapy, 4,* 273–280.

Meyer, V., Levy, R., & Schnurer, A. (1974). The behavioral treatment of obsessive-compulsive disorders. In H. R. Beech (Ed.), *Obsessional states.* London: Methuen.

Milby, J. B., Meredith, R. L., & Rice, J. (1981). Video-taped exposure: A new treatment for obsessive-compulsive disorders. *Journal of Behavior Therapy and Experimental Psychiatry, 12,* 249–255.

Mills, H. L., Agras, W. S., Barlow, D. H., & MIlls, J. R. (1973). Compulsive rituals treated by response prevention: An experimental analysis. *Archives of General Psychiatry, 28,* 524–529.

Montgomery, S. A. (1980). Clomipramine in obsessional neurosis: A placebo-controlled study. *Pharmaceutical Medicine, 1,* 189–192.

Mowrer, O. H. (1960). *Learning theory and behavior.* New York: Wiley.

O'Connor, J. (1983). Why can't I get hives: Brief strategic therapy with an obsessional child. *Family Process, 22,* 201–209.

Ong, S. B. Y., & Leng, Y. K. (1979). The treatment of an obsessive-compulsive girl in the context of Malaysian Chinese culture. *Australian and New Zealand Journal of Psychiatry, 13,* 255–259.

O'Regan, J. B. (1970). Treatment of obsessive-compulsive neurosis with haloperidol. *Canadian Medical Association Journal, 103,* 167–168.

Orvin, G. H. (1967) Treatment of the phobic obsessive-compulsive patient with oxazepam, an improved benzodiazepine compound. *Psychosomatics, 8,* 278–280.

Perse, T. L., Greist, J. H., Jefferson, J. W., Posenfeld, R., & Dar, R. (1987). Fluvoxamine treatment of obsessive-compulsive disorder. *American Journal of Psychiatry, 144,* 1543–1548.

Prasad, A. (1984). A double blind study of imipramine versus zimeldine in treatment of obsessive compulsive neurosis. *Pharmacopsychiatry, 17,* 61–62.

Prasad, A. (1986). Efficacy of trazodone as an anti-obsessional agent. *Neuropsychobiology, 15,* 19–21.

Price, L. H., Goodman, W. K., Charney, D. S., Rasmussen, S. A., & Heninger, G. R. (1987). Treatment of severe obsessive-compulsive disorder with fluvoxamine. *American Journal of Psychiatry, 144,* 1059–1061.

Rabavilas, A. D., Boulougouris, J. C., Perissaki, C., & Stefanis, C. (1979). The effect of peripheral beta-blockade on psychophysiologic responses in obsessional neurotics. *Comprehensive Psychiatry, 20,* 378–383.

Rachman, S., De Silva, P., & Roper, G. (1976). The spontaneous decay of compulsive urges. *Behaviour Research and Therapy, 14,* 445–453.

Rachman, S. J., & Hodgson, R. J. (1980). *Obsessions and compulsions.* Englewood Cliffs, NJ: Prentice-Hall.

Ramzy, I. (1967). Facteurs et traits de la névrose compulsive dans l'enfance. *Revue Française de Psychanalyse, 31,* 611–628.

Rapoport, J. L., Elkins, R., Langer, D. H., Sceery, W., Buchsbaum, M., Gillin, C., Murphy, D., Zahn, T., Lake, R., Ludlow, C., & Mendelson, W. (1981). Childhood obsessive-compulsive disorder. *American Journal of Psychiatry, 138,* 1545–1554.

Rapoport, J. L., Elkins, R., & Mikkelson, E. (1980). Clinical controlled trial of chlorimipramine in adolescents with obsessive-compulsive disorder. *Psychopharmacological Bulletin, 16,* 61–63.

Rasmussen, S. A. (1984). Lithium and tryptophan augmentation in clomipramine-resistant obsessive-compulsive disorder. *American Journal of Psychiatry, 141,* 1283–1285.

Rihmer, Z., Szanto, K., Arato, M., Szabó, M. & Bagdy, G. (1982). Response of phobic disorders with obsessive symptoms to MAO inhibitors. *American Journal of Psychiatry, 139,* 1374.

Rivers-Buckeley, N., & Hollender, M. H. (1982). Successful treatment of obsessive-compulsive disorder with loxapine. *American Journal of Psychiatry, 139,* 1345–1346.
Roper, G., Rachman, S., & Marks, I. (1975). Passive and participant modelling in exposure treatment of obsessive-compulsive neurotics. *Behaviour Research and Therapy, 13,* 271–279.
Silverman, J. S. (1972). Obsessional disorders in childhood and adolescence. *American Journal of Psychotherapy, 26,* 362–377.
Snyder, S. (1980). Amitriptyline therapy of obsessive-compulsive neurosis. *Journal of Clinical Psychiatry, 41,* 286–289.
Steiner, W., & Fontaine, R. (1986). Toxic reactions following the combined administration of fluoxetine and L-tryptophan: Five case reports. *Biological Psychiatry, 21,* 1067–1071.
Steketee, G., Foa, E. B., & Grayson, J. B. (1982). Recent advances in the behavioral treatment of obsessive-compulsives. *Australian and New Zealand Journal of Psychiatry, 39,* 1365–1371.
Stern, T. A., & Jenike, M. A. (1983). Treatment of obsessive-compulsive disorder with lithium carbonate. *Psychosomatics, 24,* 671–673.
Swedo, S. E., Rapoport, J. L., Leonard, H., Lenane, M., & Cheslow, D. (1989). Obsessive compulsive disorder in children and adolescents: I. Clinical phenomenology of 70 consecutive cases. *Archives of General Psychiatry, 46:* 335–341.
Tesar, G. E., & Jenike, M. A. (1984). Alprazolam as treatment for a case of obsessive-compulsive disorder. *American Journal of Psychiatry, 141,* 689–690.
Thorén, P., Asberg, M., Bertilsson, L., Mellström, B., Sjöqvist, F., & Träskman, L. (1980). Clomipramine treatment of obsessive-compulsive disorder: II. Biochemical aspects. *Archives of General Psychiatry, 37,* 1289–1294.
Thorén, P., Asberg, M., Cronholm, B., Jonestedt, L., & Träskman, L. (1980) Clomipramine treatment of obsessive-compulsive disorder: I. A controlled clinical trial. *Archives of General Psychiatry, 37,* 1281–1285.
Tollefson, G. (1985). Alprazolam in the treatment of obsessive symptoms. *Journal of Clinical Psychiatry, 5,* 39–42.
Trethowan, W. H., & Scott, P. A. L. (1955) Chlorpromazine in obsessive-compulsive and allied disorders. *Lancet, 51,* 781–785.
Turner, S. M., Jacob, R. G., Beidel, D. C., & Himmelhoch, J. (1985). Fluoxetine treatment of obsessive-compulsive disorder. *Journal of Clinical Psychopharmacology, 5,* 207–212.
Venkoba-Rao, A. (1964). A controlled trial with "valium" in obsessive-compulsive state. *Journal of the Indian Medical Association, 42,* 564–567.
Volavka, J., Neziroglu, F., & Yaryura-Tobias, J. A. (1985). Clomipramine and imipramine in obsessive-compulsive disorder. *Psychiatry Research, 14,* 83–91.
Walter, C. J. S. (1973). Clinical impressions on treatment of obsessional states with intravenous clomipramine. *Journal of International Medical Research, 1,* 413–415.
Walton, D. (1960). The relevance of learning theory to the treatment of an obsessive-compulsive state. In H. J. Eysenck (Ed.), *Behavior therapy and the neurosis.* Oxford: Pergamon Press.
Warneke, L. B. (1984). The use of intravenous clomipramine in the treatment of obsessive compulsive disorder. *Canadian Journal of Psychiatry, 29,* 135–141.
Warneke, L. B. (1985). Intravenous clomipramine in the treatment of obsessive compulsive disorder in adolescence: Case report. *Journal of Clinical Psychiatry, 46,* 100–103.
Weiner, I. B. (1967). Behavior therapy in obsessive-compulsive neurosis: Treatment of an adolescent girl. *Psychotherapeutic Theory Research and Practice, 4,* 27–29.
Wolff, R., & Rapoport, J. (1988). Behavioral treatment of childhood obsessive-compulsive disorder. *Behavior Modification, 12,* 252–266.
Wolpe, J. (1973). *The practice of behavior therapy* (2nd ed.). New York: Pergamon Press.
Won Kim, S. (1987). Trazodone in the treatment of obsessive–compulsive disorder: A case report. *Journal of Clinical Psychopharmacology, 7,* 278–279.
Worsley, J. L. (1986). Behavior and obsessionality. In H. Freeman (Ed.), *Progress in behavior therapy.* Bristol: John Wright.

Yamagami, T. (1978). Changes of behavior, fear and thought in the treatment by response prevention: A case study of obsessive compulsive disorder. *Folia Psychiatrica Neurologica Japonica, 32,* 77–83.

Yaryura-Tobias, J. A. (1977). L-tryptophan in obsessive-compulsive disorders. *American Journal of Psychiatry, 134,* 1298–1299.

Zohar, J., & Insel, T. R. (1987). Obsessive-compulsive disorder: Psychobiological approaches to diagnosis, treatment and pathophysiology. *Biological Psychiatry, 22,* 677–687.

# 5

# Autism and Aggression

## Magda Campbell, Richard P. Malone, and Vivian Kafantaris

### Introduction

In the past decade some progress has been achieved in the treatment of autistic children and children with a variety of psychiatric disorders whose target symptoms include aggression. Areas of progress include both psychopharmacologic and psychosocial interventions. The purpose of this chapter is to present advances in the area of pharmacotherapy for these conditions. We wish to emphasize that pharmacotherapy is never considered to be sufficient as the sole treatment modality. However, a subgroup of these children may benefit considerably from pharmacotherapy, in addition to other types of treatments.

### Autism

#### History

The syndrome of early infantile autism was first described by Kanner in 1943. In the intervening years there have been a number of diagnostic labels used to describe these children and, by some, a tendency to group together under this label a variety of serious early-onset psychiatric disorders. Kolvin (1971) differentiated two groups of children by symptomatology and age of onset. Those with an onset before the age of 3 were characterized by having symptoms more in line with the diagnosis of autism, while those with an onset after the age of 5 had symptoms of schizophrenia. Rutter's criteria for early infantile autism were: failure to develop social relationships, language delay and

---

*Magda Campbell, Richard P. Malone, and Vivian Kafantaris*   Department of Psychiatry, New York University Medical Center, New York, New York 10016.

deviance, and ritualistic activities (1972, 1978). Infantile autism was included for the first time in the third edition of the *Diagnostic and Statistical Manual of Mental Disorders* (American Psychiatric Association, 1980) as the prototype of pervasive developmental disorders, with the cardinal symptoms as defined by Kanner (1943) and Rutter (1972, 1978). The revised third edition (APA, 1987) includes major revisions in the category of autism.

Autism has a prevalence of 3 to 4 cases per 10,000 in the general population (Ritvo et al., 1989); males are affected two to three times more than females. Autism is etiologically heterogeneous (for review, see Campbell & Green, 1985; Young, Leven, Newcorn, & Knott, 1987). Subnormal intellectual functioning is commonly associated with autism: the majority of autistics have IQs under 70 (Rutter, 1972). The rate of seizure disorder is higher in autistic children than in the general population (Deykin & MacMahon, 1979; Rutter, 1972). About one-third of those who do not have seizures as young children will develop them by adolescence (Rutter & Schopler, 1978). Subnormal intellectual functioning and seizure disorders have implications for treatment with psychoactive drugs. First, psychoactive drugs can impair cognitive functioning (Platt et al., 1984), a particularly unwanted effect in those already cognitively impaired. And second, certain drugs—for example, chlorpromazine (Tarjan, Lowery, & Wright, 1957) and imipramine (Petti & Campbell, 1975)— may lower the seizure threshold and increase the frequency of seizures. While some autistic children have been able to gain enough independence to live in supervised settings away from the family as adults, many require long-term institutional settings.

## Advances in Assessment

A number of assessment instruments have been used in this population, both clinically and in research, and were recently reviewed (Campbell & Palij, 1985). The Rimland E-2 is a checklist developed to be used by parents and caretakers (Rimland, 1971). The Conners Parent-Teacher Questionnaire (PTQ), Clinical Global Impressions (CGI) (*Psychopharmacology Bulletin*, 1973), and the Children's Psychiatric Rating Scale (CPRS), a general rating instrument (*Psychopharmacology Bulletin*, 1973), have been used successfully in clinical drug trials and been shown to be sensitive to drug effects in autistic children (Campbell & Palij, 1985). Fourteen selected items of the CPRS (Campbell & Palij, 1985) and its three factors (Overall & Campbell, 1988) have been shown to be sensitive to change due to drug administration (Anderson et al., 1989; Campbell, 1987; Campbell & Spencer, 1988; Perry et al., 1989). Both the Behavioral Observation System (Freeman et al., 1980) and the Childhood Autism Rating Scale (CARS); (Schopler, Reichler, & Renner, 1985), a well-researched instrument, were designed to be clinical measures of behaviors associated with autism.

## Comprehensive and Individualized Treatment Programs

The goals of treatment in autistic children are twofold: to promote development and to decrease maladaptive behaviors, which usually interfere with learning. Autistic children are heterogeneous in regard to their behavior and level of intellectual functioning. There is a wide range in the behavioral profile and severity of their symptoms. Therefore, a treatment program has to be individualized. Treatment must include special education, behavioral work with parents, and, when indicated, pharmacological interventions. Behavioral techniques include contingency management, token economies, and engaging parents as cotherapists (for review, see Campbell & Schopler, 1989). A variety of psychoactive drugs are in use in this population (Campbell, 1987). As noted above, because these children are often intellectually subnormal and always have learning problems, caution must be used regarding possible adverse effects of drugs on cognition and learning.

## Pharmacotherapy: An Overview of the Literature

### Neuroleptics

Neuroleptics are perhaps the most extensively studied agents in this population. The high-potency neuroleptics, such as haloperidol and pimozide, have generally been found to be more beneficial than lower-potency neuroleptics, such as chlorpromazine. The lower-potency neuroleptics are generally more sedating at doses that yield only slight reduction of symptoms (Campbell, Fish, Korein, et al., 1972). Sedation is a side effect that is particularly unwanted in the cognitively impaired. Furthermore, chlorpromazine is known to lower the seizure threshold and to increase the frequency of seizures (Tarjan et al., 1957).

Of all psychoactive agents, haloperidol has been studied most systematically. The results of Faretra, Dooher, and Dowling (1970), based on a carefully conducted open clinical trial, were promising. Since that time, the efficacy of this drug has been demonstrated in well-controlled clinical trials. Haloperidol has been critically assessed in four double-blind studies involving a total of 116 subjects (Anderson et al., 1984, 1989; Campbell et al., 1978; Cohen et al., 1980). Another large placebo-controlled study represented a comparison of haloperidol and pimozide (Naruse et al., 1982). Like other neuroleptics, haloperidol is not recommended for use in exclusively hypoactive and anergic patients. In general, haloperidol has been found to be useful in reducing a number of symptoms — specifically, withdrawal and stereotypies (Campbell et al., 1978; Cohen et al., 1980), in addition to hyperactivity, angry and labile affect, and abnormal object relations (Anderson et al., 1984, 1989). Haloperidol also facilitated discrimination learning (Anderson et al., 1984) and acquisition of words when used with contingent reinforcement focusing on language (Campbell et al., 1978). In the above studies the therapeutic doses of haloperidol ranged from 0.25 to 4.0 mg/day (mean, 0.34–1.65 mg/day) or 0.016 to 0.217 mg/kg/day (Anderson et al., 1984, 1989; Campbell et al., 1978); dosage was regulated individually to achieve maximum reduction of symptoms in the absence of side effects. Side effects occurred only above optimal doses or during periods of dosage regulation; most frequent were sedation, worsening of irritability, and acute dystonic reaction (Anderson et al., 1984; Campbell et al., 1978). The dystonic reactions were relieved by diphenhydramine hydrochloride, 25 mg p.o. or i.m. Clinical experience has suggested that lower starting doses and very gradual increments may decrease the incidence of dystonic reactions or avoid them altogether. Haloperidol remains an effective drug when administered on a long-term basis (Perry, Campbell, et al., 1989).

Pimozide was studied in autistic children in a pilot study, involving four subjects, ages 5 to 16 years (Suwa et al., 1984), and in a double-blind placebo-controlled trial, involving 34 inpatients between the ages of 3 and 16 years (Naruse et al., 1982). The latter study was a comparison of pimozide (1–9 mg/d) and haloperidol (0.75–6.75 mg/d); the two drugs were equally effective and superior to placebo. In general, pimozide was particularly effective in decreasing such maladaptive behaviors as hyperactivity, labile affect, and aggressiveness.

A concern with the use of neuroleptics is the occurrence of dyskinesias associated with chronic drug administration. The neuroleptic-related dyskinesias are abnormal involuntary movements and they can involve any muscle, including the diaphragm. However, oro-buccal-lingual dyskinesias are the most common. Movements of the upper extremities and digits are also frequent; they include choreoathetotic and jerking movements of the arms, flicking movements of the fingers, and ataxia. In more severe forms, the whole body can be involved, resulting in rocking motions and thrusting of the torso. Neuroleptic-related dyskinesias can be classified (Crane & Naranjo, 1971; Gardos, Cole, & Tarsy, 1978) into those associated with decrease of dosage (covert dyskinesia) or complete drug withdrawal (withdrawal dyskinesia), and those that persist longer or remain irreversible (tardive dyskinesia).

Stereotypies, another type of abnormal movements, are often observed in autistic children, and particularly in those who are moderately to profoundly retarded (Freeman et al., 1981). The stereotypies may include chewing movements, eye blinking, lip smacking, arm twirling, and finger flicking (Campbell, 1985; Freeman et al., 1981). Because stereotypies and neuroleptic-related dyskinesias can occur in the same area and can consist of the same motions, these two types of abnormal movements can be difficult, and at times impossible, to distinguish (Meiselas et al., 1989). For this reason a careful assessment of movements on baseline should always be taken before placing a child on a psychoactive drug, particularly a neuroleptic. Every attempt should be made to carry out multiple assessments, since various movements do not necessarily occur during any given observation. Administration of neuroleptics is associated with a reduction of stereotypies (Anderson et al., 1984, 1989; Campbell et al., 1978; Cohen et al., 1980). A baseline survey of stereotypies is necessary in order to judge the effectiveness of the medication in reducing them. Once medication is begun, the presence of possible dyskinesias could be judged by comparing any new abnormal movements with the baseline stereotypies. Of course, if a patient has a history of neuroleptic exposure prior to the time the baseline is obtained, the baseline itself could include some dyskinesias as well as stereotypies. Accurate documentation of movements, preferably on an instrument like the Abnormal Involuntary Movement Scale (AIMS; Psychopharmacology Bulletin, 1985), as well as documentation of medication changes, is required.

A literature review indicates that neuroleptic-related dyskinesias occur in 0.5 to 67.6% of adults (for review, see Campbell et al., 1983). In a long-term prospective study of haloperidol in autistic children, 29% of the patients developed dyskinesias (Campbell, Adams, Perry, Spencer, & Overall, 1988). It is conceivable that the study design itself, with repeated drug withdrawal each 6 months, contributed to the high rate of dyskinesias. It is noteworthy that in this study relatively low doses of haloperidol were used (0.25–10.5 mg/day, median 1.0 mg/day, or 0.016–0.217 mg/kg/day, median 0.054 mg/kg/day). Of the 82 children who participated in this study, dyskinesias were rated in 24. Nineteen of the 24 children had withdrawal dyskinesias, and the remaining 5 developed movments while receiving haloperidol (Campbell, Adams, Perry, et al., 1988). In all children the dyskinesias were reversible (Campbell, Adams, Perry, et al., 1988). Haloperidol-related dyskinesias in the form of a Tourette-like syndrome were also reported (Perry, Nobler, & Campbell, 1989; Stahl, 1980).

*Fenfluramine*

A double-blind and placebo-controlled multicenter study was organized under the direction of Ritvo to evaluate the efficacy of fenfluramine (Ritvo et al., 1986). Fenfluramine is a potent antiserotonergic agent and a mild dopamine antagonist. Hyperserotonemia was found in about 30% of autistic children and was related to certain behavioral symptoms and to low intellectual functioning (Campbell et al., 1975; Ritvo et al., 1970; Ritvo, Freeman, Geller, & Yuwiler, 1983). This was the rationale for exploring fenfluramine (Geller, Ritvo, Freeman, & Yuwiler, 1982; Ritvo et al., 1983). While the initial reports were promising (August, Raz, & Baird, 1985; Geller et al., 1982; Ritvo et al., 1983), the results of the multicenter trial involving 81 subjects were less impressive (Ritvo et al., 1986). Some of these studies have been criticized on a methodological basis, for lack of randomization and excessive length of the study period (for review, see Campbell, 1988). More recently, carefully designed studies failed to show superiority of fenfluramine over placebo (Campbell, Adams, Small, Curren, et al., 1988; Ekman, Miranda-Linne, Gillberg, Garle, & Wetterberg, in press). The results of one report indicated that fenfluramine may have a negative effect on discrimination learning, as compared with placebo (Campbell, Adams, Small, Curren, et al., 1988). Furthermore, concern has been raised regarding the central effects of the drug: serotonin depletion of the brain (Schuster, Lewis, & Seiden, 1986).

At the present state of our knowledge, fenfluramine cannot be recommended for treatment of autistic children as a group. However, individual children have benefited and may benefit from fenfluramine. Symptoms responsive to fenfluramine administration, at daily doses ranging from 1.250 to 2.068 mg/kg, are hyperactivity, stereotypies, and withdrawal. Side effects include sleepiness, loss of weight and appetite, and increased irritability (Campbell, Adams, Small, Curren, et al., 1988; Campbell, Deutsch, Perry, Wolsky, & Palij, 1986; for review, see Campbell, 1988).

*Opioid Antagonists*

In the past 3 years, opioid antagonists have begun to be explored in this population (Campbell, Adams, Small, Tesch, & Curren, 1988; Campbell et al., 1989; Herman et al., 1986; Leboyer, Bouvard, & Dugas, 1988), because it has been hypothesized that an abnormality of the endogenous opioid system exists in autism (Panksepp, 1979). This hypothesis was based upon the observation of some analogous abnormalities in the functioning and behavior of autistic patients and those of opioid addicts and infants born to mothers who were addicts during pregnancy (Panksepp, 1979; Panksepp & Sahley, 1987). Furthermore, there is some evidence to support this hypothesis based on studies of autistic children (Gillberg, Terenius, & Lonnerholm, 1985; Weizman et al., 1984).

Naltrexone is a long-acting opioid antagonist. Results in small numbers of autistic patients suggest that this agent is effective in reducing abnormal behaviors (Herman et al., 1986) and that it has both stimulating and tranquilizing therapeutic effects (Campbell, Adams, Small, Tesch, & Curren, 1988; Campbell et al., 1989). In one of the two acute dose range tolerance trials involving 10 children, naltrexone dosages ranged from 0.5 to 2.0 mg/kg/day; side effects at these doses have been mild, consisting mainly of slight sedation of short duration. The results of short-term use of naltrexone (Leboyer et al., 1988) are similar to those with acute dosing. An ongoing double-blind and placebo-controlled study of naltrexone suggests that naltrexone is an effective and safe drug when given over a period of 3 weeks (Campbell, unpublished data). However, these are only preliminary impressions.

## Stimulants

In earlier studies administration of stimulant medication has been noted to be associated mainly with reduction of hyperactivity in the presence of severe behavioral side effects. Behavioral toxicity included worsening of preexisting stereotypies and stereotypies de novo (Campbell, Fish, David, et al., 1972; Campbell et al., 1976). Two recent reports suggest that administration of methylphenidate resulted in decreased hyperactivity without significant side effects and without worsening of stereotypies (Birmaher, Quintana, & Greenhill, 1988; Strayhorn, Rapp, Donina, & Strain, 1988). In a pilot study involving nine children, ages 4 to 16 years, dosages of methylphenidate ranged from 10 to 50 mg/day (Birmaher et al., 1988). Strayhorn et al. (1988) in a single case study found improvement in several areas, including attention and decreased activity, with worsening of mood and tantrums. These results should be looked at with caution since these were open studies and no controls were employed.

Table 1 represents an overview of the recent representative literature.

## Aggression

In children and adolescents, chronic aggressiveness directed against others and/or against self is observed in a variety of psychiatric disorders and in some of the mentally retarded. In children of normal intelligence, aggressive and explosive behavior is most frequently seen in conduct disorder (Stewart, deBlois, Meardon, & Cummings, 1980). Aggressiveness directed against self, or self-injurious behavior (SIB), is reported to be observed in 10 to 17% of the mentally retarded (Baumeister & Rollings, 1976; Schroeder, Schroeder, Smith, & Dalldorf, 1978) and in up to 66% of retarded persons (Young, personal communication). A subgroup of autistic persons also exhibits these behaviors.

Inpatient observation and evaluation of individuals with these target symptoms can be most informative. In inpatient settings one can exclude certain diagnoses, including adjustment disorder, attention deficit disorder with hyperactivity (ADHD), or psychosis, conditions that may have specific and more established treatments. In addition, the therapeutic milieu of the hospital itself can be an effective treatment in reducing aggressive behavior. For example, 19.5% of a large sample of children diagnosed as conduct disorder, and who had a profile of severe aggressiveness and explosiveness, either failed to display these symptoms following hospitalization or showed a significant reduction in these symptoms (Campbell, Small, et al., 1984). This dramatic change in behavior occurred during a 2-week baseline placebo period, and the children no longer required pharmacotherapy. The intuitive reasons for this finding may be that the environment of an acute hospital, with its predictable routine and staff who are skilled in consistent, nonpunitive limit setting, may be highly thera-

Table 1
Survey of Representative Clinical Trials in Autism

| Drug | Dose in mg/day | Reference | Sample size (and CA)[a] | Design |
|---|---|---|---|---|
| Haloperidol | 0.5–4.0 | Campbell et al., 1978 | 40 (2.6–7.2) | Double-blind, placebo-controlled, factorial (with randomization) |
| Haloperidol | 0.5–3.0 | Anderson et al., 1984 | 40 (2.33–6.92) | Double-blind, placebo-controlled, crossover (with randomization) |
| Haloperidol | 0.25–4.0 | Anderson et al., 1989 | 45 (2.02–7.58) | Double-blind, placebo-controlled, crossover (with randomization) |
| Pimozide | 1–9 | Naruse et al., 1982 | 34 (3–16) | Double-blind, placebo-controlled crossover (with randomization) |
| Fenfluramine | 1.5 mg/kg | Ritvo et al., 1986 | 81 (2.75–24) | Double-blind, placebo-controlled crossover (no randomization) |
| Fenfluramine | 1.250–2.068 mg/kg | Campbell et al., 1988[b] | 28 (2.56–6.66) | Double-blind, placebo-controlled, parallel groups (with randomization) |
| Naltrexone | 0.5–2.0 mg/kg | Campbell et al., 1989 | 10 (3.42–6.6) | Open, acute dose-range-tolerance trial |

[a]Chronological age in years.
[b]Campbell, Adams, Small, Curren et al., 1988.

peutic. Removal from home in itself also may be therapeutic for some children. The children in a therapeutic milieu are rewarded for good behavior; peer pressure to behave is also influential. Thus, at least for a subgroup, nonpharmacologic treatments could be very effective, though it is possible that the child will relapse when discharged to a suboptimal or noxious psychosocial environment. Parental or caretaker participation and cooperation is essential if the child's gains during the hospitalization are to be maintained once he is back in the community. However, in certain circumstances residential treatment is too often the only viable treatment option.

Detailed reviews of behavioral treatments are available (Baum & Forehand, 1981; Kazdin, 1975; Kazdin, Esveldt-Dawson, French, & Unis, 1987; Werry & Wollersheim, 1989; Whitman & Johnston, 1987). Attempts to measure their relative effectiveness continue. Both aggressiveness and SIB often fail to respond to psychosocial interventions, including behavior modification (Werry & Wollersheim, 1989). This chapter will focus on pharmacotherapy.

## Assessment of Aggressive Behavior and SIB

Assessment of aggressiveness and SIB can be difficult when the frequency of these behaviors is low. Videotaping, frequency counts, and using symptom rating scales are the most common methods of assessment. The Children's Psychiatric Rating Scale (CPRS), a 63-item 8-severity-point general rating scale, was specifically developed for use in clinical trials (*Psychopharmacology Bulletin*, 1973). It has a few items reflecting aggressive and explosive behaviors and was successfully used in two studies involving aggressive children (Campbell, Cohen, & Small, 1982; Campbell, Small, et al., 1984). Aman et al. (1985) developed the Aberrant Behavior Checklist specifically for the measurement of drug and other treatment effects in the mentally retarded. A well-researched instrument, it has 58 items and 5 subscales; several items reflect aggressive behaviors, including SIB. Yudofsky, Silver, Jackson, Endicott, and Williams (1986) developed a scale for patients with an aggressive profile. An instrument developed specifically to measure verbal and physical aggressiveness and its antecedents in children, the Timed Objective Rating Scale for Aggression (I. L. Cohen, unpublished data) had high interrater reliability and validity. However, it was not sensitive enough to reflect changes due to drug administration (Campbell, Small, et al., 1984).

## Pharmacotherapy: An Overview of the Literature

### Stimulants

Stimulants seem to be effective in reducing aggressive behaviors in children diagnosed as having ADHD and who are outpatients (Werry & Aman,

1975). However, they are ineffective in affecting severe aggressiveness (Aman & Werry, 1982). Stereotypic self-biting was reported to be a side effect of methylphenidate and d-amphetamine in ADHD children (Sokol, Campbell, Goldstein, & Kriechman, 1987).

*Neuroleptics*

This class of drugs has antiaggressive properties both in laboratory animals and in psychiatric patients. The limitations of chlorpromazine in disturbed and/or retarded children were discussed above. In a double-blind placebo-controlled study involving 19 severely retarded individuals who were in a residential setting, thioridazine was effective in reducing SIB (Singh & Aman, 1981). Haloperidol, a potent butyrophenone, was found to be therapeutic in aggressive and hyperactive children, both inpatients and outpatients (Campbell et al., 1982; Campbell, Small, et al., 1984; Cunningham, Pillai, & Rogers, 1968; Werry & Aman, 1975; Wong & Cock, 1971). Daily doses most commonly used ranged from 0.04 to 0.21 mg/kg (Campbell, Small, et al., 1984).

Another potent neuroleptic, pimozide, a diphenylbutylpiperidine, was also explored in children and adolescents who displayed aggressive behaviors. A multicenter trial involved 55 diagnostically heterogeneous children, ages 3 to 20 years (mean 11 years), some of whom showed physical aggressiveness and destructiveness (Reyntjens, 1972). Pimozide dosage ranged from 1 to 3 mg/day; it was calculated on the basis of body weight and it was titrated. The results of this report suggest that administration of pimozide was associated with a decrease of a variety of symptoms, including aggressiveness. At these doses, pimozide was "virtually devoid of sedative effects" (Reyntjens, 1972, p. 667). In another pilot study involving a total of 187 children, a subgroup of 114, all under 14 years of age, seemed to meet the criteria of conduct disorder (Debray, Messerschmitt, Lonchamp, & Herbault, 1972). At daily doses of 1 to 12 mg (mean 2 mg), aggressiveness directed against others and self was reported to have decreased in 85% of this subsample, in the absence of sedation. However, the criteria for improvement were not specified (Debray et al., 1972). It should be noted that both studies had serious methodological flaws.

Naruse et al. (1982) compared pimozide with haloperidol, employing placebo as a control. Theirs was a multicenter double-blind crossover study. The sample consisted of 87 children who were diagnostically heterogeneous: 34 were autistic, 17 were retarded and 27 were hyperkinetic. The remaining 9 were neurotic or psychotic. Their ages ranged from 3 to 16 years. Pimozide, at doses ranging from 1 to 9 mg/d, was significantly superior to placebo in reducing aggressiveness ($p<.05$), injury and violence to others, and furniture breaking ($p<.01$). Self-mutilation was not significantly reduced by either drug. Excessive sedation was the most common side effect with both drugs, and it was significantly greater with active drugs than with placebo (Naruse et al., 1982).

Less encouraging were the findings of White and Aman (1985) involving eight severely retarded and disruptive persons (mean age 15.7 years, $SD$ 3.42) who received pimozide under double-blind placebo-controlled conditions, employing a crossover design. In this carefully designed study with a washout period between treatments and using multiple assessments, daily doses of pimozide ranged from 0.09 to 0.18 mg/kg (mean 0.12). On the Aberrant Behavior Checklist (ABC; Aman, Singh, Stewart, & Field, 1984), there was a significant decrease on two dimensions: irritability and hyperactivity/noncompliance. Although this small sample of patients was described as displaying both SIB and aggressiveness, it is not specified whether these maladaptive behaviors decreased in response to pimozide (White & Aman, 1985).

The limitations of haloperidol, as of other neuroleptics, are parkinsonian side effects (Campbell, Green, & Deutsch, 1985; Campbell et al., 1985), possible negative effects on performance and cognition in the laboratory (Platt, Campbell, Green & Grega, 1984; Werry & Aman, 1975), and their association with dyskinesias when administered on a long-term basis (Campbell et al., 1983; Campbell, Adams, Perry, et al., 1988; Sprague & Newell, 1987). It should be noted that in this young age group most information on neuroleptic-related dyskinesias is based on autistic and retarded populations; there is practically no knowledge involving children and adolescents who are of normal intelligence and free of psychosis. However, the association of neuroleptic administration with tardive dyskinesia led to exploration of other types of psychoactive agents.

## Lithium Carbonate

Lithium is a psychoactive agent with specific antiaggressive properties, as demonstrated in laboratory animals (Sheard & Aghajanian, 1970) and in young aggressive humans (Sheard, Marini, Bridges, & Wagner, 1976). There is some evidence suggesting that lithium is effective when aggressiveness or SIB is accompanied by explosive affect (Campbell, Fish, Korein, et al., 1972; Campbell et al., 1982; Campbell, Small, et al., 1984; Dostal, 1972). A clinically and statistically significant reduction of aggressiveness and explosiveness was reported in treatment-resistant hospitalized children, ages 5.2 to 12.9 years (Campbell, Small et al., 1984). Most common side effects were nausea, vomiting, weight gain, and tremor of hands. Optimal doses of lithium ranged from 500 mg/d to 2000 mg/d, and serum levels were 0.32 to 1.51 mEq/l, mean 0.993 (Campbell, Small, et al., 1984).

The studies of Campbell, Small, et al. (1984) and Sheard et al. (1976) were carefully designed and well controlled, involving individuals of normal intelligence. Two additional reports, one positive, the other negative, are based on open administration of lithium. Ziring and Teitelbaum (1980) found that lithium, under careful clinical and laboratory monitoring, was very effective in reducing severe aggressiveness and/or SIB in profoundly retarded individuals in a residential setting. The findings of DeLong and Aldershof (1987) are much less encouraging. These authors, who have the most extensive experience with lithium in disturbed children (total $N = 196$), reported that of 33 patients, ages 5.3 to 17.4 years, diagnosed as conduct disorder, only 5 (or 15%) responded to lithium. Even in a somewhat different type of child, with "angry aggressiveness" and explosiveness ($N = 9$), ages 6.8 to 16 years (mean 12.3), only 5 were "dramatic responders" (DeLong & Aldershof, 1987).

Lithium administration requires a careful baseline laboratory assessment (including differential cell count, thyroid and kidney function studies, and electrocardiogram) and careful clinical and laboratory monitoring. Side effects as well as safety in children are discussed elsewhere (Campbell, Perry, & Green, 1984; Campbell, Small, et al., 1984; Platt et al., 1984; Reisberg & Gershon, 1979; Spencer & Campbell, 1990).

Clearly, there is some disagreement as to the efficacy of lithium in children and adolescents with symptoms of aggressiveness and/or SIB. The positive studies await replication. More effective and safe novel drugs, or old drugs with new indications, are sought for the treatment of these populations.

*Carbamazepine*

Carbamazepine is a tricyclic anticonvulsant with antiaggressive and other psychoactive properties (Post, 1987). Some of its clinical effects are similar to those of lithium. The antiaggressive properties of this agent may be related to its ability to increase plasma total and free tryptophan (Pratt, Jenner, Johnson, Shorvon, & Reynolds, 1984). In adults, carbamazepine was reported to be effective in affective disorders (see Post, 1987), in psychotic patients with symptoms of assaultiveness and excitement, and in episodic dyscontrol syndrome (for review, see Spencer & Campbell, in press).

In children, carbamazepine was reported to be helpful in a variety of disorders, with or without brain damage, mainly characterized by aggressiveness and explosiveness. However, most evidence is based on small samples of patients or on case reports (for review, see Evans, Clay, & Gualtieri, 1987; O'Donnell, 1985). Birkmayer (1976) published the papers presented at a symposium. Remschmidt (1976) summarized results of 28 clinical trials, 21 open and 7 double-blind, which included a total of more than 800 children. These studies, including those of Groh (1976), Kuhn-Gebhart (1976), and Puente (1976), suggest that target symptoms responsive to carbamazepine are impulsivity, aggressiveness, and emotional lability. In children, therapeutic doses of carbamazepine range from 400 to 600 mg/day, and in adolescents, to 800 mg/day. Therapeutic plasma levels range from 4 to 12 µg/ml (Gamstorp, 1976; Sillanpaa, 1981). Side effects include behavioral toxicity, nausea, sleepiness, ataxia, elevated liver-function tests, blood dyscrasias, diplopia, and vertigo (Gamstorp, 1976; Sillanpaa, 1981). In children, however, allergic skin rash and drowsiness are most common (Gamstorp, 1976). Psychosis, mania, worsening of seizure disorder, and development of seizures were also associated with carbamazepine administration (Leviatov et al., 1976; Pleak, Birmaher, Gavrilescu, Abichandani, & Williams, 1988; Sillanpaa, 1981, pp. 83 & 85; Silverstein, Parrish, & Johnston, 1982).

Thus, carbamazepine seems to be a potentially effective agent in children with symptoms of aggressiveness. However, the efficacy and safety of carbamazepine should be critically assessed in carefully designed studies involving well-defined and diagnostically homogeneous patient samples.

*Beta-Blockers*

The beta-blockers—propranolol, nadolol, and atenolol—were explored in patients with treatment-resistant rages, aggressiveness, or SIB. The reports are based on open pilot studies, with small sample sizes and concomitant use (continuation) of other psychoactive agents, usually one or two neuroleptics. The study of Williams, Mehl, Yudofsky, Adams, and Roseman (1982) included 26 children and adolescents and 4 adults; 25 of the 30 patients were diagnosed as conduct disorder, unsocialized aggressive. Seventy-five percent of the patients responded to propranolol by moderate to marked reduction of rages. In another study, 15 of 19 retarded adults who displayed aggressiveness or SIB had a marked to moderate response to propranolol (Ratey et al., 1986). Eight autistic adults with the same target symptoms showed a similar good response to beta-blockers (Ratey, Bemporad, et al., 1987, Ratey, Mikkelson, et al., 1987).

These are encouraging reports, and the beta blockers await a critical assessment under controlled conditions.

*Opiate Antagonists*

Abnormalities of endogenous opioids were implicated in SIB (for review, see Deutsch, 1986; Spencer & Campbell, in press). This was the rationale for administering the opioid antagonists, naloxone or naltrexone, to individuals with SIB. The reports of Richardson and Zaleski (1983) and Sandman et al. (1983) on the efficacy of naloxone were promising. However, other investigators reported less positive (Davidson, Kleene, Carroll, & Rockowitz, 1983) or negative results (Beckwith, Couk, & Schumacher, 1986) with the parenteral use of naloxone. Bernstein, Hughes, Mitchell, and Thompson (1987) and Herman et al. (1987) found naltrexone to be effective in reducing SIB. Naltrexone is a potent and long-acting oral opiate antagonist, and it appears to be relatively free of serious side effects (for review, see Campbell, Adams, Small, Tesch, & Curren, 1988; Campbell et al., 1989; Herman et al., 1987, 1988).

All data on the efficacy of naltrexone in SIB are based on very small sample sizes or on single-case reports, and usually involve open studies. Clearly, naltrexone awaits a critical assessment in reasonable sample sizes of patients under well-controlled conditions.

Table 2 represents an overview of the recent representative literature.

## Summary and Conclusions

This chapter has focused on the pharmacological treatment of autism and aggression. However, medications are but one part of the total treatment of these disorders and are used concurrently with educational, behavioral, cognitive, family, and other psychosocial therapies.

In autism, research has demonstrated the efficacy and safety of the high-potency neuroleptics in both short- and long-term studies. Haloperidol decreases stereotypies, hyperactivity, anger, labile affect, and abnormal object relations, and facilitates learning in the laboratory. Pimozide has shown similar efficacy. Fenfluramine, while initially promising, has failed in recent studies to show superiority over placebo. The opioid antagonist naltrexone appears to be a promising agent in acute dosage tolerance studies and brief clinical trials with small numbers of patients. Stimulants reduce hyperactivity but can have a deleterious effect on mood and increase stereotypies.

There is supportive evidence that neuroleptics are beneficial in a subgroup of children and adolescents with target symptoms of aggressiveness and/or SIB. The best studies have been with haloperidol and pimozide. Despite the effectiveness of neuroleptics, different agents are being sought because of neuroleptic-related side effects, including adverse effects on cognition and tardive and withdrawal dyskinesias. No definite statement can be made about the efficacy of lithium in these populations. It has been found to be safe and effective in two well-controlled studies, but other reports indicate less success. Carbamazepine deserves more attention, since there have been a few encouraging controlled studies. Beta-blockers and naltrexone are other promising agents that await further critical assessment in aggression and SIB.

There is a paucity of research comparing pharmacological therapies with behavioral interventions. Questions to be answered in future work include these: (1) Are the different modalities equally effective? (2) What are the interactive effects of these modalities?

ACKNOWLEDGMENTS. This work was supported in part by NIMH Grants MH-32212, MH40177, and T3 MH18915 to Dr. Campbell.

## Table 2
### Survey of Representative Clinical Trials in Aggression

| Drug | Dose in mg/day | Reference | Sample size (and CA)[a] | Design | Diagnosis |
|---|---|---|---|---|---|
| Haloperidol | 1–6 | Campbell et al., 1984 | 61 (5.2–12.9) | Double-blind placebo-controlled parallel groups | Hospitalized aggressive children with conduct disorder |
| Haloperidol | 0.75–5.75 | Naruse et al., 1982 | 87 (3–16) | Double-blind placebo-controlled crossover | Children with behavioral disorders |
| Pimozide | 1–9 | Naruse et al., 1982 | 87 (3–16) | Double-blind placebo-controlled crossover | Children with behavioral disorders |
| Lithium | 1212–1691 (0.6–1.0 mEq/L) | Sheard et al., 1976 | 66 (16–24) | Double-blind placebo-controlled | Aggressive, non-psychotic prisoners |
| Lithium | 500–2,000 (0.32–1.51 mEq/L) | Campbell et al., 1984 | 61 (5.2–12.9) | Double-blind placebo-controlled parallel groups | Hospitalized children with conduct disorder |
| Carbamazepine | 200–300 | Puente, 1976 | 27 (5–13) | Double-blind placebo-controlled crossover | Cerebral damage or dysfunction with behavioral disorders |
| Carbamazepine | Not specified | Groh, 1976 | 20 (8–14) | Double-blind placebo-controlled crossover | Behavioral disorder; abnormal EEG in 19/20, but nonepileptic |
| Propranolol | 60–320 | Williams et al., 1982 | 30 (7–35) | Open trial | Uncontrolled rage outbursts associated with organic brain dysfunction |
| Propranolol | 80–280 | Kuperman and Stewart, 1987 | 16 (4–24) | Open trial | Children with physically aggressive behavior; not schizophrenic |
| Naltrexone | 0.5–1.5 mg/kg | Herman et al., 1987 | 3 (10–17) | Double-blind placebo-controlled | Self-injurious behavior in mentally retarded |

[a]Chronological age in years.

## References

Aman, M. G., Singh, N. N., Stewart, A. W., & Field, C. J. (1984). The Aberrant Behavior Checklist: A behavior rating scale for the assessment of treatment effects. *American Journal of Mental Deficiency, 89,* 485–491.

Aman, M. G., Singh, N. N., Stewart, A. W., & Field, C. J. (1985). The Aberrant Behavior Checklist. *Psychopharmacology Bulletin, 21,* 845–850.

Aman, M. G., & Werry, J. S. (1982). Methylphenidate and diazepam in severe reading retardation. *Journal of the American Academy of Child Psychiatry, 21,* 31–37.

American Psychiatric Association. (1980). *Diagnostic and statistical manual of mental disorders* (3rd ed.). Washington, DC: Author.

American Psychiatric Association. (1987). *Diagnostic and statistical manual of mental disorders* (3rd ed., rev.). Washington, DC: Author.

Anderson, L. T., Campbell, M., Adams, P., Small, A. M., Perry, R., & Shell, J. (1989). The effects of haloperidol on discrimination learning and behavioral symptoms in autistic children. *Journal of Autism and Developmental Disorders, 19,* 227–239.

Anderson, L. T., Campbell, M., Grega, D. M., Perry, R., Small, A. M., & Green, W. H. (1984). Haloperidol in the treatment of infantile autism: Effects on learning and behavioral symptoms. *American Journal of Psychiatry, 141,* 1195–1202.

August, G. J., Raz, N., & Baird, T. D. (1985). Brief report: Effects of fenfluramine on behavioral, cognitive, and affective disturbances in autistic children. *Journal of Autism and Developmental Disorders, 15,* 97–107.

Baum, C. G., & Forehand, R. (1981). Long-term follow-up assessment of parent training by use of multiple outcome measures. *Behavior Therapy, 12,* 643–652.

Baumeister, A. A., & Rollings, J. P. (1976). Self-injurious behavior. In N. R. Ellis (Ed.), *International review of research in mental retardation* (Vol. 8, pp. 1–34). New York: Academic Press.

Beckwith, B. E., Couk, D. I., & Schumacher, K. (1986). Failure of naloxone to reduce self-injurious behavior in two developmentally disabled females. *Applied Research in Mental Retardation, 7,* 183–188.

Bernstein, G. A., Hughes, J. R., Mitchell, J. E., & Thompson, T. (1987). Effects of narcotic antagonists on self-injurious behavior: A single case study. *Journal of the American Academy of Child and Adolescent Psychiatry, 26,* 886–889.

Birmaher, B., Quintana, H., & Greenhill, L. L. (1988). Case study: Methylphenidate treatment of hyperactive autistic children. *Journal of the American Academy of Child and Adolescent Psychiatry, 27,* 248–251.

Birkmayer, W. (Ed.). (1976). *Epileptic seizures—behaviour—pain.* Bern: Hans Huber.

Campbell, M. (1985). Timed Stereotypies Rating Scale. *Psychopharmacology Bulletin* (Special Feature: Rating scales and assessment instruments for use in pediatric psychopharmacology research), *21,* 1082.

Campbell, M. (1987). Drug treatment of infantile autism: The past decade. In H. Y. Meltzer (Ed.), *Psychopharmacology: The third generation of progress* (pp. 1225–1231). New York: Raven Press.

Campbell, M. (1988). Fenfluramine treatment of autism. Annotation. *Journal of Child Psychology and Psychiatry, 29,* 1–10.

Campbell, M., Adams, P., Perry, R., Spencer, E. K., & Overall, J. E. (1988). Tardive and withdrawal dyskinesia in autistic children: A prospective study. *Psychopharmacology Bulletin, 24,* 251–255.

Campbell, M., Adams, P., Small, A. M., Curren, E. L., Overall, J. E., Anderson, L. T., Lynch, N., & Perry, R. (1988). Efficacy and safety of fenfluramine in autistic children. *Journal of the American Academy of Child and Adolescent Psychiatry, 27,* 434–439.

Campbell, M., Adams, P., Small, A. M., Tesch, L. M., & Curren, E. L. (1988). Naltrexone in infantile autism. *Psychopharmacology Bulletin, 24,* 135–139.

Campbell, M., Anderson, L. T., Meier, M., Cohen, I. L., Small, A. M., Samit, C., & Sachar, E. J. (1978). A comparison of haloperidol, behavior therapy and their interaction in autistic children. *Journal of the American Academy of Child and Adolescent Psychiatry, 17,* 640–655.

Campbell, M., Cohen, I. L., & Small, A. M. (1982). Drugs in aggressive behavior. *Journal of the American Academy of Child and Adolescent Psychiatry, 21,* 107–117.

Campbell, M., & Deutsch, S. I. (1985). Neuroleptics in children. In G. D. Burrows, T. Norman, & B. Davies (Eds.), *Drugs in psychiatry, Vol. 3, Antipsychotics* (pp. 213–238). Amsterdam: Elsevier Biomedical Press.

Campbell, M., Deutsch, S. I., Perry, R., Wolsky, B. B., & Palij, M. (1986). Short-term efficacy and safety of fenfluramine in hospitalized preschool-age autistic children: An open study. *Psychopharmacology Bulletin, 22,* 141–147.

Campbell, M., Fish, B., David, R., Shapiro, T., Collins, P., & Koh, C. (1972). Response to Triiodothyronine and dextroamphetamine: A study of preschool schizophrenic children. *Journal of Autism and Childhood Schizophrenia, 2,* 343–358.

Campbell, M., Fish, B., Korein, J., Shapiro, T., Collins, P., & Koh, C. (1972). Lithium and chlorpromazine: A controlled crossover study of hyperactive severely disturbed young children. *Journal of Autism and Childhood Schizophrenia, 2,* 234–263.

Campbell, M., Friedman, E., Green, W. H., Collins, P. J., Small, A. M., & Breuer, H. (1975). Blood serotonin in schizophrenic children. A preliminary study. *International Pharmacopsychiatry, 10,* 213–221.

Campbell, M., & Green, W. H. (1985). Pervasive developmental disorders of childhood. In H. I. Kaplan & B. J. Sadock (Eds.), *Comprehensive textbook of psychiatry* (4th ed., Vol. 2, pp. 1672–1683). Baltimore: Williams & Wilkins.

Campbell, M., Green, W. H., and Deutsch, S. I. (1985). *Child and Adolescent Psychopharmacology.* Beverly Hills: Sage Publications.

Campbell, M., Overall, J. E., Small, A. M., Sokol, M. S., Spencer, E. K., Adams, P., Foltz, R. L., Monti, K. M., Perry, R., Nobler, M., & Roberts, E. (1989). Naltrexone in autistic children: An acute open dose range tolerance trial. *Journal of the American Academy of Child and Adolescent Psychiatry, 28,* 200–206.

Campbell, M., & Palij, M. (1985). Behavioral and cognitive measures used in psychopharmacological studies of infantile autism. *Psychopharmacology Bulletin, 21,* 1047–1053.

Campbell, M., Perry, R., Bennett, W. G., Small, A. M., Green, W. H., Grega, D., Schwartz, V., & Anderson, L. (1983). Long-term therapeutic efficacy and drug-related abnormal movements: A prospective study of haloperidol in autistic children. *Psychopharmacology Bulletin, 19,* 80–83.

Campbell, M., Perry, R., & Green, W. H. (1984). The use of lithium in children and adolescents. *Psychosomatics, 25,* 95–106.

Campbell, M., & Schopler, E. (Cochairmen). (1989). Pervasive developmental disorders. In *Psychiatric Treatment Manual I (PTM-I)* (APA Task Force on Treatment of Psychiatric Disorders, T. Byram Karasu, Chairman). Washington, DC: American Psychiatric Press.

Campbell, M., Small, A. M., Collins, P. J., Friedman, E., David, R., & Genieser, N. (1976). Levodopa and levoamphetamine: A crossover study in young schizophrenic children. *Current Therapeutic Research, 19,* 70–86.

Campbell, M., Small, A. M., Green, W. H., Jennings, S. J., Perry, R., Bennett, W. G., & Anderson, L. (1984). Behavioral efficacy of haloperidol and lithium carbonate: A comparison in hospitalized aggressive children with conduct disorder. *Archives of General Psychiatry, 41,* 650–656.

Campbell, M., & Spencer, E. K. (1988). Psychopharmacology in child and adolescent psychiatry: A review of the last five years. *Journal of the American Academy of Child and Adolescent Psychiatry, 27,* 269–279.

Cohen, I. L., Campbell, M., Posner, D., Small, A. M., Triebel, D., & Anderson, L. T. (1980). Behavioral effects of haloperidol in young autistic children: An objective analysis using a within-subjects reversal design. *Journal of the American Academy of Child Psychiatry, 19*, 665–677.

Crane, G. E., & Naranjo, E. R. (1971). Motor disorders induced by neuroleptics. *Archives of General Psychiatry, 24, 179–184*.

Cunningham, M. A., Pillai, V., & Rogers, W. J. B. (1968). Haloperidol in the treatment of children with severe behaviour disorders. *British Journal of Psychiatry, 114*, 845–854.

Davidson, P. W., Kleene, B. M., Carrol, M., & Rockowitz, R. J. (1983). Effects of Naloxone on self-injurious behavior: A case study. *Applied Research in Mental Retardation, 4*, 1–4.

Debray, P., Messerschmitt, P., Lonchamp, D., & Herbault, M. (1972). The use of pimozide in child psychiatry. *La Nouvelle Presse Medicale, 43*.

Delong, G. R., & Aldershof, A. L. (1987). Long-term experience with lithium treatment in childhood: Correlation with clinical diagnosis. *Journal of the American Academy of Child and Adolescent Psychiatry, 26*, 389–394.

Deutsch, S. I. (1986). Rationale for the administration of opiate antagonists in treating infantile autism. *American Journal of Mental Deficiency, 90*, 631–635.

Deykin, E. Y., & MacMahon, B. (1979). The incidence of seizures among children with autistic symptoms. *American Journal of Psychiatry, 136*, 1310–1312.

Dostal, T. (1972). Antiaggressive effect of lithium salts in mentally retarded adolescents. In A. L. Annell (Ed.), *Depressive states in childhood and adolescence* (pp. 491–498). Stockholm: Almquist & Wiskell.

Ekman, G., Miranda-Linne, F., Gillberg, C., Garle, M., & Wetterberg, L. (in press). Fenfluramine treatment of 20 autistic children. *Journal of Autism and Developmental Disorders*.

Evans, R. W., Clay, T. H., & Gualtieri, C. T. (1987). Carbamazepine in pediatric psychiatry. *Journal of the American Academy of Child and Adolescent Psychiatry, 26*, 2–8.

Faretra, G., Dooher, L., & Dowling, J. (1970). Comparison of haloperidol and fluphenazine in disturbed children. *American Journal of Psychiatry, 126*, 1670–1673.

Freeman, B. J., Ritvo, E. R., Schroth, P. C., Tonick, I., Guthrie, D., & Wake, L. (1981). Behavioral characteristics of high- and low-IQ autistic children. *American Journal of Psychiatry, 138*, 25–29.

Freeman, B. J., Schroth, P., Ritvo, E., Guthrie, D., & Wake, L. (1980). The Behavior Observation Scale for Autism (BOS): Initial results of factor analyses. *Journal of Autism and Developmental Disorders, 10*, 343–346.

Gamstorp, I. (1976). Carbamazepine in the treatment of epileptic disorders in infancy and childhood. In W. Birkmayer (Ed.), *Epileptic seizures—behaviour—pain* (pp. 98–103). Bern: Hans Huber.

Gardos, G., Cole, J. O., & Tarsy, D. (1978). Withdrawal syndromes associated with antipsychotic drugs. *American Journal of Psychiatry, 135*, 1321–1324.

Geller, E., Ritvo, E. R., Freeman, B. J., & Yuwiler, A. (1982). Preliminary observations on the effects of fenfluramine on blood serotonin and symptoms in three autistic boys. *New England Journal of Medicine, 307*, 165–169.

Gillberg, C., Terenius, L., & Lonnerholm, G. (1985). Endorphin activity in childhood psychosis: Spinal fluid levels in 24 cases. *Archives of General Psychiatry, 42*, 780–783.

Groh, C. (1976). The psychotropic effect of Tegretol in non-epileptic children, with particular reference to the drug's indications. In W. Birkmayer (Ed.), *Epileptic seizures—behaviour—pain* (pp. 259–263). Baltimore: University Park Press.

Herman, B. H., Egan, J., Hammock, M. K., Chatoor, I., Arthur-Smith, A., Chamberlain, R., Herrmann, G., & Hartzler, J. (1988, December). *Evidence for a role of proopiomelanocortin peptides in self-injurious behavior*. Paper presented at the Annual Meeting of the American College of Neuropsychopharmacology, San Juan, Puerto Rico.

Herman, B. H., Hammock, M. K., Arthur-Smith, A., Egan, J., Chatoor, I., Werner, A., & Zelnik, N. (1987). Naltrexone decreases self-injurious behavior. *Annals of Neurology, 22*, 550–552.

Herman, B. H., Hammock, M. K., Arthur-Smith, A., Egan, J., Chatoor, I., Zelnik, N., Appelgate, K., & Boeckx, R. L. (1986). Effects of naltrexone in autism: Correlation with plasma opioid concentrations. *American Academy of Child and Adolescent Psychiatry* (Scientific Proceedings for the Annual Meeting), *2*, 11–12.

Kanner, L. (1943). Autistic disturbances of affective contact. *Nervous Child, 2,* 217–250.

Kazdin, A. E. (1975). *Behavior modification in applied settings* (1st ed.). Homewood, IL: Dorsey Press.

Kazdin, A. E., Esveldt-Dawson, K., French, N. H., & Unis, A. S. (1987). Effects of parent management training and problem-solving skills training combined in the treatment of antisocial child behavior. *Journal of the American Academy of Child and Adolescent Psychiatry, 26,* 416–424.

Kolvin, I. (1971). Psychoses in childhood—A comparative study. In M. Rutter (Ed.), *Infantile autism: Concepts, characteristics and treatment* (pp. 7–26). London: Churchill-Livingstone.

Kuhn-Gebhart, V. (1976). Behavioural disorders in non-epileptic children and their treatment with carbamazepine. In W. Birkmayer (Ed.), *Epileptic seizures—behaviour—pain* (pp. 264–267). Bern: Hans Huber.

Kuperman, S., & Stewart, M. A. (1987). Use of propranolol to decrease aggressive outbursts in younger patients. *Psychosomatics, 28,* 315–320.

Leboyer, M., Bouvard, M. P., & Dugas, M. (1988). Effects of naltrexone on infantile autism. *Lancet, 1,* 715.

Leviatov, V. M., Veselovskaja, T. D., Marienko, G. Ph. and Chtchegoleva, A. P. (1976). Psychoses au Tegretol chez des epileptiques. *Ann. med. psychol., 1,* 473.

Meiselas, K. D., Spencer, E. K., Oberfield, R. A., Peselow, E. D., Angrist, B., & Campbell, M. (1989). Differentiation of stereotypies from neuroleptic-related dyskinesias in autistic children. *Journal of Clinical Psychopharmacology, 7.*

Naruse, H., Nagahata, M., Nakane, Y., Shirahashi, K., Takesada, M., & Yamazaki, K. (1982). A multicenter double-blind trial of pimozide (Orap), haloperidol and placebo in children with behavior disorders, using crossover design. *Acta Paedopsychiatrica, 48,* 173–184.

O'Donnell, D. J. (1985). Conduct disorders. In J. M. Wiener (Ed.), *Diagnosis and psychopharmacology of childhood and adolescent disorders* (pp. 249–287). New York: Wiley.

Overall, J. E., & Campbell, M. (1988). Behavioral assessment of psychopathology in children: Infantile autism. *Journal of Clinical Psychology, 44,* 708–716.

Panksepp, J. (1979). A neurochemical theory of autism. *Trends in Neuroscience, 2,* 174–177.

Panksepp, J., & Sahley, T. L. (1987). Possible brain opioid involvement in disrupted social intent and language development in autism. In E. Schopler & G. B. Mesibov (Eds.), *Neurobiological issues in autism* (pp. 357–372). New York, Plenum Press.

Perry, R., Campbell, M., Adams, P., Lynch, N., Spencer, E. K., Curren, E. L., & Overall, J. E. (1989). Long-term efficacy of haloperidol in autistic children: Continuous vs. discontinuous drug administration. *Journal of the American Academy of Child Psychiatry, 28,* 87–92.

Perry, R., Nobler, M. S., & Campbell, M. (1989). Case report: Tourette-like symptoms associated with chronic neuroleptic therapy in an autistic child. *Journal of the American Academy of Child and Adolescent Psychiatry, 28,* 93–96.

Petti, T. A., & Campbell, M. (1975). Imipramine and seizures. *American Journal of Psychiatry, 132,* 538–540.

Platt, J. E., Campbell, M., Green, W. H., & Grega, D. M. (1984). Cognitive effects of lithium carbonate and haloperidol in treatment-resistant aggressive children. *Archives of General Psychiatry, 41,* 657–662.

Pleak, R. R., Birmaher, B., Gavrilescu, A., Abichandani, C., & Williams, D. T. (1988). Mania and neuropsychiatric excitation following carbamazepine. *Journal of the American Academy of Child and Adolescent Psychiatry, 27,* 500–503.

Post, R. M. (1987). Mechanisms of action of carbamazepine and related anticonvulsants in affective illness. In H. Y. Meltzer (Ed.), *Psychopharmacology: The third generation of progress* (pp. 567–576). New York: Raven Press.

Pratt, J. A., Jenner, P., Johnson, A. L., Shorvon, S. D., & Reynolds, E. H. (1984). Anticonvulsant drugs alter plasma tryptophan concentrations in epileptic patients: Implication for antiepileptic action and mental function. *Journal of Neurology, Neurosurgery and Psychiatry, 47,* 1131–1133.

*Psychopharmacology Bulletin, Special Issue:* Pharmacotherapy of Children. (1973).

*Psychopharmacology Bulletin.* Special Feature: rating scales and assessment instruments for use in pediatric psychopharmacology research. *21* (4): (1985).

Puente, R. M. (1976). The use of carbamazepine in the treatment of behavioral disorders in children. In W. Birkmayer (Ed.), *Epileptic seizures—behavior—pain* (pp. 243–252). Bern: Hans Huber.

Ratey, J. J., Bemporad, J., Sorgi, P., Bick, P., Polakoff, S., O'Driscoll, G., & Mikkelsen, E. (1987). Brief report: Open trial effects of beta-blockers on speech and social behaviors in 8 autistic adults. *Journal of Autism and Developmental Disorders, 17,* 439–445.

Ratey, J. J., Mikkelsen, E. J., Bushnell Smith, G., Upadhayaya, A., Zuckerman, H. S., Martell, D., Sorgi, P., Polakoff, S., & Bemporad, J. (1986). B-blockers in the severely and profoundly mentally retarded. *Journal of Clinical Psychopharmacology, 6,* 103–107.

Ratey, J. J., Mikkelsen, E. J., Sorgi, P., Zuckerman, S., Polakoff, S., Bemporad, J., Bick, P., & Kadish, W. (1987). Autism: The treatment of aggressive behaviors. *Journal of Clinical Psychopharmacology, 7,* 35–41.

Reisberg, B., & Gershon, S. (1979). Side effects associated with lithium therapy. *Archives of General Psychiatry, 36,* 879–887.

Remschmidt, H. (1976). The psychotropic effect of carbamazepine in non-epileptic patients, with particular reference to problems posed by clinical studies in children with behavioural disorders. In W. Birkmayer, (Ed.), *Epileptic seizures—behaviour—pain* (pp. 253–258). Bern: Hans Huber.

Reyntjens, A. M. (1972). A series of multicentric pilot trials with pimozide in psychiatric practice. *Acta Psychiatrica Belgica, 72,* 662–670.

Richardson, J. S., & Zaleski, W. A. (1983). Naloxone and self-mutilation. *Biological Psychiatry, 18,* 99–101.

Rimland, B. (1971). The differentiation of childhood psychoses: An analysis of checklists for 2,218 psychotic children. *Journal of Autism and Childhood Schizophrenia, 1,* 161–174.

Ritvo, E. R., Freeman, B. J., Geller, E., & Yuwiler, A. (1983). Effects of fenfluramine on 14 outpatients with the syndrome of autism. *Journal of the American Academy of Child Psychiatry, 22,* 549–558.

Ritvo, E. R., Freeman, B. J., Pingree, C., Mason-Brothers, A. Jorde, L., Jenson, W. R., McMahon, W. M., Petersen, P. B., Mo, A., & Ritvo, A. (1989). The UCLA-University of Utah epidemiologic survey of autism: Prevalence. *American Journal of Psychiatry, 146,* 194–199.

Ritvo, E. R., Freeman, B. J., Yuwiler, A., Geller, E., Schroth, P., Yokota, A., Mason-Brothers, A. August, G. J., Klykylo, W., Leventhal, B., Lewis, K., Piggott, L., Realmuto, G., Stubbs, E. G., & Umansky, R. (1986). Fenfluramine treatment of autism: UCLA collaborative study of 81 patients at nine medical centers. *Psychopharmacology Bulletin, 22,* 133–140.

Ritvo, E. R., Yuwiler, A., Geller, E., Ornitz, E. M., Saeger, K., Plotkin, S. (1970). Increased blood serotonin and platelets in early infantile autism. *Archives of General Psychiatry, 23,* 566–572.

Rutter, M. (1972). Childhood schizophrenia reconsidered. *Journal of Autism and Childhood Schizophrenia, 2,* 315–337.

Rutter, M. (1978). Diagnosis and definition. In M. Rutter & E. Schopler (Eds.), *Autism: A reappraisal of concepts and treatment* (pp. 1–25). New York: Plenum Press.

Rutter, M., & Schopler, E. (Eds.). (1978). *Autism: A reappraisal of concepts and treatment.* New York, Plenum Press.

Sandman, C. A., Datta, P. C., Barron, J., Koehler, F. K., Williams, C., & Swanson, J. M. (1983). Naloxone attenuates self-abusive behavior in developmentally disabled clients. *Applied Research in Mental Retardation, 4,* 5–11.

Schopler, E., Reichler, R. J., & Renner, B. R. (1985). *The Childhood Autism Rating Scale—CARS.* New York: Irvington Publications.

Schroeder, S. R., Schroeder, C. S., Smith, B., & Dalldorf, J. (1978). Prevalence of self-injurious behaviors in a large state facility for the retarded: A three-year follow-up study. *Journal of Autism and Childhood Schizophrenia, 8,* 261–269.

Schuster, C. R., Lewis, M., & Seiden, L. S. (1986). Fenfluramine: Neurotoxicity. *Psychopharmacology Bulletin, 22,* 148–151.

Sheard, M. H., & Aghajanian, G. K. (1970). Neuronally activated metabolism of serotonin; effect of lithium. *Life Science, 9,* 285–290.

Sheard, M. H., Marini, J. L., Bridges, C. I., & Wagner, E. (1976). The effects of lithium on impulsive aggressive behavior in man. *American Journal of Psychiatry, 133,* 1409–1413.

Sillanpaa, M. (1981). Carbamazepine. Pharmacology and clinical uses. *Acta Neurologica Scandinavica* (Suppl. 88), *64,* 1–202.

Silverstein, F. S., Parrish, M. A., & Johnston, M. V. (1982). Adverse behavioral reactions in children treated with carbamazepine (Tegretol). *Journal of Pediatrics, 101,* 785–787.

Singh, N. N., & Aman, M. G. (1981). Effects of thioridazine dosage on the behavior of severely mentally retarded persons. *American Journal of Mental Deficiency, 85,* 580–587.

Sokol, M. S., Campbell, M., Goldstein, M., & Krechman, A. M. (1987). Attention deficit disorder with hyperactivity and the dopamine hypothesis: Case presentation with theoretical background. *Journal of the American Academy of Child and Adolescent Psychiatry, 26,* 428–433.

Spencer, E. K., & Campbell, M. (in press). Aggressiveness directed against self and others: Psychopharmacologic intervention. In S. L. Harris & J. S. Handleman (Eds.), *Life threatening behavior: Aversive vs. nonaversive interventions.*

Sprague, R. L., & Newell, M. K. (1987). Toward a movement control perspective of tardive dyskinesia. In H. Y. Meltzer (Ed.), *Psychopharmacology: The third generation of progress* (pp. 1233–1238). New York: Raven Press.

Stahl, S. M. (1980). Tardive Tourette syndrome in an autistic patient after long-term neuroleptic administration. *American Journal of Psychiatry, 137,* 1267–1269.

Stewart, M. A., deBlois, C. S., Meardon, J., & Cummings, C. (1980). Aggressive conduct disorder of children: The clinical picture. *Journal of Nervous and Mental Disease, 168,* 604–610.

Strayhorn, J. M., Jr., Rapp, N., Donina, W., & Strain, P. S. (1988). Randomized trial of methylphenidate for an autistic child. *Journal of the American Academy of Child and Adolescent Psychiatry, 27,* 244–247.

Suwa, S., Naruse, H., Ohura, T., Tsuruhara, T., Takesada, M., Yamazaki, K., & Mikuni, M. (1984). Influence of pimozide on hypothalamo-pituitary function in children with behavioral disorders. *Psychiatry Endocrinology, 9,* 37–44.

Tarjan, C., Lowry, V. E., & Wright, S. W. (1957). Use of chlorpromazine in two hundred seventy-eight mentally deficient patients. *A.M.A. Journal of Disturbed Children, 94,* 294–300.

Weizman, R., Weizman, A., Tyano, S., Szekely, G., Weissman, B. A., & Sarne, Y. (1984). Humoral-endorphin blood levels in autistic, schizophrenic and healthy subjects. *Psychopharmacology, 82,* 368–370.

Werry, J. S., & Aman, M. G. (1975). Methylphenidate and haloperidol in children. *Archives of General Psychiatry, 32,* 790–795.

Werry, J. S., & Wollersheim, J. P. (1989). Behavior therapy in children and adolescents: A twenty-year overview. *Journal of the American Academy of Child and Adolescent Psychiatry, 28,* 1–18.

White, T. J. R., & Aman, M. G. (1985). Pimozide treatment in disruptive severely retarded patients. *Australian and New Zealand Journal of Psychiatry, 19,* 92–94.

Whitman, T. L., & Johnston, M. B. (1987). Mental retardation. In M. Hersen & B. B. Van Hasselt (Eds.), *Behavior therapy with children and adolescents* (pp. 184–223). New York: Wiley.

Williams, D. T., Mehl, R., Yudofsky, S., Adams, D., & Roseman, B. (1982). The effects of propranolol on uncontrolled rage outbursts in children and adolescents with organic brain dysfunction. *Journal of the American Academy of Child Psychiatry, 21,* 129–135.

Wong, G. H., & Cock, R. J. (1971). Long-term effects of haloperidol on severely emotionally disturbed children. *Australian and New Zealand Journal of Psychiatry, 5,* 296–300.

Young, J. G., Leven, L. I., Newcorn, J. H., & Knott, P. J. (1987). Genetic and neurobiological approaches to the pathophysiology of autism and the pervasive developmental disorders. In H. Y. Meltzer (Ed.), *Psychopharmacology: The third generation of progress* (pp. 825). New York: Raven Press.

Yudofsky, S. C., Silver, J. M., Jackson, W., Endicott, J., & Williams, D. (1986). The overt aggression scale for the objective rating of verbal and physical aggression. *American Journal Psychiatry, 143,* 35–39.

Ziring, P. R., & Teitelbaum, L. (1980). Affiliation with a university department of psychiatry: Impact on the use of psychoactive medication in a large public residential facility for mentally retarded persons. Paper presented at the Conference on use of medications in controlling the behavior of the mentally retarded. September 22–24, 1980, University of Minnesota, Minneapolis, Minnesota.

# 6

# Treatment of Children and Adolescents with Substance Abuse Disorders

## Nicholas L. Rock

### Introduction

Alcohol and substance abuse is a worldwide problem. In 1950 the World Health Organization (WHO) reported international concerns about alcoholism as a disease and as a social problem. In 1979 WHO declared that problems related to alcohol ranked among the world's major public health problems and constituted serious hazards for human health, welfare, and life (Moser, 1985). Many countries reported that patients with primary or secondary diagnosis of alcoholism or alcoholic psychosis accounted for 20 to 30% of all first-time admissions to both psychiatric and general hospitals. In addition, WHO surveys of many countries revealed significant drug use (Johnson, 1980). For example, in 12- to 19-year-olds, 12% (Thailand and Pakistani) to 16% (Canada) used or experimented with substances such as marijuana, LSD, stimulants, and narcotics.

The large size of nonstudent youth populations in developing countries has resulted in a high risk for drug abuse (Smart et al., 1981). Nonstudent youths used more cannabis, amphetamines, barbiturates, and hallucinogens than students. This survey was done in Chandigarh, Islamabad, Penang, and Toronto on 15- to 23-year-olds. In the United States, it is projected that in future years, nonmedical use of drugs will have the greatest incidence in young adults 18 to 25 years old, with peak use at 18 to 21 (Richards, 1981). Reports by the U.S. Department of Justice on American high school seniors over a 10-year period (1975–1986) showed the following trends on drug use in the previous year:

---

*Nicholas L. Rock*   Department of Psychiatry, Louisiana State University Medical Center, New Orleans, Louisiana 70112.

marijuana, similar 40 to 39%; hallucinogens, downward 11 to 6%; cocaine, upward 6 to 13%; alcohol, same 85 to 85%. During the same time period, high school seniors, both male and female, who received one or more traffic tickets or warnings for driving while under the influence in the previous year was as follows: alcohol, fairly constant rate of 13 to 11%; drugs downward of 8 to 3% (Flanagan & Jamieson, 1988).

Treatment programs for adults have been developed in most countries over the past two decades, but only in recent years for children and adolescents. A review of 5515 psychiatric hospital admissions throughout the United States during 1985 for ages 0 to 19 years with the CHAMPUS (Civilian Health and Medical Program of the Uniformed Services) revealed all types of psychiatric problems. Inpatient treatment of primary substance abuse was 9% of the total. This rate was the same as for schizophrenia, but higher than for adjustment disorders (6%). Therefore, it is important that professionals, particularly child psychiatrists, know how to identify and treat these common endemic worldwide problems of substance abuse disorders in our children. More and better treatment programs are a priority.

Competent treatment requires the basic medical skills of a physician. Complete medical work-ups include close monitoring of mental, nutritional, metabolic, and physiological functions. An empathic attitude along with a motivation to treat individuals with these disorders is essential.

## Treatment Program

Since drug abuse causes not only mental health problems but also physical disorders and injuries due to accidents, treatment must be comprehensive. It involves primary, secondary, and tertiary prevention strategies.

Primary prevention includes education and training in the problems of substance abuse and addiction. Consultation and coordination of medical personnel with schools, courts, law enforcement, and parent organizations is essential (U.S. Department of Education, 1987). Secondary prevention is early identification and treatment. Initiation of counseling and continued education, consultation, and liaison of other professionals is important (American Academy of Pediatrics, 1988). Tertiary prevention comprises the direct medical and psychological interventions needed to return the person to healthy functioning with minimal impairments (Schuckit, 1981).

Specific requirements to be considered for a professional entering this area is their level of knowledge, skills, and attitudes. The biggest and most difficult barrier to overcome is the professional's attitude toward identifying and treating individuals with substance abuse problems. Knowledge and skills are generally acquired in medical school, internship, and residency training.

## Attitude

Prior to 1970, there was little emphasis in American medical training programs for the treatment of substance abuse outside of severe complications and of the end stages of the disease, such as liver failure and Korsakoff syndrome. Further, it was illegal to treat narcotic addicts outside of the very limited federal facilities. After 1971 with alcohol treatment legislation in the United States, and in 1972 with its extension to include drug abuse, medical treatment was mandated and hospitals began to provide programs. However, American training programs, particularly in child psychiatry, did not focus on treating psychiatric complications of substance abuse or rehabilitation for nonaddicted patients. Only in the past several years has the U.S. Accreditation Council for Graduate Medical Education required for accredited residencies instruction in the clinical management of patients with alcoholism and drug abuse. Therefore, it is not surprising that a reluctance exists to treat children, adolescents, or adults in medical settings.

When an adolescent inpatient program is initiated, there is a predictable panic by administrators, nursing personnel, and other professionals. The general attitude prevails that the adolescent will "tear up" the unit, drug use will become rampant, young girls will "seduce" the staff, and other patient care will suffer. Much of this resistance is due to the limited experience and training in adolescent medicine and substance abuse for the majority of professionals.

Attitudes of physicians can be changed. During the 1970s most military physicians were drafted from a cross section of medical schools. Most had a negative attitude toward identifying, treating, and rehabilitating soldiers with substance abuse problems. A 2-day course was set up on basic psychiatric and medical principles as they applied to substance abuse. Follow-up reports indicated that their negative attitude was dependent on the physicians' obtaining the necessary knowledge and the skills needed to treat the substance abuser, many of whom were older adolescent soldiers.

## Knowledge and Skills

Almost two decades of experience by the U.S. military medical staff with substance abuse problems has shown that treatment principles learned in the general medical and psychiatric programs for adults were easily extended to children and adolescents (Rock & Donley, 1975).

The general modalities of diagnosis and treatment for acute admissions will be presented in detail. Specific areas of treatment revolve around the initial use of the medical skills of detoxification and pharmacological therapy. The management of medical complications caused by substance abuse, treatment of underlying psychiatric problems, and follow-up therapy and rehabilitation programs will be reviewed.

The initial effort to make the individual drug-free is best done in a hospital setting. Rehabilitation is better done in outpatient or specialized programs. With children and young adolescents, the major problem is the treatment of acute intoxications or unacceptable behavior resulting from the use of various substances. With older adolescents, there may be an additional addictive state requiring a withdrawal procedure. Programs should be prepared to handle the worst case.

The general categories of diagnosis and treatment are related to the following substances: (1) alcohol; (2) opiates; (3) CNS depressants and sedative hypnotics; (4) CNS sympathomimetics and stimulants, including cocaine, caffeine, and nicotine; (5) special substances, such as cannabinoids (marijuana), psychedelics (LSD, PCP), inhalants (gasoline), volatile solvents (glue sniffing), bromides; (6) over-the-counter drugs (OTC), particularly the anticholinergics.

Treatments should be used to prevent various physical and mental complications resulting from the use of the following substances:

- Alcohol: acute brain syndromes, seizures, vitamin deficiencies, aggravation of existing medical conditions.
- Narcotics: respiratory arrest, pulmonary edema, malnutrition.
- Sedative hypnotics: coma, convulsions, delirium.
- Stimulants: generalized convulsions, delirium, psychosis, self-destructive behavior.
- Solvents: multiple pulmonary problems.
- Hallucinogens: psychosis.

The combination of multiple drugs, including OTC and prescribed medications, can cause severe organicity, psychosis, and physical complications.

The most important factor for successful treatment is continuity of care. Inpatient and outpatient units must interact with each other. Other psychosocial and maintenance systems, such as Alcoholics Anonymous (AA) and Narcotics Anonymous (NA) and residential/halfway houses, provide additional support. With adolescents, the cooperation of schools, courts, police, and other agencies may be useful.

## *Diagnosis*

The initial suspicion that substance abuse is present in any patient is important. A specific diagnosis may not be possible without laboratory or collateral information. Physical findings are the key to treatment. A continuous update on what drugs are currently in use in the community will help. This information can be found in poison control centers, community rehabilitation programs, police, emergency rooms, and the patient's peers. There is an emergency room computer program called "Poisondex,"* which contains recent information on diagnosis, drug identification, and treatment of all substances currently known.

The general characteristics of significant use or acute reactions of substances abusers that lead to a diagnosis and treatment are as follows:

- Alcohol: general physical changes, odor of the breath, general nervousness, gastrointestinal problems, various marks on the body due to accidents, chronic cough, denial of problems, ability to tolerate high quantities of alcohol, depression.
- Opioids: depressed respiration, temperature, and blood pressure; constipation; pulmonary difficulties; constricted pupils; gastrointestinal problems; euphoria; anxiety; depression.
- Sedative/hypnotics: symptoms similar to those of the opioids, but the pupils are dilated; slurred speech; nystagmus; ataxia; tremulousness; anxiety; disorientation; convulsions.
- Stimulants: elevated temperature, heart rate, blood pressure, and respiration; hyperactivity; hyperalertness; paranoia, or suspiciousness; dysphoria; dry mouth; sweating; tremors.
- Other substances: combination of all the above physical problems plus additional psychiatric problems ranging from organicity to psychosis.

It is important to suspect that any changes in behavior, school performance, prevalence of accidents, or physical condition are due to substance abuse until proven otherwise.

## *Treatment*

Each treatment unit should develop a written policy of procedures in order to provide consistent care. A sample of such procedures is shown in Appendix 1 for alcohol. For other substances, specifics can be substituted or added, as illustrated in Appendixes 2 and 3. The basic care program is essentially the same for all substance abuse. The medical treatment procedures are basically centered around the management of alcohol, narcotics, and depressants, while the standard psychiatric treatments for organic brain syndromes and mental dysfunctions cover the other substances.

Initially, the emergency treatment must ensure an open airway, spontaneous breathing, and adequate blood pressure and heart rate. The staff should periodically review and participate in a Basic Cardiac Life Support (BCLS, CPR) program, or any emergency care program such as those sponsored by the

*Micromedex, Inc., 660 Bannock Street, Denver, Colorado 80204-4506. Telephone: 1-800-525-9083.

American Heart Association. This practice will ensure that lifesaving skills are there when needed. Pharmacotherapy can be initiated when the patient is medically stable.

## Detoxification

After the general physical stabilization of the individual, detoxification is initiated if indicated. The safe withdrawal or removal of the substance from the body can be better controlled and more safely done in a hospital setting. This usually takes 3 to 7 days. Initially, patients need close medical monitoring to prevent death from intoxification. Patients abusing substances need close psychiatric observation to prevent self-inflicted injuries due to mental and behavioral changes.

Controlled pharmacological substitution or pharmacotherapy is the treatment of choice. The rationale for such an approach is the cross-tolerance of drugs, which allows substitution of one drug for another to prevent severe withdrawal reactions.

Drug-induced anxieties and psychoses can be controlled by various specific psychotropic drugs. Care must be taken not to overuse medications, especially in the acute intoxicated state, in debilitated patients, or in markedly elevated drug levels. For example, if blood alcohol levels are over 100 to 150 mg per deciliter, any further CNS depressants should be administered with caution. Oral medication is preferred over injection, owing to the fear of needles or the symbolism of this intrusion. However, rapid need for medication or noncompliance is an overriding factor.

Psychotropic drugs are needed in most cases. Doses are hard to determine in children and adolescents because of differences in body mass. Experience has shown that with psychotropics, most doses are similar to those in adults. Children metabolize drugs faster and this allows them to handle adult doses.

Major tranquilizers are important and basic to the treatment process. It is useful to be thoroughly familiar with a few drugs in each of the major categories. As a general rule, it is best to start with low doses of any drug, and then add, rather than use high initial doses, which may be excessive and hard to control. Tranquilizers will be beneficial in most cases. The following two are available in all forms: (1) Haloperidol (Haldol) is an excellent neuroleptic and is available in oral (liquid and tablets), I.M., and I.V. preparations. Low doses of around 2 to 5 mg every 2 hours are effective. Side effects are easily treated with diphenhydramine (Benadryl), which also comes in all forms. (2) Chlorpromazine HCL (Thorazine) is still a favorite neuroleptic with both oral and injectable forms, but hypotension and excessive sedation can be a serious problem. Doses of 50 to 75 mg every 6 hours are usually adequate.

Minor tranquilizers, such as benzodiazepine anxiolytics, are generally the drugs of choice. They act rapidly and can prevent withdrawals. The non-benzodiazepine buspirone may not be effective since it has limited antiseizure activity and questionable cross-tolerance. When an I.M. benzodiazepine is needed, the drug of choice is lorazepam (Ativan), 2 to 4 mg, because diazepam (Valium) and chlordiazepoxide (Librium) are both poorly absorbed by this route. Lorazepam 1 mg is roughly equivalent to diazepam 5 mg. Oral diazepam is preferred, owing to its long action and antiseizure activity; it is also available in different forms. Its use is described in Appendix 1.

Benzodiazepines can be used in the management of alcohol, narcotic, or sedative/hypnotic withdrawal, as shown in Appendix 2. Once the patient is symptom-free, daily doses should be reduced by 20% or less each day. Benzodiazepines must never be stopped abruptly since seizures may occur. The following symptoms may indicate the need for further benzodiazepine therapy: tremulousness, fever, hyperreflexia, nausea, vomiting, tachycardia, diaphoresis, systolic and diastolic hypertension, irritability, anxiety, malaise, incoherent speech, illusions, hallucinations, memory impairment, disorientation, psychomotor slowing, disturbance of sleep–wake cycle with insommia or daytime drowsiness.

For barbiturate withdrawal, pentobarbital or phenobarbital procedures can be used. The short-acting drug, pentobarbital, can be used to determine the level of drug dependence. Appendix 2 describes a specific procedure to follow.

Narcotic withdrawal can be initiated by a narcotic antagonist such as naloxone HCL (Narcan) or may be used to treat acute intoxications (Appendix 3). Methadone overdoses must be watched for 24 hours because of the long-acting effect of methadone. Narcotic withdrawal is characterized by pain, gastrointestinal symptoms, insomnia, and nervousness. Effective treatments are noted in Appendix 3.

The alpha and beta adrenergic blockers are effective in dealing with motor restlessness and anxiety. Clonidine HCL (Catapres) can be effective with narcotic and cocaine withdrawal (Appendix 3). Propranolol HCL (Inderal) is longer acting than clonidine and can be effective in controlling anxiety. Carbamazepine (Tegretol) should be considered if explosive behavior is a problem. Tricyclic antidepressants help reduce craving and relapse in some cases of stimulant abuse, and they alleviate dysphoria and hypersomnia.

Sleeping medications at bedtime should be used with least interference of REM sleep stages and CNS alerting mechanism. Triazolam (Halcion), 0.25 to 0.5 mg at bedtime, is helpful with debilitated patients, but the dose must be kept low. Chloral hydrate, 500 mg to 1 g, is still a good drug and comes in syrup form.

Anticonvulsants should not be used routinely unless seizures are present or the patient has a history of seizures. IV fluids are needed only if the patient is severly dehydrated, vomiting, or debilitated. Vitamin administration, particularly thiamine, folic acid, and vitamin K, is essential owing to possible vitamin deficiencies and slow prothrombin times.

Acidification of the urine increases excretion of many drugs, particularly the stimulants, and thereby shortens duration of effect. Vital signs and sensorium must be monitored closely, at least four times a day for 3 to 5 days.

Laboratory tests should include screening for HIV virus infection since drug abusers are at high risk. Urine and blood tests to detect abused substances should be repeated regularly to ensure no further abuse while the patient is hospitalized and during follow-up rehabilitation. Urine drug testing can be used effectively instead of a locked ward.

Nursing care must include weight checks, supplement feedings, and familiarization to the unit. There should be a standard mental status orientation checklist to be used daily. Persistent or impaired mental status must be reviewed.

## Rehabilitation

Rehabilitation should start as soon as detoxification is completed. Other psychiatric conditions, such as attention deficit disorders, learning disabilities, and depression, must be identified and treated. Other consultations must be considered, such as neurology for possible organic brain syndromes, or neuropsychological testing for cognitive impairments. Special education should be pursued if needed in regular school setting, day treatment, or residential programs. Long-term intensive treatment programs may be needed because of the patients' inability to function outside a structured environment. Individual and family psychotherapy and other supportive programs, such as AA, Al-Anon, AlaTeen, and drug abuse groups, should be started in the hospital as part of the required program.*

Alcoholics Anonymous is a self-help support group for the adult alcoholic, while AlaTeen is directed more to the younger person. Al-Anon is for family support and help in dealing with the alcohol abuser. Narcotic Anonymous (NA) is similar to AA but focused on substance abuse. Family support groups for substance abuse include programs like Tough Love and Family Anonymous. All these programs are generally voluntary, autonomous, confidential, and free of cost, and are not considered medical treatment services. Their advantage is the social/community involvement and support, which can and does go on for years or a lifetime.

---

*Information about such support groups can be obtained from the local chapters or throughout the United States by writing to The National Clearinghouse for Alcohol and Drug Information, P.O. Box 2345, Rockville, Maryland 20852.

## Summary

A successful treatment program for substance abuse disorders begins by developing a positive attitude that such programs are in the patient's best interest. An inpatient admission is not the total program but is a prerequisite to a drug-free beginning for the patient.

A review of basic medical skills will lead to a standard policy and protocols for care in a particular facility. It is important to initiate diagnostic procedures to identify underlying psychiatric conditions in order to prescribe proper follow-up therapy. Multidisciplinary teams are needed to initiate comprehensive programs as soon as the patient is physically and mentally capable. Successful recovery for many children and adolescents make any substance program cost-effective for the patients, their families, and society.

## Appendix 1

### A Model Alcohol Withdrawal Procedure

Each clinic or inpatient unit needs to develop a set of guidelines or procedures (Standard Operation Procedures, SOP) that can be updated regularly. This will provide a basis for a quality assurance program and consistency within the institution. Any new staff can then be oriented to the unit program.

The following represents an "ideal" SOP for an alcohol withdrawal program and can be modified for any other substance. A separate SOP for each major category of substance use disorder should be on file.

I. *Purpose.* To prevent medical and withdrawal complications such as (1) organic brain syndrome, (2) vitamin deficiency, (3) neuropathic and encephalopathic disease, and (4) aggravation of existing medical problems. Withdrawal symptoms can begin within hours of the last drink, but may not emerge until up to 7 days.

II. *Medications.* All medications, if possible, should be given orally to avoid activating psychological needs and symbolism of injections. Doses are based on the average 70-kg adolescent. Higher or lower amounts should be based on actual physical status.

   A. *Vitamins.* Initially it is extremely important to start the debilitated patient on parental vitamins (i.e., thiamine HCL, Berocca Parental Nutrition) immediately on admission to avoid the possibility of one of the permanent organic brain syndromes or peripheral neuropathies. However, if oral intake is adequate, high doses of oral vitamins should be used for the first week. After that, an adequate diet should suffice.

     1. Berocca Parental: 4 ml I.M. (for 1 or 2 doses).

2. Vitamin K: 5–10 mg I.M. (for 1 or 2 times if prothrombin time is prolonged more than 3 seconds beyond the control).
3. Thiamine HCL: 50–100 mg I.M. Start P.O. vitamins as soon as possible.
4. Ascorbic acid: 500 mg per day.
5. Pyridoxine HCL: 100 mg per day.
6. Folic acid: 1–5 mg per day × 5 days.
7. Multiple vitamins: 1 twice a day.
8. Thiamine: 100 mg 3 times a day.

B. *Tranquilizers.* Type should be based on several factors of which physician's experience, drug, and patient characteristics are of paramount importance. These can be used during the first few days of "detox" if needed. Care should be taken not to overuse tranquilizers or other sedatives in the acute intoxication phase or with markedly elevated alcohol blood levels, e.g., 100–150 mg/dl or above. BDZs are the drugs of choice, but major tranquilizers can be used if necessary. If IM BDZs are needed, use lorazepam (Ativan).

1. Diazepam (Valium): Initial loading dose of 20 mg P.O. every 1 hour until symptom-free and mildly sedated. Usually 1–3 doses over the 1–6 hours are needed, but up to 12 doses over 48 hours may be required. Determination of the need for continued dosing should be made 45 minutes after the previous dose. Thereafter, no more is needed owing to its long half-life.
2. Chlordiazepoxide (Librium): Similar to diazepam schedule especially if more sedation is desirable. Doses of 50–100 mg every 1 to 1½ hours.
3. Lorazepam (Ativan): 2–4 mg I.M. as above if oral medication cannot be tolerated or I.M. medication is required. 1 mg of lorazepam is equivalent to about 5 mg of diazepam.
4. Haloperidol (Haldol): 2–5 mg oral or I.M. every 2 hours or more often for agitation.
5. Chlorpromazine (Thorazine): 50–75 mg oral or I.M. every 4–6 hours for agitation. Check BP in standing position ½ hour before medication. Do not use if BP less than 80mm Hg systolic. Hypovolemic individuals or liver problems need special precautions.
6. Diphenhydramine (Benadryl): 25–50 mg I.M. STAT for EPS, followed by any oral antiparkinsonian agent if major tranquilizer is required.
7. Other major and minor tranquilizers can be used depending upon clinical experience.

C. *Sleeping medications (barbiturates).* Should be avoided because of the probability of prior abuse.

## Substance Abuse Disorders

1. Flurazepam (Dalmane): 15–30 mg HS. Fewer problems with interference of the REM stages of sleep and alerting mechanisms.
2. Triazolam (Halcion): 0.25–0.5 mg HS. In debilitated patients, 0.125–0.25 mg HS.
3. Chloral Hydrate (Noctec): 500 mg to 2 g HS. In younger children or those needing lower doses, a syrup, 500 mg per 5 cc, is available.

D. *Anticonvulsive medications.* Should not be used routinely but only if seizures have been a factor in the past. If a severe withdrawal has resulted in seizurelike activity despite diazepam use, the following can be used for 7–10 days:
1. Phenytoin (Dilantin): 200 mg I.M., then:
2. Phenytoin: 100 mg, 4 times a day P.O. Do not exceed blood levels of 1 to 2 mg/dl therapeutic range.

E. *Intravenous fluids.* Only if severe dehydration, orthostatic hypotension, hemoconcentration, vomiting, or debilitation is present. The rapid administration of 1–2 liters of balanced IV fluids with vitamins added, infused over several hours, should reduce morbidity.

III. Laboratory tests:
  A. Within 24 hours or sooner: initial blood alcohol, blood sugar, CBC (to include mean blood cell volume, MCV), urine analysis (including drug screen), SMA group for liver screen (at least SGOT, LDH, Alkaline phosphatase, Bilirubin), albumin, serology, chest Xray (PA and lateral). A MCV increase may indicate folate deficiency, liver disease, or reticulocytosis.
  B. In high-risk groups, blood antibodies for HIV.
  C. EEG and EKG should be done initially only if clinically indicated and best repeated after 7 to 10 days of return to a fairly normal physiological status.
  D. Other tests to consider: electrolytes (sodium, potassium, chloride), BUN, creatinine, amylase, bromsulphalein (for hepatocellular damage), fasting and 2-hour postprandial bloodsugar, sputum for culture and sensitivity.

IV. Nursing care:
  A. Vital signs:
    1. TPR and BP four times a day for 3 days, then routine. Pulse and blood pressure, supine then after 3 minutes standing, for 48 hours, then routine.
    2. Weight: Admission and then on Monday, Wednesday, and Friday.
  B. Diet: Initially patients may need assistance, encouragement, and direction in obtaining an adequate diet.
    1. Fluids: Large oral intake is necessary because of various degrees of dehydration. Orange juice is a good source of potassium.

2. Supplementary feedings, if indicated.
C. Orientation: Patients should be oriented and familiarized to the unit. Orientation should be checked and noted daily. A standard orientation checklist is desirable.
V. Neurological evaluation: Focus on EMG studies to pick up early neuropathy. Brain mapping and other recent procedures used to study brain structure and functions (CAT scan, PET, MRI) should be considered.
VI. Psychological testing: Consult may be general in nature with a routine test battery. If specific, questions should be asked—e.g., evaluate degree of organicity, learning disabilities, mental retardation.
VII. Other: Physical, occupational, recreational, and art therapy programs need to be specified. Group meetings to include AA-type programs for individual and family. Educational needs depending on school requirements. Psychotherapy based on individual needs. Antabuse therapy, behavior modification, or hypnotherapy may be of value.
VIII. Follow-up: Discharge planning should be started shortly after admission. Extended care programs such as residential, halfway houses, and other specialized units should be considered. Family members and others involved in the care of the individual must be involved in the planning process.

## Appendix 2

### Specific Sedative/Hypnotic Withdrawal

Generally, most of the alcohol SOP applies. Insert a specific section for this category of substances.

II. *Medications.*
F. *Tranquilizer withdrawal.* For oral drugs use diazepam. If I.M. needed, use lorazepam—1 mg lorazepam = 5 mg diazepam.
 1. Loading dose: 10–20 mg diazepam, or 2–5 mg lorazepam I.M.
 2. Maintenance dose: Repeat dose every hour over next 6 to 48 hours until symptom-free and mildly sedated. Determine next dose after 45 minutes of previous dose. Once stability is achieved, no further diazepam is needed owing to its long half-life.
G. *Barbiturate withdrawal.* Check for level of tolerance with use of short-acting drug. Thereafter a long-acting drug can be used for withdrawal.
 1. Test dose: Pentobarbital. 50–200 mg P.O. every ½ to 1 hour over 6-hour period to point of intoxication: ataxia, nystagmus, slurred speech. If less than 100–200 mg produces intoxication, then a detox schedule is not needed.

## Substance Abuse Disorders

2. Stabilization dose: The 6-hour test dose is given 4 times a day for the next 1–3 days. 30 mg of phenobarbital can be substituted for 100 mg pentobarbital and given once or twice a day because of its long half-life.
3. Withdrawal dose: Decrease 100 mg pentobarb or 30 mg phenobarb, or less, per day over the next 10 to 20 days.
4. If withdrawal symptoms occur, slow down reducing dose. Consider blood and urine for barb levels and other drugs.

### Appendix 3

### Narcotic Withdrawal Procedures

As with sedative/hypnotics, use the alcohol SOP as it is basically similar. Additional medications are needed for narcotics because of physical difficulties.

II. *Medications.*
   F. *Narcotic withdrawal.* A narcotic antagonist will start the withdrawal abruptly or reverse an acute overdose. Methadone and clonidine can be used to prevent withdrawal symptoms; however, withdrawal by itself is not life-threatening.
1. Acute overdose: Naloxone 0.4 mg I.M., I.V., or S.C. every 5 minutes until awake. Usually 0.8–1.2 mg (2–3 vials) is adequate. Infants and young children, use 0.01 mg per kg, repeat every 10 minutes.
2. Initiate withdrawal dose: As above, but less frequent to produce physical withdrawal symptoms.
3. Methadone dose: This long-acting narcotic can be used for withdrawal. Its purity may cause more of an addiction than the street doses.
   a. Initial dose: 15–20 mg PO, for both inpatients and outpatients.
   b. Withdrawal dose: Inpatients, repeat dose when symptoms return over 24 hours. Reduce daily dose by 5–10 mg per day. Outpatients, give only a 24-hour dose, usually 30–40 mg divided for twice-a-day intake, and decrease dose as with inpatients.
   c. Methadone maintenance: Not generally accepted for children because doses of 100 mg plus or minus 25 mg per day are used.
4. Clonidine: This alpha 2-adrenergic agonist has been found effective because it replaces opiate-mediated inhibition of brain noradrenergic activity.
   a. Initial dose: 5 ug/kg/day in 2 equal doses (0.35 mg/day for average 70-kg adolescent).

b. Withdrawal dose: Taper dose over 6–10 days to avoid rebound hypertension.
5. Infant withdrawal:
   a. Phenobarbital: 8–10 mg/kg/day in 4 divided doses,
   b. or Chlorpromazine: 2.8 mg/kg/day in 4 divided doses,
   c. or Paregoric: 3–5 drops orally before each meal.

G. *Pain.*
   1. Propoxyphene (Darvon): 65–103 mg every 3 or 4 hours.
   2. ASA (aspirin): or phenacetin.

H. *Muscle spasms.*
   1. Diazepam: 10 mg.
   2. Chlorzoxazone (Paraflex): 500–700 mg or
   3. Chlorzoxazone: 250 mg plus acetaminophen 300 mg (Parafon Forte) every 4–6 hours.

I. *Nausea.*
   1. Prochlorperazine (Compazine): 10 mg. If extrapyramidal effects, diaphenydramine, 25–50 mg I.M. If vomiting a problem, use 5 mg I.M. or suppositories, 5-mg or 25-mg size.
   2. Trimethobenzamide (Tigen): 250 mg every 4 hours.

J. *Diarrhea, cramps.*
   1. Diphenoxylate with atropine (Lomotil): 2.5–5 mg every 4 hours.
   2. Propantheline (Pro-Banthine): 15–30 mg every 4–6 hours.
   3. Dicyclomine (Bentyl): 10 mg every 4–6 hours.

K. *Constipation.* Deimpaction and oil retention enemas.

## *References*

American Academy of Pediatrics. (1988). *Substance abuse: A guide for health professionals.* Elk Grove Village, IL: Author.

American Medical Association. (1986). *Drug evaluations* (6th ed.). Chicago: Author.

Bayless, T. M., & Brain, M. C. (1984). *Current therapy in internal medicine.* St. Louis: C. V. Mosby.

Behrman, R. E., & Vaughan, V. C. (Eds.). (1983). *Nelson textbook of pediatrics* 12th ed.). Philadelphia: W. B. Saunders.

Blum, K. (1984). *Handbook of abusable drugs.* New York: Gardner Press.

Flanagan, T. J., & Jamieson, K. M. (1988). *Sourcebook of criminal justice statistics—1987.* Washington, DC: U.S. Government Printing Office.

Gilman, A. G., Gilman, L. S., Rall, T. W., & Murad, F. (1985). *Goodman and Gilman's: The pharmacological basis of therapeutics* (7th ed.). New York: Macmillan.

Johnson, L. D. (1980). *Review of general population surveys on drug abuse* (WHO Offset Publication No. 52). Geneva: World Health Organization.

Medical Economics Co. (1989). *Physician's desk reference* (43rd ed.). Dradell, NJ: Author.

Moser, J. (1985). *Alcohol policies in national health and development planning.* (WHO Offset Publication No. 89). Geneva: World Health Organization.

Richards, L. G. (1981). *Demographic trends and drug abuse, 1980–1985* (NIDA Research Monograph No. 35). Washington, DC: U.S. Government Printing Office.
Rock, N. L., & Donley, P. J. (1975). Treatment program for military personnel with alcohol problems, Part II. The program. *International Journal of Addictions, 3,* 467–476.
Rock, N. L., & Silsby, H. D. (1975). The attitude of American physicians stationed with the U.S. Army Europe in regard to alcohol and drug abuse. *Military Medicine, 11,* 781–783.
Schuckit, M. A. (1989). *Drug and alcohol abuse: A clinical guide to diagnosis and treatment* (3rd ed.). New York: Plenum.
Smart, R. G., Arif, A., Hughes, P., & Mora, M. E. M., Navaratnam, V., Varma, V. K., & Wadud, K. A. (1981). *Drug use among non-student youth* (WHO Offset Publication No. 60). Geneva: World Health Organization.
U.S. Department of Education. (1987). *What works—schools without drugs.* Washington, DC: U.S. Government Printing Office.

# 7

# Treatment of Anorexia Nervosa Current Status

## Kai Tolstrup

### Introduction

Two recent handbooks (Brownell & Foreyt, 1986; Garner & Garfinkel, 1985) give evidence of the many current methods of treatment of eating disorders. In this chapter some selected facts, personal descriptions, and considerations will be presented.

Diagnostically, the eating disorders cover nearly the same main syndromes in the American DSM-III (American Psychiatric Association, 1980) and the World Health Organization's draft of ICD 10 (World Health Organization, 1987) — that is, anorexia nervosa (AN), bulimia nervosa (BN), and cases of obesity that are caused by, or result in, psychological disturbances. Clinically, a more adequate term would be eating *and weight* disorders, because their own weight always is of great personal emotional concern to these patients, and because the consequences of undernourishment and fatness, respectively, indicate essential practical problems of treatment. Apart from this, a few traits are common to the underweight and the overweight syndromes, but the differences are important: AN and BN are linked to the crisis of puberty and nearly always occur in late childhood and adolescence, while obesity usually is a lifelong problem. The underweight syndromes often require acute somatic treatment and longterm psychiatric effort, whereas the treatment of obesity, although tough and protracted, is not so dramatic. Obese patients relatively rarely come to the attention of a psychiatrist. Therefore, the treatment of psychogenic obesity is not dealt with here.

---

*Kai Tolstrup*  University Clinic of Child Psychiatry, Rigshospitalet University Hospital, Copenhagen, Denmark 2100,Ø.

## The Treatment of Anorexia Nervosa

It is well known that anorectic patients are often unwilling, or unable, to explain their opinions and feelings. But sometimes they express themselves very vividly in drawings (Figure 1). One can understand this series in both directions, as growing either ill and thin or healthy and fat. The picture also expresses the problems about finding the right balance of bodily appearance.

In a survey of the treatment of AN, Hsu (1986) states that there is no specific treatment, because the etiology is unknown and because patients' needs differ. Therefore, treatment must be pragmatic. In my personal experience, the treatment should be empirically determined and, in each case, dependent on the stage of illness, the individual need of the patient, and the resources of the therapist.

Some of the treatment models of AN that have been described (e.g., Bruch, 1978; Minuchin, Rosman, & Baker, 1978; Palazzoli, 1974) are based on specific theories of psychogenesis. The results of the more comprehensive studies, which also fulfill demands for a long catamnestic period (e.g., Morgan, Purgold, & Welbourne, 1983; Santonastaso, Favaretto, & Canton, 1987; Theander, 1985; Tolstrup et al., 1985) do not point to simple etiological explana-

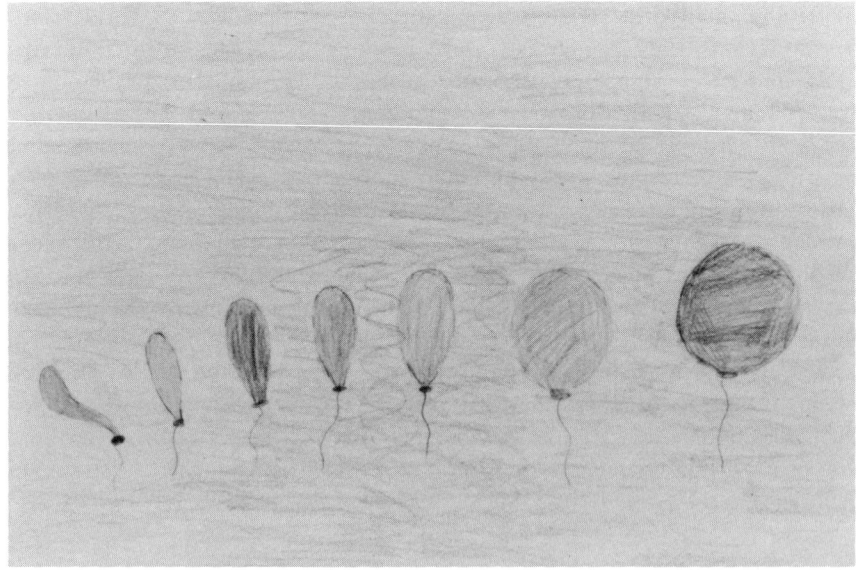

*Figure 1.* Drawing by a 13-year-old girl with anorexia nervosa in the middle of her treatment—and she feels like one of the middle balloons.

## Anorexia Nervosa

tions. However, whether the different forms of treatment described are theoretically founded or based on clinical experience only, a series of common traits can be found in the descriptions, which allows, I think, the following characteristics to be summarized:

1. The simultaneous physical and psychological disturbances of the anorectic patient mean that the therapist must have both medical-biological and psychotherapeutic competence. The consequences of the undernourishment, possibly a state that threatens life, must be abolished, but the disease is not cured before the psychical complaints also are gone. Therefore, the therapy should be saturated by a deliberate psychotherapeutic attitude.

2. As the course of the disease may be spread over many years, or even decades, treatment should have a long-range perspective, be characterized by continuity, and preferably be carried out by the same therapist.

3. The denial of disease by the patient or by the family, as well as resistance to treatment, often makes it difficult to motivate the patient, and the family, for treatment. If therapy is established, consequence, flexibility, and firmness to an unusually high degree are required by the therapist.

4. The fully developed syndrome is rather uniform, and on the whole independent of sex and age, within the wide limits of puberty and adolescence. This uniformity concerns the outer appearance, which is to a great extent superficial and caused by the undernourishment and the reactions by the environment, reactions that the anorectic behavior has brought about. Therefore, it is only apparently a paradox to maintain that

5. The patients and the families differ individually from each other and, especially in the later therapeutic phases, require individualized treatment.

### A Model for Integrated Treatment

This model, which I try to visualize in the form of a tree, a trunk with branches, builds on my experiences through 39 years in the treatment of more than 200 patients with AN and/or BN, and describes the current practice in the department of child psychiatry at Rigshospitalet in Copenhagen. This setting is a university clinic, and it admits patients of all psychiatric categories from all over Denmark. Treatment is carried out in a child psychiatry framework, but with no upper age limit, and the philosophy is offered in the treatment of young adults, too.

There are no definite etiological or therapeutic theories behind the treatment. I have, however, developed the following conception of AN:

AN is a disturbance of the bodily and mental functions of puberty, reflecting the vulnerability and the conflicts of this developmental period, most often associated with the female sex, but universally human and fundamentally independent of sex. Cases requiring treatment are pathological variants of normal crisis phenomena in puberty, but in severe cases it is an illness threatening health and life. A tendency to spontaneous cure is obvious, but there is a remarkable liability to relapse and chronicity. The most important therapeutic purpose is to *promote the tendency to healing* and *counteract the liability to death, chronicity, and relapse*.

As to the much-debated question of the relation between anorexia and bulimia, one can look upon the different forms of AN and BN as a continuum or a spectrum spread from cases of pure food restriction at one end, through cases with bulimic episodes in an otherwise classical AN, and patients with pure bulimia at the other end. They all have in common the fear of growing fat, and a distorted image and feeling of their own body. The continuity in "bulimic variants" (Tolstrup, 1982) may be seen as an indicator of more or less effective defense mechanisms against strong eating impulses. For practical reasons one cannot treat pure food refusal and pure eating binges in exactly the same way, but I find it natural that the basic psychotherapeutic point of view and attitude should be the same. Moreover, the subdivision of bulimia nervosa in underweight and normal-weight patients is practical for therapeutic reasons.

The elements of treatment can be represented in the form of a tree (Figure 2). The trunk is an individual supportive psychotherapy combined with an eating-weight regime. The therapeutic trunk can be expanded according to need and resources. The branches are family contact, group therapy (for patients or parents), admission to hospital with milieu-treatment in the ward, art therapy, specific motoric training and, rarely, psychotropic drugs.

The term *model* in this connection does not mean a theory but is only a schematic representation of those forms of therapy that are parts of our therapeutic programs determined by the traditions of the department and by present resources. *Integrated* means that we strive to use in each case the mixture of therapeutic handling and methods that is suitable to the individual patient, and that we aim at a balanced approach.

The basic treatment is a simultaneous bodily and psychotherapeutic supportive therapy carried out by the same therapist, in principle a physician. The starting point is, if possible, outpatient treatment. Sessions with talk about weight control are from 30 minutes to 1 hour. Frequency can vary from twice a week to once a month, or even more seldom. In the beginning the talks consist of *information, support*, and *demands*. All three aspects are present at the same time, although in varying degrees in the course of treatment. Later on *discussion* and *interpretation* may be more prominent.

*Information* is very important, particularly in the opening stages. At the first consultation, lasting usually 1 to 2 hours, the patient is presented with today's essential knowledge about AN. She is informed of the dangerousness of the illness, but also of the good chances of total cure. The aim is to give her a feeling of confidence that is therapeutically decisive, and to make her understand the rational and detailed program offered her and the family.

# Anorexia Nervosa

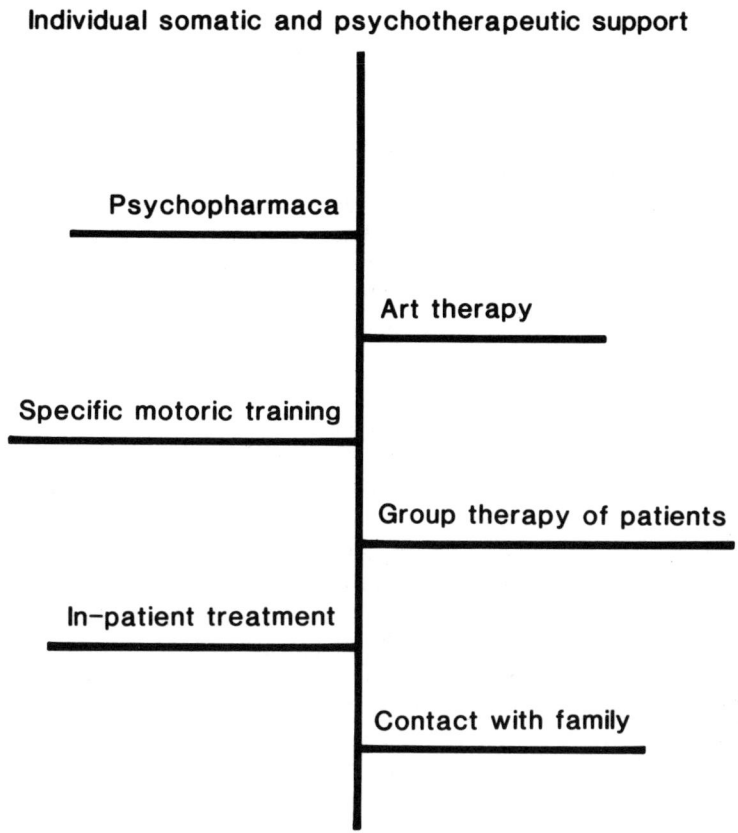

*Figure 2.* The model represents the different forms of treatment of anorexia nervosa used in the Department of Child Psychiatry at Rigshospitalet, Copenhagen. (Stem treatment with possible branches.)

*Supportive* therapy means making the patient feel that her disease is taken seriously but is not accepted as the right solution of her problems. The therapist is looking for the healthy person who was there before she became ill, now hidden in the disease, and who will reappear when she has recovered. This attitude may be illustrated by the comments sometimes made by the therapist about her looks. More than once I have seen an anorectic patient in a state of cachexy feeling shocked, encouraged, and supported by being told that she is now awful-looking, but that she will be helped to regain her former beautiful and healthy look, only on a more mature stage of development. This frankly expressed statement is also an appeal to her feminine feeling and female identity, currently impaired by the disease.

At the same time, the therapist makes *demands* as to eating and weight. A continuous increase of weight is demanded by the therapist as an indispensable part of the therapeutic contract. Disagreement and conflict with the patient often follows because this demand is relentless and is looked upon as the patient's contribution in return for the therapist's commitment. The therapeutic starting point addresses the main symptoms—that is, weight-phobia and refusal to eat. The therapist must figuratively "shake hands with the symptoms."

The patient's denial of disease and need for help may make the beginning of the treatment most difficult. Often, however, behind a superficial denial one finds a real wish, and a call for help, to emerge from a life situation in which the patient has lost control. It does not matter so much that she shouts and scolds and cries, if only at last she cooperates with the therapeutic conditions given her, and in reality accepted by her.

If the treatment is successful, the emphasis is gradually and continuously shifted from eating-weight problems to the feelings behind. Even if food, weight, and appearance are still now and then at issue, the patient's other thoughts and feelings, and their background will increasingly stand out. Various themes give occasion for talking about conflicts associated with puberty, such as her own looks and that of other girls; perhaps the overweight of other members of the family, their beauty or less good looks; the anxiety of growing and developing conflicting with the wish to become an adult, a woman, a sexual partner and perhaps a mother; insecurity about possibly again having menstruations, for the youngest patients with the beginning of menstruations at all; relationships with close family and friends; the everlasting quarrels with mother; rivalry with an elder sister; admiration and insecurity toward the father and all other males.

In the treatment of an anorectic girl one must be prepared to meet silence, and often not to *speak with* so much as *talk to* the girl. It is, however, not seldom that both somatic and mental symptoms disappear during treatment without any thorough working through or an open discussion of the personal problems.

It is a well-founded fact that most AN patients cannot be treated with a classical conflict-solving, psychoanalytically oriented psychotherapy. It may be practical to characterize some of the AN personalities according to their similarities with either hysterical, obsessive–compulsive, borderline psychotic or depressive patients. However, their personalities differ very much and cannot be characterized as uniform. In terms of modern ego- or self-psychology (Goodsit, 1985), many of the severe cases can be considered narcissistic or alexithymic personalities, and the psychotherapy can be undertaken accordingly. It may be fruitful to regard their reactions and attitudes as expressions of the defense mechanisms of *splitting* and *projective identification*. Perhaps these latter personality characteristics are more conspicuous in the bulimic cases. It has been said by Goodsit (1985) that in self-supporting therapy the therapist offers himself as a self-object or transitional object. Some key words for the therapy are *structure with dynamic understanding* and *authority without aggression*.

## Core Therapy

The core treatment can be carried out with the girl alone if an older patient insists on her family not being involved. But as a rule, and for the younger without exception, it is essential to establish and keep family contact. This contact can have varying degrees of intensity: family therapy proper, talks with parents, parental groups, or a looser contact where the main aim is to motivate the parents to facilitate the treatment.

### Family Contact

In recent years many child psychiatrists have considered family therapy proper to be the standard method for treatment of AN. Although family therapy must have a central position in the therapeutic armament, it should, like other specific forms of therapy, be used only in selected and appropriate cases (Russell, Szmukler, Dare, & Eisler, 1987).

From the outset, the possibility or need for family therapy proper must be evaluated. There are patients referred to our clinic who have had family therapy elsewhere, but without success, so that we must try other branches of the "treatment tree." (It also happens, of course, that our treatment fails, and the patient and family must be treated elsewhere.) In some cases, motivation for family therapy develops during the course of the basic treatment. At times family therapy is not possible because the family is too weak, the conflicts are too deep and entangled, or the members simply do not want it.

The parents' acceptance of the treatment plan is essential. Parents of the most severely disabled patients are apparently also the best motivated. They have often become stuck because of the troubles with the patient at home. Even if they seem primarily well motivated, however, this attitude may change in the course of treatment, when the most imminent dangers have disappeared and the immediate pressure on the family has been relieved through admission of the patient to the hospital. They may then yield to pressure from the patient, who mobilizes the parents' feelings of guilt to strengthen her own resistance to treatment. As a result, parents may terminate therapy prematurely.

In connection with the many problems that the family contact may bring up, it should never be forgotten, first, that it is very difficult to have an anorectic girl in the family, second, that many of the problems are created by the illness, and third, in my opinion, that many of these families are strong and good and were "normal" before the disease started.

## Group Therapy

### Patient Groups

We do group therapy either in patient groups or in parental groups.

The group of AN patients is an open one, unselected inasmuch as all AN patients in the clinic are expected to participate, consists of 6 to 11 in- or outpatients, and is carried out by a trained group therapist who is under "live supervision." The group therapy is independent of all other therapy carried out in the same period for the same patients in the department, but we try to integrate the different forms of therapy with the therapist running the core treatment responsible for integration.

One of the advantages of the patient group is its efficiency due to the mutual influence between participants. Status in the group may depend on biological age, the duration of the disease, and time of hospital stay. A new, severely emaciated patient will get a frank and merciless message from the other group members about her appearance, and they will tell her all about the characteristics of her illness (including the common tricks) and the local conditions of treatment. The girls, and occasionally a boy, show each other a sincerity, care, and criticism that they would not tolerate from any therapist or adult.

Patient groups, including self-help groups, may contribute to the solution of a quantitative problem if there are many patients and few therapists. But it is a therapy form in its own right (Hall, 1985). It may be especially efficient in the treatment of bulimia (Mitchell et al., 1985).

### Parent Groups

We conduct parent groups in simultaneous sessions of one and a half hours in two open groups meeting once a month. Six to 12 parents participate in each group, with three therapists present. This therapy, too, is principally independent of other therapy given to the same parents and children in the department. Attendance is very high, although the parents, who come from all over Denmark, often have to travel a long way for the session. The purpose of the group is to let the parents exchange their experiences and express and discuss feelings, thoughts, and attitudes relating to the children and their disease. The activity level of the group members is high, and accordingly interference from the three therapists is discreet. Typical themes have been responsibility and powerlessness, guilt feelings in relation to their child, criticism of and aggressions against the treating team, and insecurity in the roles of parents, children, and grandparents. Indulgence and firmness have been discussed, and so have problems about denial of disease and the question of whether the anorectic girls behave provocatively. We have seen the formation of subgroup alliances—for instance, between mothers (women) on one side and fathers (men) on the other. The groups have discussed how marital relations are influenced by the daughter's AN, and examples have shown that the disease can uncover problems in the parents' relationships and thus perhaps indirectly lead to improvement or aggravation. Further, these groups have given the therapists the opportunity of comparisons that again emphasize how different the parents of the AN patients are behind the superficial uniform reaction pattern caused by the illness. A most vivid description of experience with parental groups is given by Jeammet and Gorge (1980).

## Art Therapy

Art therapy has been undertaken in a weekly group with four or five patients suffering from AN. It is led by a trained psychologist. The participants may draw whatever they want and can afterwards comment on their own or the other group members' work. The drawings belong to the group and are not mentioned or referred to in other parts of the integrated treatment program.

The meaning of art therapy is well formulated in a remark by one of the girls: "I like drawing therapy because you become aware, in another way, of what is going on inside yourself through your own drawings and those of other group members. So you are also 'compelled' to think over your own situation." In this form of therapy it is perhaps most clearly confirmed that behind their smooth and rejecting facade these girls hide a rich life of feelings with strong affects and tensions. For instance, a very withdrawn and contact-rejecting girl, who is very "neutral" in daily life, showed in her art passionate colors and bodies of a very sensual character. Some of the common topics are a longing for the far-off and unattainable; an endeavor for, and, at the same time, anxiety of, freedom and display; also a simultaneous urge to, and a dislike of, isolation. The pictures may be clear and naturalistic, or they may be more vague and symbolic. They often represent human figures, usually children and young women, but also plants and animals, flying birds, rainbows, and sprouting herbs in blurred outline. They are either colored or in shades from gray to black.

Art therapy of AN systematically performed in any clinic is not reflected in the literature. A single case followed up through many years is described by Veyrat and Bogert (1986).

## Motoric Training

Specific motoric training is performed by a specialist in movement therapy who is attached to the department to treat all our patients, including the AN patients. The AN patients are often very tense and excited, and display a bodily hyperactivity that can take grotesque forms. Motoric training can be established when the pathological hyperactivity is moderated as a part of the general improvement, so that simple exercises of relaxation can be conducted by the movement therapist. The girls will then often benefit from a skilled and gentle modification of their pattern of movements.

## Pharmacological Treatment

### Pharmacotherapy

We seldom use drugs in the treatment of AN. When we do, the aim is to influence symptoms other than the anorectic ones. Occasionally, sadness can look like endogenous depression, and in these cases tricyclic antidepressants are used with some effect. A borderline personality AN patient may benefit from neuroleptics. In the rare cases of physically aggressive boys with AN, it has been necessary to give sedative neuroleptics.

It is generally accepted that psychopharmaceuticals are not specifically efficient in the treatment of AN (Bond, Crabbe, & Sanders, 1986). Antidepressants are stated to be effective for bulimia in controlled studies, but it has not been our experience that improvement can be expected if the patient has no obvious signs of severe depression.

All the "branches on the treatment tree" are in principle applicable both to outpatient therapy and in the ward.

### Hospitalization

When should an AN patient be sent to a hospital? The most important indications are (1) emaciation, with resulting or imminent complications that cannot be treated outside the hospital, (2) need for relief of the family and the patient when the situation is deadlocked because of her anorectic behavior and the pressure of feelings, (3) need for milieu therapy performed in a (child) psychiatry ward with special experience in this field.

The stay in hospital must give 24-hour control of eating and weight and must make the girl feel confident and safe. Professionals who are familiar with the illness, in all its strange varieties, behave professionally without losing their human and personal attitudes.

The inpatient treatment has two main elements: the core treatment (perhaps continued from the outpatient therapy), and a structured milieu therapy based on the experience and traditions of the ward, where usually four to eight patients are in treatment. All the above-mentioned forms of therapy may be added according to need and resources. The patient's weight and eating indicate continuously the state of the disease. The aim of milieu therapy is to help the girl out of the tyranny of food and weight, and to promote development toward normal life. This means attending school, in the ward or outside; participating in activities according to her age; and being with other children and adults.

If free eating of the meals usually served in the ward is not followed by a sufficient weight gain, the next step will be a prescribed diet with a detailed discussion with dieticians and the patient. The diet has a surplus of calories, which should secure weight gain — if it is eaten, of course. Patient observation in the first hour after the meal may be necessary to prevent established or suspected vomiting. If eating, weight, and status as a whole are still not satisfactory, bed rest with a watch night and day for at least a few weeks will be established. This 24-hour watch is aimed at preventing all possible tricks and cheating, but it may also have the advantage of relaxation and comfort on the level of a younger child. If improvement fails to appear, the last step is tube feeding at each meal, with the tube removed between meals, never *á demeure*. Only rarely do we reach the step of tube feeding in the ladder of treatment, the main reason being that the girl quickly realizes the strictness of the regime, and acknowledges the sincerity of our promise neither to let her die nor to let her get stuck in her illness.

A contact, most often a nurse, is assigned to the patient during the stay in the ward. Together with the psychiatrist, who is in charge of the core treatment, the nurse is responsible for the accomplishment of the regime. She is the primary contact in all aspects of the girls' daily life, such as preparation for school, and clothes and makeup, and she may take her to town for shopping or to attend concerts. It is a success, of course, if they develop a relationship of confidence that may help the anorectic girl to reestablish a natural female identification.

The hospital inpatient stay will be rarely less than 3 months, and it often lasts for about 1 year.

## Discharge

When is it time for discharge from the hospital? It may be difficult to find the balance between a premature discharge, before the patient is strong enough to continue the core treatment outside the hospital, and a discharge that is too late, when she has become too dependent on the protective ward milieu (Figure 3). Some patients return home, while others must be transferred to a residential school or a residential treatment-home because of unsolved problems at home. Practically all continue to attend the outpatient clinic, usually for at least 1 year.

This sort of treatment requires a highly qualified and specially trained staff and demands many resources. It is hard work even for a clinic with a long and

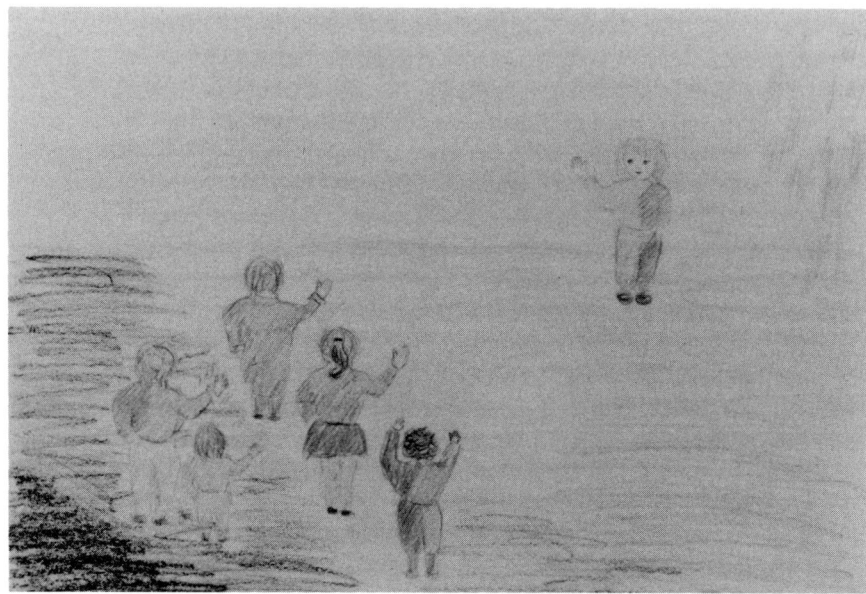

*Figure 3.* "Leaving the hospital." Drawing by a 15-year-old girl with anorexia nervosa. These small children in reality represent 14- to 16-year-old patients.

continuous tradition of treating AN. The staff must be prepared to be "cheated" without too much personal disappointment, and they must at all times be both firm and flexible, yet neither rigid nor too easily influenced. Communication within the team about the status of treatment and the latest problems should be open, direct, and fast. One of the greatest difficulties is the risk that the therapist and the contact person be caught by the demand for secondary gains by the patient, with the consequence that the therapist feels either too compassionate or too aggressive. On the other hand, the staff must be able to adequately express their feelings to the patient. The long duration of treatment and frequent relapses easily give rise to feelings of severe disappointment. The staff has to realize that the time-consuming therapy and the deep personal commitment do not always result in a constant or enduring improvement. The dangers of countertransference are always present. Support and supervision are very much needed, even for the most competent therapist, since even the best staff may have the experience of being stuck in this treatment. On the other hand, successes are frequent, and it is very rewarding when the therapists have the satisfaction of seeing the development of a valuable human being released from her illness.

Aspects of this empirical model of integrated treatment could be interpreted partially in terms of behavior theory, cognitive therapy, psychoanalysis, or object relations. These and other theories have indeed influenced and inspired the treatment model. What I find more important, however, is the actual similarity with treatment models described by other clinicians in light of their experience with large numbers of patients (Andersen, 1985; Crisp, 1980; Garner, 1986; Jeammet, 1982; Russell et al., 1987; Schutze, 1980). The similarities in the treatment interventions of everyday clinical life, often dictated by necessity, are more impressive than the differences in theoretical explanations.

## Treatment Outcome

From long-term follow-up studies we know a little about the course of AN, but until now, knowledge about the efficacy of different forms of treatment has been scanty. Short-term efficacy is high in most forms of treatment. An evaluation of long-term results is especially relevant in an illness with such an established tendency of long duration, relapse, and death. At present, we have to conclude that we do not know to what extent the outcome is determined by the treatment given, or whether the "natural history" (Tolstrup, Brinch, & Isager, 1984) of the disease is the most important determinant factor.

Long-term studies confirm that AN is a serious disease (Theander, 1985). The follow-up results from Copenhagen (Tolstrup et al., 1985) are typical: 4 to 22 years after the initial treatment about half of the surviving patients had recovered and one-quarter still suffered from AN or had relapsed. One-quarter had signs of another mental disease and 6 % had died. Although it is a sample of severe cases—and, as emphasized by Szmukler and Russell (1986), the selection of patients is always to be considered when evaluating outcome—these figures underline the seriousness of the illness.

Thus, none of the treatment methods described in the literature has been proven superior to others. The longer the follow-up periods, the more similar and uniform the results of different forms of treatment. The same is true as far as the outcome in the follow-up study from Copenhagen (Isager, Brinch, & Tolstrup, 1985; Tolstrup et al., 1985) is concerned. Table 1 shows that the outcome after an average of 12 years does not differ significantly in three different departments at Rigshospitalet, one of which is the clinic of child psychiatry using the treatment model described above. Although the results have not yet been fully statistically analyzed, this lack of difference in results seems to be true also as to physical stage and other criteria of relevance for evaluation. And the three departments treated AN in rather different ways. In the department of internal medicine, duration of treatment was much shorter and consisted of a strictly maintained diet, and there was usually no psychiatric assistance. The duration of treatment in the department of adult psychiatry was in between, and psychotherapy was less intensive. The reader will find more

*Table 1*
Copenhagen Anorexia Nervosa Study

| Department | N of patients | No mental disorder | Anorexia (including bulimic variations) | Neurosis | Other |
|---|---|---|---|---|---|
| Child psychiatry | 54 | 55 | 25 | 11 | 9 |
| Adult psychiatry | 35 | 38 | 30 | 14 | 18 |
| Internal medicine | 27 | 56 | 19 | 11 | 14 |

about the differences in Tolstrup et al. (1985). In the evaluation of results it should be considered, however, that patients treated in psychiatric departments generally have a worse prognosis than those treated in medical wards, probably because of selection for admission (Szmukler & Russell, 1986).

## Indications for and Need of Treatment—Resources

Since the efficiency of treatment is so uncertain, the choice of therapy in each case must depend on some simple criteria, such as (1) severity of disease, physically and psychologically, (2) the character of the dominant symptoms, (3) the age of the patient, and (4) the therapeutic resources available.

In cases with severe loss of weight and long duration of illness it is especially important that treatment is expressly medically directed and concentrated upon the fight against undernourishment. A first and incontestable aim of treatment, of course, is the prevention of death and the consequences of undernourishment. In some cases threatened by death, commitment to a mental hospital may be necessary. This question has been discussed in a German paper (Lehmkuhl & Schmidt, 1986).

If bulimic elements are dominant, the painful and violent binges usually are a better motivation for treatment than for the patient with a purely restrictive AN. The therapist should be aware of the possibility that vomiting without binges may be used as a means of reducing weight. Also, it should cause a modification of the treatment when purging, diuretics, or extreme hyperactivity are the preferred means of losing weight. The importance of age for choice of therapy is mainly due to need of coordinated work with the family. Family therapy proper is more effective with the younger patient (Russell et al., 1987).

The use of specific therapeutic methods such as milieu therapy, group therapy, behavior therapy, and art therapy depends on, and is limited by, the availability of trained therapists (psychiatrists, psychologists). Specific motoric training, too, must be performed by a trained staff member. Pharmacotherapy can be given only by a psychiatrist.

How great is the need for treatment? The figures of prevalence are questionable (Schleimer, 1983). The tendency to denial of the disease probably means that several patients are untreated in the early stages of the illness. Even though the incidence of the registered severe cases is increasing, the figures are still rather small, between 1 in 10,000 and 1 in 100,000.

## Who Should Treat AN?

The great public interest in AN and BN at present, possibly combined with a higher incidence, results in a strong pressure on treatment resources. The above outlined "core treatment" in the early stages and lighter cases ought to be carried out primarily by the family doctor, perhaps helped by a consulting psychiatrist. The school doctor has a role to play at the diagnostic level. If the disease has lasted for more than half a year, or if the girl becomes very ill, the responsibility should be taken over by a psychiatrist. Local circumstances should determine whether a short stay in a pediatric or internal medicine ward is appropriate. Severe cases must be treated in a child or adolescent psychiatry ward with special experience in AN. For a population of 5 million people—the size of Denmark—there ought to be one special clinic for treatment and research of AN and BN exclusively, with close cooperation between child and adult psychiatrists, pediatricians, and specialists in internal medicine and in gynecology.

## What About Prevention?

Primary prevention, in the sense of eradicating the causes of eating disorders, is unrealistic because we do not know the origin. It is also undesirable, because the only certain precondition is a surplus of food, which at the same time is a fundamental benefit of our civilization.

It has become fashionable in recent decades for girls and young women to reduce weight and look slim—a trend emphasized for commercial reasons in books, magazines, and TV to a very unsound and excessive degree. However, slimming as such does not make a girl anorectic (Schleimer, 1983). We need much more popular, well-formulated, and professional sober information to counteract the commercialization of slim fashion, and the too-easy solutions for eating and weight problems now offered to the public.

At present, the most efficient preventive measures are to try and influence the children and young people at risk—that is, to do secondary prevention. The key groups are schoolgirls just before and during puberty and adolescents who are beginning to lose weight extraordinarily and who have irregular menstruations. Teachers, school doctors, and school nurses should be taught about the risks and must be ready to intervene with counseling to control weight and diet.

## Conclusion

Many different forms of therapy for eating disorders have been used, but none of them, alone or combined, are proven definitely the best. The long-term outcome of AN and BN is insufficiently known, and the results of treatment are uncertain. This is partly because differently selected cases and treated patients cannot be compared, and partly because we know too little about the natural history of the disease. It should not be concluded that it is needless to treat these patients, or that it does not matter which form of therapy is used. However, it should be emphasized that the form of therapy must be in accordance with your patient population and appropriate for your resources and philosophy. Therapy will often last for years, but it is rewarding if done with the commitment that these often fascinating personalities deserve. Sometimes we have to face the fact that an older patient has become a chronic anorectic. Our therapeutic task is to help her live with that condition, though we also know that seemingly chronic patients may recover after many years (Theander, 1985). Szmukler and Russell are right: "The prediction of outcome in an individual case is generally believed to remain something of a guess" (Szmukler & Russell, 1986). But I prefer to end this chapter in the optimistic spirit that an anorectic girl expressed by drawing a series of flowers: The first was seemingly broken, while the sequence showed the power of a young flower to straighten and right itself.

## References

American Psychiatric Association. (1980). *Diagnostic and statistical manual of mental disorders* (3rd ed.) Washington, DC.

Andersen, E. A. (1985). *Practical comprehensive treatment of anorexia nervosa and bulimia*. Baltimore: Johns Hopkins University Press.

Bond, W. S., Crabbe, S., & Sanders, M. C. (1986). Pharmacotherapy of eating disorders: A critical review. *Drug Intelligence and Clinical Pharmacy. 20*, 659–665.

Brownell, K.D., & Foreyt, J. P. (1986). *Handbook of eating disorders*. New York: Basic Books.

Bruch, H. (1978). *The golden cage*. London: Open Books.

Crisp, A. H. (1980). *Let me be*. London: Academic Press.

Garner, D. M. (1986). Cognitive therapy for anorexia nervosa. In K. D. Brownell & J. P. Foreyt (Eds.), *Handbook of eating disorders*. New York: Basic Books.

Garner, D. M., & Garfinkel, P. E. (Eds.). (1985). *Handbook of psychotherapy for anorexia nervosa and bulimia*. New York: Guilford Press.

Goodsit, A. (1985). Self-psychology and the treatment of anorexia nervosa. In D. M. Garner & P. E. Garfinkel (Eds.), *Handbook of psychotherapy for anorexia nervosa and bulimia* (pp. 55–83). New York: Guilford Press.

Hall, A. (1985). Group psychotherapy for anorexia nervosa. In D. M. Garner & P. E. Garfinkel (Eds.), *Handbook of psychotherapy for anorexia nervosa and bulimia* (pp. 213–239). New York: Guilford Press.
Hsu, L. K. G. (1986). The treatment of anorexia nervosa. *American Journal of Psychiatry, 143*, 573–581.
Isager, T., Brinch, M., & Tolstrup, K. (1985). Death and relapse in anorexia nervosa: Survival analysis of 151 cases. *Journal of Psychiatric Research, 19*, 515–521.
Jeammet, P. (1982). *Comment adapter le traitement de l'anorexie mentale aux données tirées de l'évolution à long terme des patientes?* Paper presented at the 10th International Congress of the IACP, Dublin.
Jeammet, P., & Gorge A. (1980). Une forme de thérapie familiale: Le group de parents. *Psychiatrie de l'Enfant, 23*, 587–636.
Lehmkuhl, G., & Schmidt, M. H. (1986). Wie freivillig kann die Behandlung von jugendlichen Patienten mit anorexia nervosa sein? *Psychiatrishe Praxis, 13*, 236–241.
Minuchin, S., Rosman, B. L., & Baker, L. (1978). *Psychosomatic families*. Cambridge: Harvard University Press.
Mitchell, J. E., Hatsukami, D., Goff, G., Pyle, R. L., Eckert, E. D., & Davis, L. E. (1985). Intensive outpatient group treatment for bulimia. In D. M. Garner & P. E. Garfinkel (Eds.), *Handbook of psychotherapy for anorexia nervosa and bulimia* (pp. 240–253). New York: Guilford Press.
Morgan, H. G., Purgold, J., & Welbourne, J. (1983). Management and outcome in anorexia nervosa. *British Journal of Psychiatry, 143*, 282–287.
Palazzoli, M. S. (1974). *Self-starvation*. London: Human Context Books.
Russell, G. F. M., Szmukler, G. I., Dare, C., & Eisler, I. (1987). An evaluation of family therapy in anorexia nervosa and bulimia nervosa. *Archives of General Psychiatry, 44*, 1047–1056.
Santonastaso, P., Favaretto, G., & Canton, G. (1987). Anorexia nervosa in Italy. *Psychopathology, 20*, 8–17.
Schleimer, K. (1983). Dieting in teen-age school-girls. *Acta Paediatrica Scandinavica, 312*(Suppl.), 1–54.
Schutze, G. (1980). *Anorexia nervosa*. Bern: Huber.
Szmukler, G. I., & Russell, G. F. M. (1986). Outcome and prognosis of anorexia nervosa. (1986). In K. D. Brownell & J. P. Foreyt (Eds.), *Handbook of eating disorders* (pp. 283–301). New York: Basic Books.
Theander, S. (1985). Outcome and prognosis in anorexia nervosa and bulimia. *Journal of Psychiatric Research, 19*, 493–508.
Tolstrup, K. (1982). Anorexia nervosa—A typical psychosomatic disease of puberty and adolescence. *Triangle, 21*, 85–88.
Tolstrup, K., Brinch, M., & Isager, T. (1984). Therapie und vuerlauf der anorexia nervosa. In H. Remschmidt (Ed.), *Psychotherapie mit Kindern* (Vol. 2; pp. 45–53). Stuttgart: Enke.
Tolstrup, K., Brinch, M., Isager, T., Nielsen, S., Nystrup, J., Severin, B., & Olesen, N. S. (1985). Long-term outcome of 151 cases of anorexia nervosa. *Acta Psychiatrica Scandinavica, 71*, 380–387.
Veyrat, J. G., & Bogaert, E. (1986). Evolution sur 20 ans d'un cas d'anorexie mentale á travers l'analyse de sa production picturale. *Société Medico-Pscyhologique*, 294–309.
World Health Organization. (1987). *ICD 10*. Draft of chapter V. Geneva: Author.

# 8

# Child and Adolescent Psychopharmacology

## Jovan G. Simeon

### Introduction

Pediatric psychopharmacology is a rapidly growing new field linking medicine, behavioral sciences, and neurosciences to child psychiatry. Its development has significantly lagged behind that of adult psychopharmacology. The widening acceptance of drug therapy in pediatric psychiatry by psychiatrists, pediatricians, and general practitioners has been accompanied by increasing concerns among therapists, parents, educators, and the public over the potential hazards of medications and their prolonged use. Probably the most general problem has been whether drugs alleviate a disorder, or whether children's behaviors are modified because they are perceived as unacceptable or undesirable by parents, teachers, and society. Are children treated because they are disturbed, or because they are disturbing? Criticisms that some of the drugs used in children are undesirable, dangerous, and misused as chemical "straightjackets" are usually based on the inability of doctors to diagnose and evaluate by objective scientific criteria (Werry, 1978).

Extrapolations from adult to child psychopharmacology can be difficult and misleading because drug effects and indications differ significantly. In contrast to adult psychiatry, evaluations of therapeutic and adverse effects are more complicated in children. Pharmacotherapy in child psychiatry is based more on a symptomatic than a disease model, and maladaptive behaviors are more often based on variations of temperament or interactions with the environment. Drug therapy and research in children depend on parents, teachers, and institutions, while in adolescents they are also influenced by such factors as marked biological growth, family and social factors, and drug compliance.

---

*Jovan G. Simeon*  Department of Psychiatry, University of Ottawa, Ottawa, Ontario K1Z 7K4 Canada.

Many psychiatric disorders occur in particular in children and adolescents, such as attention deficit and conduct disorders, childhood autism, separation anxiety, learning disability, enuresis, parasomnias, and anorexia nervosa. Since there are no comparable adequate models in adult psychiatry, drug trials in children and adolescents are necessary to continue making advances in pediatric psychopharmacology.

Our knowledge of psychotropic drug effects in children and adolescents is still inadequate for a rational and consistent clinical approach. This is especially true for various adolescent disorders such as depression, dysthymia, anorexia and bulimia nervosa, borderline conditions, and substance and alcohol abuse. There has been very little systematic clinical psychopharmacology research in these disorders. Therapy of these disorders has been remarkably unsuccessful and difficult; since their incidence has been on the increase, research on their treatment remains urgently needed.

Nevertheless, recent research in pediatric psychopharmacology has contributed to significant progress in the areas of hypothesis testing, study design, development of interview techniques and rating scales, diagnostic classification, new drugs, and new indications for existing medications (Campbell, Green, & Deutsch, 1985; *Psychopharmacology Bulletin*, 1985; Simeon & Saletu, 1979; Werry, 1982a, 1982b, 1982c). Drugs have also been useful as tools in increasing our knowledge of the biological, cognitive, and social manifestations of child psychiatry disorders, especially of hyperactivity, depression, autism, and Tourette's disease. Owing to these advances, an ever-increasing number of effective psychotropic drugs has been used in the therapy of child psychiatric patients.

The uses of drugs and diets are also discussed in other chapters of this book by W. Shekim, S. Kutcher, and P. Marton; B. Garfinkel; M. Campbell, R. Malone, and V. Kafantaris; M. Flament and L. Vero; and B. Ferguson. In addition, information on pediatric psychopharmacology is available in extensive publications elsewhere (Campbell et al. 1985; Conners & Werry, 1979; Klein, Gittelman, Quitkin, & Rifkin, 1980; Meltzer, 1987; Rifkin, Wortman, Reardon, & Siris, 1986; Simeon, 1976; *Psychopharmacology Bulletin*, 1975; Werry, 1977, 1978; White, 1977).

## General Guidelines of Prescribing

The reasons for therapy, goals, methods, and possible outcomes must be honestly and openly discussed with the parents and the patient. Children with identical diagnoses often show different responses to the same medications. Therefore, each time a patient is medicated, the treatment should be considered as a clinical trial. Prior to any drug therapy it is essential that a detailed baseline clinical assessment be undertaken. Assessments during therapy must be frequent, especially during the initial phases. Evaluations must include overt behavior, cognitive functions (attention, memory, learning) (Ferguson & Simeon, 1984), mood, self-esteem, social behavior, family dynamics, and physiological symptoms. Information obtained from different sources (child, parents, teachers) must be integrated. A comprehensive package of assessment instruments and ratings scales has been developed for use in pediatric psychopharmacology (*Psychopharmacology Bulletin*, 1985).

The clinician's interview of the child is seldom sufficient to detect therapeutic effects but is important to detect adverse and toxic effects. Teachers, on the other hand, are the best informants of drug effects on attention, memory, and learning.

Initial dosages should be low, and increases gradual, until either significant improvement or adverse effects occur. Recommended dosages are often too high (for example, for stimulants) or too low (for example, tricyclic antidepressants in depressive disorders). Initial improvements are not necessarily due to the medication given, since improvement may be due to reassurance, spontaneous recovery, or a placebo effect. In the opinion of this author, "drug holidays" are often overused; they can often be detrimental, and they are seldom beneficial. Periodic reassessments without medication, however, are indicated. To determine if a drug is still needed, placebo administration or a gradual withdrawal is recommended. Best results are achieved by a comprehensive therapeutic approach, where medication facilitates other types of therapy.

### *Stimulants*

About 70% of children with attention deficit hyperactivity disorder (ADHD) treated with psychostimulants show significant improvement of behavioral symptoms (inattention, hyperactivity, impulsivity), academic and psychometric performance, and social interaction with parents, teachers, and peers. The clinical effects of psychostimulants are neither paradoxical nor specific for ADHD. Stimulants are also useful in children with unsocialized aggressive conduct disorders and in those who are shy, withdrawn, or overanxious (Werry, 1978). Beneficial responses to stimulants have been shown also by preschool and adolescent ADHD patients (Conners, 1975). Hyperactive children treated with stimulants seem to have a better outcome as adults (Hechtman, Weiss, & Perlman, 1984). The behavioral and autonomic effects of d-amphetamine in normal children are similar to those in hyperkinetic children (Rapoport et al., 1978). A marked behavioral rebound occurs about 5 hours after d-amphetamine is given in both normal and hyperkinetic children.

Improvement of the target symptoms with methylphenidate and d-amphetamine generally occurs within 1 hour; drug effects last 4 to 6 hours, and most patients require a second dose around noon. The average daily dose of methylphenidate is 10 mg to 20 mg, and that of d-amphetamine 5 mg to 10 mg. The matter of dosage for the stimulants is a very controversial area (Cantwell & Carlson, 1978). The total amount of medication required by an individual child is very idiosyncratic. A general principle is to use the smallest dosage possible initially; dosage increments should be gradual, titrated individually, until optimal effects on behavior and learning are achieved. Magnesium pemoline (Cylert) has a longer half-life and, therefore, is given once daily. The initial daily dose is 37.5 mg, increments of 18.75 mg are weekly, and the usually therapeutic dose is 56.25 mg to 75 mg daily. In contrast to methylphenidate and d-amphetamine, significant clinical improvement may be seen only after 3 or 4 weeks of treatment. The duration of therapeutic efficacy of the recently developed slow-release methylphenidate, to be given once daily, appears to have shown significant interindividual variability (Fried, Greenhill, Torres, Martin, & Solomon, 1987).

Behavioral and cognitive therapies fail to add to the therapeutic effects of stimulants used alone (Gittelman-Klein, 1987). Methylphenidate is not useful in treating children with severe specific reading retardation (Aman & Werry, 1982). The reading performance of developmentally dyslexic children, however, appears to be favorably influenced by piracetam, representative of a new "nootropic" drug class (Rudel & Helfgott, 1984; Volavka, Simeon, Simeon, Cho, & Reker, 1981; Wilsher, 1987). In addition to the psychostimulants, a variety of antidepressants (tricyclic, nontricyclic, MAOIs) (Casat, Pleasants, & Van Wyck Fleet, 1987; Cox, 1982; Gastfriend, Biederman, & Jellinek, 1984; Simeon, Ferguson, & Van Wyck Fleet, 1986; Zametkin, Rapoport, Murphy, Linnoila, Karoum, et al., 1985), neuroleptics and clonidine (Hunt, Minderaa, & Cohen, 1985) have been reported effective in the treatment of hyperkinetic and conduct disorders. Combined pharmacotherapy (for example, methylphenidate and imipramine, clonidine, or thioridazine) also appears useful in certain patients. Further research is needed to evaluate these newer drugs and drug combinations. Such therapeutic trials may be especially warranted in patients who are nonresponders to stimulants, those who relapse, and those who suffer from significant adverse effects.

Methylphenidate serum levels in hyperkinetic children show wide interindividual as well as intraindividual variations. These levels do not seem to differ in clinical responders versus nonresponders, suggesting that nonresponse to methylphenidate is not due to pharmacokinetic differences but rather to pharmacodynamic differences (Gualtieri et al., 1982). Adverse effects of psychostimulants are dose-related. These consist of increased heart rate, increased blood pressure, gastrointestinal irritability, nausea and vomiting, anorexia and weight loss, mood alterations, irritability, restlessness, insomnia, and, very rarely, psychosis. Tics and stereotypies may also occur. Findings on growth suppression are contradictory: In one study, reductions of height and weight growth rates were temporary and minor, and any growth retardation in the first year was recovered by a height gain in the second year (Satterfield, Cantwell, Schell, & Blaschke, 1979); in another study, decreases of height and weight percentiles were significant (Mattes & Gittelman, 1983). No development of drug abuse or dependence occurs (Beck, Langford, MacKay, & Sum, 1975; Hechtman et al. 1984; Weiss, 1975). Stimulants can exacerbate symptoms in children with autism, schizophrenia, and borderline personality disorders (Campbell et al. 1985). Their use is contraindicated in depression and anorexia nervosa (Cantwell & Carlson, 1978). In vulnerable children, Tourette's disorder may be accelerated (Lowe, Cohen, Detlor, Kremenitzer, & Shaywitz, 1982).

ADHD appears to be a heterogeneous syndrome, frequently coexisting with conduct or oppositional disorders, and infrequently with anxiety disorders. The specific nature of the "attention deficit" has never been defined, nor have the specific effects of stimulants on cognition. Response or nonresponse to psychostimulants cannot be used as a diagnostic confirmation of any specific disorder. The evidence for the noradrenergic, dopaminergic, and serotonergic hypotheses of ADHD has been inconclusive and contradictory (Zametkin & Rapoport, 1987; Sokol, Campbell, Goldstein, & Kriechman, 1987). Methylphenidate, d-amphetamine, and magnesium pemoline increase dopamine and norepinephrine at the synapse. Several dopamine agonists, however, have been clinically ineffective in open clinical trials (Gittelman-Klein, 1987). Improvement of ADHD children treated with clonidine (Hunt et al., 1985) suggests the importance of norepinephrine in the pathophysiology of this syndrome. Psychostimulant administration is associated with significant changes of norepinephrine and its metabolites, but correlations with clinical change are not consistent (Zametkin, Rapoport, Murphy, Linnoila, Karoum, Potter, & Ismond, 1985; Zametkin, Karoum, et al., 1985). Further research is needed to determine whether these behavioral syndromes have distinct biochemical abnormalities responding to different and more specific psychotropic drugs.

## Antidepressants

Antidepressant drugs are used for a variety of child and adolescent psychiatric disorders, such as enuresis; insomnia and parasomnias; attention deficit, conduct, depressive, obsessive–compulsive, and panic disorders; school phobias; and bulimia (Flament et al. 1985; Gittelman-Klein & Klein, 1971; Rapoport & Mikkelsen, 1978; Rapoport et al. 1980; Simeon & Ferguson, 1985; *Psychopharmacology Bulletin*, 1987; Zametkin & Rapoport, 1983). Most of these disorders persist, in some form, into adulthood. The majority of reported studies with children have used tricyclic compounds, particularly imipramine. Tricyclics are long-acting drugs. Their adverse effects are anticholinergic symptoms, weight loss, stomachache, irritability, and tearfulness. Higher doses can result in seizures and cardiotoxicity. There appears to be no relationship between imipramine oral dose and plasma levels (Puig-Antich, Perel, Lupatkin, & Chambers, 1987). Imipramine plasma levels are related to antidepressant, antienuretic, and adverse effects (Geller, Perel, Knitter, Lycaki, & Farooki, 1983; Lake, Mikkelsen, Rapoport, Zavadil, & Kopin, 1979; Preskhorn, Weller, & Weller, 1982; Preskhorn, Weller, Weller, & Glotzbach, 1983; Rapoport et al. 1980). As a general guideline, imipramine daily dosage of 5 mg per kg of body weight should not be exceeded. However, in view of the wide interindividual variability of plasma tricyclic levels, doses based on body weight can be misleading. Measurements of plasma levels may be more useful, especially in nonresponders. When this drug is prescribed, careful clinical and EKG evaluations must be undertaken until the optimal dose is established and the patient is stabilized. Gradual tapering of dosage is recommended.

*Enuresis*

Although imipramine is the drug of choice for symptomatic treatment of enuresis, the mode of action of tricyclics in enuresis is not known. Recent data do not support theories of anticholinergic or alpha-adrenergic action (Shaffer, Hedge, & Stephenson, 1978; Stephenson, 1979). Antidepressants are an effective short-term intervention with enuresis, but withdrawal usually leads to relapse. Since the effects of long-term drug treatment of children are unknown, continued drug treatment should be considered only when other interventions have failed, and when the child or parents are extremely distressed by the bedwetting (Rapoport et al., 1980). The usual effective dose of imipramine is 25 to 50 mg at bedtime.

*Attention Deficit and Conduct Disorders*

Controlled trials of imipramine (Rapoport & Mikkelsen, 1978), desipramine (Donnelly, Zametkin, & Rapoport, 1986) and clomipramine (Garfinkel, Wender, Sloman, & O'Neill, 1983) have shown beneficial therapeutic effects in childhood behavior disorders. Although less effective than stimulants, these antidepressants showed a different therapeutic profile and seemed more useful when affective pathology was present. In open trials with nontricyclic antidepressants, such as maprotiline (Simeon, Maguire, & Lawrence, 1981), mianserin (Langer, Rapoport, Ebert, Lake, & Nee, 1984), and bupropion (Simeon et al., 1986), generally positive results have been reported. These findings need to be replicated in placebo-controlled trials. MAOIs (Clorgyline and tranylcypromine) have been reported to have behavioral and cognitive effects equal to those of d-amphetamine (Zametkin, Rapoport, Murphy, Linnoila, & Ismond, 1985). While antidepressants appear to have a role in the management of attention and/or conduct disorders, their more precise therapeutic profiles and indications require further research.

*Separation Anxiety and School Phobia*

In a double-blind study published in 1971, imipramine was reported superior to placebo in the treatment of school-phobic children (Gittelman-Klein & Klein, 1971). This study has not been replicated, possibly because of concerns over the high average daily doses (100 to 200 mg). Relatively low doses of clomipramine (40 to 75 mg daily) were no better than placebo in school-phobic children (Berney et al., 1981). Imipramine and alprazolam in conjunction with psychotherapy were found effective in chronic school refusers with anxiety and depressive symptoms (Garfinkel, 1989; Garfinkel & Bernstein, 1984). The role of antidepressants in separation anxiety as well as in panic disorder in adolescents needs to be further investigated.

*Depression*

Recent research has resulted in significant progress in the areas of diagnosis, assessment, epidemiology, family pathology, study design, pharmacokinetics, and psychopharmacology of depressive disorders in children (Chapter 2, this volume; Puig-Antich et al., 1982). Such disorders in children and adolescents are valid clinical entities that can be identified using diagnostic criteria similar to those for adults. Depressive episodes are usually of long duration, with high rates of relapse, and are usually associated with school, family, and social failure. There is a significant excess of affective illness and alcoholism in the families of depressed adolescents, and a high rate of behavioral impairment among children of parents with affective disorders (Strober, 1984). Biological manifestations of depressive disorders may be significantly affected by developmental and hormonal changes. During depressive episodes, prepubertal children show abnormalities of growth hormone and cortisol secretion, while dexamethasone suppression test (DST) and sleep EEG findings are contradictory (Puig-Antich et al., 1982).

The findings of controlled studies of tricyclic antidepressants and placebo in children and adolescents are difficult to interpret because of the high improvement rates of depressed children with placebo (about two-thirds), and relatively small sample sizes (Ambrosini, 1987; Kramer & Feiguine, 1981; Puig-Antich et al., 1987). In prepubertal children, high total maintenance plasma levels of imipramine plus desipramine (over 150 mg/ml was reported to be associated with good clinical response (Preskhorn et al., 1982; Puig-Antich et al., 1987). In adolescents, imipramine seemed ineffective, and no association with plasma levels was found (Ryan et al., 1986). Tricyclic antidepressants should not be prescribed routinely; they should be given when depression persists, with careful clinical and EKG monitoring of the patient, and preferably in inpatient settings.

More recent research has suggested therapeutic efficacy of MAOIs (tranylcypromine and phenelzine), and a combination of lithium and a tricyclic antidepressant in adolescent depressions resistant to tricyclics (Ryan, 1988a, 1988b). In a preliminary pilot study, fluoxetine (a nontricyclic antidepressant) was effective and safe in depressed adolescents (Simeon & Ferguson, 1986). In a recently completed double-blind fluoxetine placebo-controlled study by the author, about two-thirds of the adolescents showed marked or moderate short-term improvements with both fluoxetine and placebo; global, symptom, and self-ratings showed statistical trends in favor of fluoxetine (Simeon, Ferguson, Copping, & DiNicola, 1988). The daily dosages used (60 mg) may have been too high: The optimal daily dosage currently recommended is 20 mg.

In the treatment of childhood and adolescent depression, individual and family therapy seems essential, indicating the need for careful research of psychosocial interventions as well. Psychosocial adaptation and mood disturbances remain ongoing problems in this population (DiNicola & Simeon, 1988).

### *Obsessive—Compulsive Disorder*

Obsessive–compulsive disorder of adults frequently has its onset in childhood (Rapoport, 1987), and, therefore, effective management during childhood is most important. In a placebo-controlled trial, clomipramine in daily doses of 100 to 200 mg has been reported to be very effective in the treatment of obsessive–compulsive children and adolescents (Chapter 4, this volume). Marked decreases of obsessions and compulsions were independent of depression, and improvement was not related to the plasma levels of clomipramine or its metabolites. The data lend support to a serotonin hypothesis (Flament, Rapoport, Murphy, Berg, & Lake, 1987), suggesting trials with other serotonin reuptake blockers, such as fluoxetine and fluvoxamine.

### *Eating Disorders*

Recent reviews on the therapy of eating disorders indicate that in anorexia nervosa, drug and other somatic therapies seem of no specific value, while antidepressants seem useful in bulimia nervosa (*Psychopharmacology Bulletin*, 1987; Yager, 1988). Antidepressants, low-dose neuroleptics, and other drugs have been used on an empirical basis in anorexia nervosa. Symptoms of bulimia nervosa seem to be controlled by imipramine, desipramine, and phenelzine. Newer nontricyclic antidepressants (e.g., fluoxetine) also appear promising in bulimia nervosa. Antidepressants should be given to bulimic patients if they suffer from concurrent depressive and/or anxiety disorders, have family histories of affective disorders, or are nonresponders to prior therapy (Yager, 1988).

### Antipsychotics

A variety of child psychiatric disorders are treated with antipsychotics. In general, these drugs should be given only to very disturbed children or to those who have not responded to other types of medication. Most of the children receiving antipsychotic drugs in clinical practice are not psychotic. Antipsychotics are used for the relief of symptoms in children with various types of psychoses and to facilitate other forms of therapy, but their role in altering the basic course of the disorder is limited (Campbell et al., 1984, 1985; Campbell, Malone, & Kafantaris, 1989). These drugs are also used in the management of aggression, temper tantrums, psychomotor excitement, stereotypies, and hyperactivity unresponsive to other therapy. Their calming effect is due to general central nervous system depression. The high-potency antipsychotics—haloperidol, thiothixene, fluphenazine, and pimozide—are about equally effective. Antipsychotics should not be prescribed to children with sleep disorders such as insomnia. Chlorpromazine is contraindicated in children with epilepsy.

If treatment is effective, the drug should be given for at least 2 to 3 months, then gradually reduced or discontinued within 6 months to determine whether the drug is still required, or whether withdrawal dyskinesia will develop. Rebound behavioral worsening has been observed following drug withdrawal, and it usually lasts about 1 week. Withdrawal symptoms following discontinuation of long-term antipsychotic administration also may occur and may consist of a transient extrapyramidal rebound syndrome characterized by nausea, vomiting, diaphoresis, ataxia, dyskinesia, and dystonia (Polizos, Engelhardt, Hoffman, & Waizer, 1973). Behavioral toxicity usually appears early and is frequent in children treated with high doses of antipsychotics. It manifests by worsening of symptoms or the appearance of hyperactivity, hypoactivity, irritability, apathy, impairment of learning, stereotypies, tics, or hallucinations. Extrapyramidal side effects include acute dystonic reactions, akathisia, and parkinsonism. Acute dystonic reactions can be avoided if the initial dose is very low and increases are very gradual. Extrapyramidal symptoms are best treated by reduction of the dose rather than administration of anticholinergic drugs. Long-term adverse effects consist of rapid perioral muscle movements (rabbit syndrome) and tardive dyskinesias, which can be reversible or permanent (Gualtieri, Quade, Hicks, Mayo, & Schroeder, 1984).

## Infantile Autism

The efficacy of antipsychotics in autism is symptomatic and limited. High doses of drugs like chlorpromazine and thioridazine often cause excessive sedation. High-potency neuroleptics are recommended, such as haloperidol, which appears to improve hyperactivity, stereotypies, affect, motivation, social relating and withdrawal, and learning in the laboratory (Campbell et al., 1984, 1989). Autistic children sustain their gains with haloperidol maintenance therapy on a long-term basis. One week after drug discontinuation there is significant worsening of stereotypies, withdrawal, hyperactivity, fidgetiness, and abnormal object relations (Campbell et al., 1983). A good baseline evaluation is therefore essential, since it may be very difficult to differentiate the withdrawal dyskinetic movements from reemerging stereotypies that had been suppressed by the medication. Prolonged and heavy use of antipsychotics in children has been increasingly associated with tardive dyskinesia.

Fenfluramine, an antiserontonergic drug, was initially reported beneficial in autism (Klykylo, Feldis, O'Grady, Ross, & Halloran, 1985; Ritvo, Freeman, Geller, & Yuwiler, 1983). More recent data, however, suggest that fenfluramine is no better than placebo, and that it may even adversely affect learning (Campbell et al., 1987).

## Tourette's Syndrome

This disorder must be distinguished from the transient tic disorder in children. In the latter, drugs must not be used (Bruun, 1984). Haloperidol and pimozide, dopamine-blocking neuroleptics, are the most effective drugs in Tourette's syndrome (Shapiro & Shapiro, 1984). In a recent study, half of the Tourette patients treated with clonidine, an alpha-adrenergic agonist, were reported to have had long-term symptomatic improvement (Leckman et al., 1983). Stimulants exacerbate the symptoms in some Tourette patients, and the complexity of their responses indicates both biological and clinical heterogeneity of the syndrome (Caine, Ludlow, Polinsky, & Ebert, 1984). There is controversy whether stimulants can provoke a full-blown syndrome that persists after drug discontinuation.

## Anxiolytics

While benzodiazepines and other anxiolytics are used frequently in child psychiatry practice, data about their efficacy are very limited. This is due to a lack of recognition of anxiety in children, the heterogeneity of clinical samples, lack of reliable assessment methods, and theoretical biases about the nature of childhood anxiety and its management. The probable indications for anxiolytics are insomnia, night waking, night terrors, and somnambulism, whereas anxiety is a possible indication (Gittelman, 1986; Simeon & Ferguson, 1985, 1987b; Werry, 1978). Diazepam (Glick, Schulman, & Turecki, 1971; Reid & Gutnik, 1980), flurazepam (Reimao & Lefevre, 1982), and midazolam (Popoviciu & Corfariu, 1983) have been found effective in the treatment of insomnia and parasomnias.

Benzodiazepines are metabolized faster in children than in adults and are, therefore, remarkably nontoxic in therapeutic doses. Adverse effects of benzodiazepines include sedation and disinhibition (irritability, aggression, euphoria, incoordination). Disinhibition can be also therapeutic in pathologic behavioral inhibitions (avoidant disorders) and may facilitate social learning. Withdrawal of benzodiazepines must be gradual in order to prevent a sudden relapse, withdrawal symptoms, or rebound anxiety. The risk of withdrawal reactions is greater with the short- and intermediate-acting drugs (for example, triazolam, alprazolam). Owing to the lack of safety and proven efficacy, the use of nonbenzodiazepines, such as barbiturates, meprobamate, tybamate, and antipsychotics, should be strongly discouraged in childhood anxiety disorders. The anxiolytic efficacy of antihistamines in children has not been demonstrated, but they appear to be widely used in the control of sleep problems.

When anxiety is symptomatic of another disorder, the primary disorder must be treated first. There are no published controlled benzodiazepine studies in which the criteria for selection were primarily related to one of the childhood anxiety disorders. While panic attacks and separation anxiety (school phobia) may respond to imipramine, clinical practice suggests that the addition of a benzodiazepine could alleviate the anticipatory anxiety. Preliminary findings with alprazolam suggest a good response in separation anxiety (Garfinkel, 1989; Garfinkel & Bernstein, 1984) and in overanxious and/or avoidant disorders (Simeon & Ferguson, 1987a). Controlled studies of anxiolytics alone and combined with antidepressants and psychotherapy are needed (Simeon & Ferguson, 1985)

Diazepam in very high dosages had a sedative but not an antipsychotic effect in adolescent schizophrenics (Weizman, Tyano, Wijsenbeck, & Ben, 1984); given intravenously it is rapidly effective and safe in treating drug-induced extrapyramidal symptoms in children (Ranier-Pope, 1979). In children, benzodiazepines are also often used in the prophylaxis and therapy of epileptic seizures, during surgery, and in dentistry.

## Antiaggressive Drugs

Different psychotropic drugs are widely used to treat pathological aggression in children, but indications are vague and mechanisms of action unclear (Simeon, 1979). The drugs listed below may be useful in the treatment of borderline disorders; the choice of drug should depend on the predominant symptomatology. Antipsychotic drugs are effective in reducing aggressiveness, but sedation, cognitive impairment, and long-term adverse effects limit their usefulness. They may be necessary for severely disturbed patients, but they are frequently overused.

Available findings demonstrate the efficacy of lithium in chronic aggressive conduct disorders, bipolar disorders, and periodic mood or behavior disorders with a family history of bipolar disorder (Campbell, Cohen, & Small, 1982; Campbell et al., 1984). The antiaggressive properties of lithium need further assessment in children with poor long-term prognosis. Lithium is not useful in hyperactivity (Greenhill, Rieder, Wender, Buchsbaum, & Zahn, 1973)

Stimulants may reduce aggressive behavior in most hyperactive children (Amery, Minichiello, & Brown, 1984). Propranolol, a beta-adrenergic blocking agent effective in controlling explosive rage outbursts in adults, has recently been found to produce a moderate to marked improvement in the control of rage outbursts and aggressive behavior in children and adolescents with organic brain dysfunction (Williams, Mehl, Yudofsky, Adams, & Roseman, 1982). Anticonvulsants such as phenytoin, carbamazepine, sulthiam, and sodium valproate are well-established antiepileptics, but their beneficial effects on behavior and cognition as psychotropic agents is speculative and anecdotal. They appear ineffective in childhood aggression and other behavior disorders unless these are associated with epilepsy (Stores, 1978). Evidence has been accumulating, however, that carbamazepine and valproic acid are effective in treatment-resistant adult patients with bipolar or major depressive disorders. The role of anticonvulsants in child psychiatry ought to be researched methodically.

## Conclusion

Modern pediatric psychopharmacology began over 50 years ago with the introduction of amphetamine to disturbed children (Bradley, 1937). Existing drug therapies are far from ideal, and a great deal remains to be accomplished. Research and clinical practice are complicated by significant medical, psychological, social, ethical, and legal factors. There are marked differences in the uses of psychotropic drugs in children between different centers and countries (Simeon, Utech, Simeon, & Itil, 1974). Drug prescription practices are to a great extent determined by many nonmedical factors. One of the main problems is in deciding whether drugs treat a disorder or modify behaviors unacceptable to others: Disturbing children may not be disturbed, and vice versa. As a result of this dilemma, many children and adolescents are deprived of the benefits of pharmacotherapy. Drugs alone without other types of therapy, however, are seldom sufficient; applications of pharmacotherapy and psychotherapy must complement each other and not compete. While progress toward a more rational psychopharmacology continues, child psychiatrists will meanwhile need to treat children on the basis of current knowledge. Optimal results will be obtained by those clinicians who can integrate theoretical knowledge, experience, skills, determination, and commitment to their patients.

ACKNOWLEDGMENT. This chapter is an expanded version of an article published in the *Canadian Journal of Psychiatry, 34,* 115–122 (1989).

## References

Aman, M. G., & Werry, J. S. (1982). Methylphenidate and diazepam in severe reading retardation. *Journal of the American Academy of Child and Adolescent Psychiatry, 21,* 31–37.

Ambrosini, P. J. (1987) Pharmacotherapy in child and adolescent major depressive disorder. In H. Y. Meltzer (Ed.), *Psychopharmacology: The third generation of progress* (pp. 1247–1254). New York: Viking Press.

Amery, B., Minichiello, M. D., & Brown, G. L. (1984). Aggression in hyperactive boys: Response to d-amphetamine. *Journal of the American Academy of Child and Adolescent Psychiatry, 23,* 291–294.

Beck, L., Langford, W., MacKay, M., & Sum, G. (1975). Childhood chemotherapy and later drug abuse and growth curve: A follow-up study of 30 adolescents. *American Journal of Psychiatry, 132,* 436–438.

Berney, T., Kolvin, T., Bhate, S. R., Garside, R. F., Kay, B., & Scarth, L. (1981). School phobia: A therapeutic trial with clomipramine and short-term outcome. *British Journal of Psychiatry, 138,* 110–118.

Bradley, C. (1937) The behavior of children receiving benzedrine. *American Journal of Psychiatry, 94,* 577–585.

Bruun, R. D. (1984). Gilles de la Tourette's syndrome: An overview of clinical experience. *Journal of the American Academy of Child and Adolescent Psychiatry, 23,* 126–133.

Caine, E. D., Ludlow, C. L., Polinsky, R. J., & Ebert, M. H. (1984). Provocative drug testing in Tourette's syndrome: d- and l-amphetamine and haloperidol. *Journal of the American Academy of Child and Adolescent Psychiatry, 23,* 147–152.

Campbell, M., Cohen, I. L., & Small, A. M. (1982). Drugs in aggressive behavior. *Journal of the American Academy of Child and Adolescent Psychiatry, 21,* 107–117.

Campbell, M., Green, W. H., & Deutsch, S. I. (1985). In A. E. Kazdin (Ed.), *Child and adolescent psychopharmacology.* Beverly Hills, CA: Sage Publications.

Campbell, M., Malone, R. P., & Kafantaris, V. (1989). Autism and aggression. In J. G. Simeon & H. B. Ferguson (Eds.), *Advances in the treatment of child psychiatric disorders.* New York: Plenum Publishing Corporation.

Campbell, M., Perry, R., Bennett, W. G., Small, A. M., Green, W. H., Grega, D., Schwartz, V., & Anderson, L. (1983). Long-term therapeutic efficacy and drug-related abnormal movement: A

prospective study of haloperidol in autistic children. *Psychopharmacology Bulletin, 19*(1), 80–83.
Campbell, M., Small, A. M., Green, W. H., Jennings, S. J., Perry, R., Bennett, W. G., & Anderson, L. (1984). Behavioral efficacy of haloperidol and lithium carbonate: A comparison in hospitalized aggressive children with conduct disorder. *Archives of General Psychiatry, 41*(7), 650–656.
Campbell, M., Small, A. M., Palij, M., Perry, R., Polonsky, B. B., Lukashok, D., & Anderson, L. T. (1987). The efficacy and safety of fenfluramine in autistic children: Preliminary analysis of a double-blind study. *Psychopharmacology Bulletin, 23*(1), 123–127.
Cantwell, D. P., & Carlson, G. A. (1978). Stimulants. In J. S. Werry (Ed.), *Pediatric psychopharmacology: The use of behavior modifying drugs in children*, 171–207. New York: Brunner/Mazel.
Casat, C. D., Pleasants, D. Z., & Van Wyck Fleet, J. (1987). A double-blind trial of bupropion in children with attention deficit disorder. *Psychopharmacology Bulletin, 23*(1), 120–122.
Conners, C. K. (1975). A controlled trial of methylphenidate in preschool children with minimal brain dysfunction. *International Journal of Mental Health, 4*, 61–74.
Conners, C. K., & Werry, J. S. (1979). Pharmacotherapy. In H. C. Quay, & J. S. Werry (Eds.), *Psychopathological disorders of childhood*, (2nd ed.) (pp. 336–386). New York: John Wiley & Sons.
Cox, W. H. (1982). An indication for use of imipramine in attention deficit disorder. *The American Journal of Psychiatry, 139*(8), 1059–1060.
DiNicola, V. F., & Simeon, J. G. (1988, October). *Managing adolescent depression: A follow-through study*. Paper presented at the meeting of the American Academy of Child and Adolescent Psychiatry, Seattle, Washington.
Donnelly, M., Zametkin, A. J., Rapoport, J. L., Ismond, D. R., Weingartner, H., Lane, E., Oliver, J., Linnoila, M., & Potter, W. Z. (1986). Treatment of hyperactivity with desipramine: Plasma drug concentration, cardiovascular effects, plasma and urinary catecholamine levels, and clinical response. *Clinical Phramacology and Therapeutics, 39*, 72–81.
Ferguson, H. B., & Simeon, J. G. (1984). Evaluating drug effects on children's cognitive functioning. *Progress in Neuropsychopharmacology, 8*, 683–686.
Flament, M. F., Rapoport, J. L., Berg, C. B., Sceery, W., Kilts, C., Mellstrom, B., & Linnoila, M. (1985). Clomipramine treatment of childhood obsessive compulsive disorder: A double-blind controlled study. *Archives of General Psychiatry, 42*(10), 977–983.
Flament, M. F., Rapoport, J. L., Murphy, D. S., Berg, C. J., & Lake, R. (1987). Biochemical changes during clomipramine treatment of childhood obsessive-compulsive disorder. *Archives of General Psychiatry, 44*, 219–225.
Fried, J., Greenhill, L., Torres, D., Martin, J., & Solomon, N. (1987, October). *Sustained-release methylphenidate: Long-term clinical efficacy in ADDH males*. Paper presented at the meeting of the American Academy of Child and Adolescent Psychiatry, Washington, D.C.
Garfinkel, B. D. (1989). Psychopharmacological treatment of school phobia. In J. G. Simeon & H. B. Ferguson (Eds.), *Advances in the treatment of child psychiatry disorders*. New York: Plenum Publishing Corporation.
Garfinkel, B. D., & Bernstein, G. A. (1984, October). *The pharmacological treatment of separation anxiety*. Paper presented at the American and Canadian Academies of Child Psychiatry, Toronto, Ontario.
Garfinkel, B. D., Wender, P. H., Sloman, L., & O'Neill, I. (1983). Tricyclic antidepressant and methylphenidate treatment of attention deficit disorder in children. *Journal of the American Academy of Child and Adolescent Psychiatry, 22*(4), 343–348.
Gastfriend, D. R., Biederman, J., & Jellinek, M. S. (1984). Desipramine in the treatment of adolescents with attention deficit disorder. *The American Journal of Psychiatry, 141*, 906–908.
Geller, B., Perel, J. M., Knitter, E. F., Lycaki, H., & Farooki, Z. Q. (1983). Nortriptyline in major

depressive disorder in children: Response, steady state plasma levels, predictive kinetics and pharmacokinetics. *Psychopharmacology Bulletin, 19*, 62–65.

Gittelman, R. (1986). *Anxiety disorders of childhood*. New York: Guildford Press.

Gittelman-Klein, R. (1987). Pharmacotherapy of childhood hyperactivity: An update. In H. Y. Meltzer (Ed.), *Psychopharmacology: The third generation of progress* (pp. 1215–1224). New York: Raven Press.

Gittelman-Klein, R., & Klein, D. (1971). Controlled imipramine treatment of school phobia. *Archives of General Psychiatry, 23*, 204–207.

Glick, G. S., Schulman, D., & Tureck, S. (1971). Diazepam treatment in childhood sleep disorders. *Diseases of the Nervous System, 32*(8), 565–566.

Greenhill, L. L., Rieder, R. O., Wender, P. H., Buchsbaum, M., & Zahn, T. P. (1973). Lithium carbonate in the treatment of hyperactive children. *Archives of General Psychiatry, 28*, 636–640.

Gualtieri, C. T., Quade, D., Hicks, R. E., Mayo, J. P., & Schroeder, S. R. (1984). Tardive dyskinesia and other clinical consequences of neuroleptic treatment in children and adolescents. *The American Journal of Psychiatry, 141*(1), 20–23.

Gualtieri, C. T., Wargin, W., Kanoy, R., Patrick, K., Shen, C. D., Youngblood, W., Mueller, R. A., & Breese, G. R. (1982). Clinical studies of methylphenidate serum levels in children and adults. *Journal of the American Academy of Child and Adolescent Psychiatry, 21*(1), 19–26.

Hechtman, L., Weiss, G., & Perlman, T. (1984). Young adult outcome of hyperactive children who received long-term stimulant treatment. *Journal of the American Academy of Child and Adolescent Psychiatry, 23*(3), 261–269.

Hunt, R. D., Minderaa, R. B., & Cohen, D. J. (1985). Clonidine benefits children with attention deficit disorder and hyperactivity: Report of a double-blind placebo-crossover therapeutic trial. *Journal of the American Academy of Child and Adolescent Psychiatry, 24*(5), 617–629.

Klein, D. F., Gittelman, R., Quitkin, F., & Rifkin, A. (1980). *Diagnosis and drug treatment of psychiatric disorders: Adult and children*, (2nd ed.). Baltimore: Williams and Wilkins.

Klykylo, W. M., Feldis, D., O'Grady, D., Ross, D. L., & Halloran, C. (1985). Brief report: Clinical effects of fenfluramine in ten autistic subjects. *Journal of Autism and Developmental Disorders, 15*(4), 417–423.

Kramer, A. D., & Feiguine, R. J. (1981). Clinical effects of amitriptyline in adolescent depression. *Journal of the American Academy of Child and Adolescent Psychiatry, 20*(3), 636–644.

Lake, C. R., Mikkelsen, E. J., Rapoport, J. L., Zavadil, A. P., & Kopin, I. J. (1979). Effect of imipramine on norepinephrine and blood pressure in enuretic boys. *Clinical Pharmacology and Therapeutics, 26*, 647–653.

Langer, D. H., Rapoport, J. L., Ebert, M., Lake, C. R., & Nee, L. (1984). Pilot trial of mianserin hydrochloride for childhood hyperactivity. In B. Shopsin, & L. Greenhill (Eds.), *The psychobiology of childhood: A profile of current issues* (pp. 197–210). New York: Spectrum Publications.

Leckman, J. G., Leekman, Detlor, J., Harcherik, D. F., Young, J. G., Anderson, G. M., Shaywitz, B. A., & Cohen, D. J. (1983). Acute and chronic clonidine treatment in Tourette's syndrome: A preliminary report on clinical response and effect on plasma and urinary catecholamine metabolites, growth hormone and blood pressure. *Journal of the American Academy of Child and Adolescent Psychiatry, 22*(5), 433–440.

Lowe, T. L., Cohen, D. J., Detlor, J., Kremenitzer, M. W., & Shaywitz, B. A. (1982). Stimulant medications precipitate Tourette's syndrome. *Journal of the American Medical Association, 247*, 1729–1731.

Mattes, J., & Gittelman, R. (1983). Growth of hyperactive children on maintenance methylphenidate. *Archives of General Psychiatry, 40*, 317–321.

Meltzer, H. Y. (Ed.). (1987). *Psychopharmacology: The third generation of progress*. New York: Raven Press.

Polizos, P., Engelhardt, D. M., Hoffman, S. P., & Waizer, J. (1973). Neurological consequences of psychotropic drug withdrawal in schizophrenic children. *Journal of Autism and Childhood Schizophrenia, 3*(3), 247-253.

Popoviciu, L., & Corfariu, O. (1983). Efficacy and safety of midazolam in the treatment of night terrors in children. *British Journal of Psychiatry, 16*, 97-102.

Preskhorn, S., Weller, E., & Weller, R. A. (1982). Depression in children: Relationship between plasma imipramine levels and response. *Journal of Clinical Psychiatry, 43*(11), 450-453.

Preskhorn, S., Weller, E., Weller, R. A., & Glotzbach, E. (1983). Plasma levels of imipramine and adverse effects in children. *The American Journal of Psychiatry, 140*, 1332-1335.

Puig-Antich, J., Goetz, R., Hanlon, C., Tabrizi, M. A., Davies, M., & Weitzman, E. D. (1982). Sleep architecture and REM sleep measures in prepubertal major depressives. *Archives of General Psychiatry, 39*, 932-939.

Puig-Antich, J., Perel, J. M., Lupatkin, W., & Chambers, W. J. (1987). Imipramine in prepubertal major depressive disorders. *Archives of General Psychiatry, 44*, 81-89.

Ranier-Pope, C. R. (1979). Treatment with diazepam of children with drug-induced extrapyramidal symptoms. *South African Medical Journal, 55*, 328-330.

Rapoport, J. L. (1987). Pediatric psychopharmacology: The last decade. In H. Y. Meltzer (Ed.), *Psychopharmacology: The third generation of progress* (pp. 1211-1214). New York: Raven Press.

Rapoport, J. L., Buchsbaum, M., Zahn, T., Weingartner, H., Ludlow, C., & Mikkelsen, E. (1978). Dextroamphetamine: Cognitive and behavioral effects in normal prepubertal boys. *Science, 199*, 560-562.

Rapoport, J. L., & Mikkelsen, E. J. (1978). Antidepressants. In J. S. Werry (Ed.), *Pediatric psychopharmacology: The use of behavior modifying drugs in children* (pp. 208-233). New York: Brunner/Mazel.

Rapoport, J. L., Mikkelsen, E. J., Zavadil, A., Nee, L., Cruenau, C., Mendelsen, J., & Gillin, J. (1980). Childhood enuresis. II. Psychopathology, tricyclic concentration in plasma, and antienuretic effect. *Archives of General Psychiatry, 37*, 1146-1152.

Reid, W. H., & Gutnik, D. (1980). Case report: Treatment of intractable sleepwalking. *Psychiatric Journal of the University of Ottawa, 5*(2), 86-88.

Reimao, R., & Lefevre, A. (1982). Evaluations of flurazepam and placebo on sleep disorders in childhood. *Arquivos De Neuro-Psiquiatria, 40*, 1-13.

Rifkin, A., Wortman, R., Reardon, G., & Siris, S. G. (1986). Psychotropic medication in adolescents: A review. *Journal of Clinical Psychiatry, 47*(8), 400-408.

Ritvo, E. R., Freeman, B. J., Geller, E., & Yuwiler, A. (1983). Effects of fenfluramine on 14 outpatients with the syndrome of autism. *Journal of the American Academy of Child and Adolescent Psychiatry, 22*(6), 549-558.

Rudel, R. G., & Helfgott, E. (1984). Effect of piracetam on verbal memory of dyslexic boys. *Journal of the American Academy of Child and Adolescent Psychiatry, 23*(6), 695-699.

Ryan, N. (1988a). Li/TCA augmentation adolescent MDD. *Journal of the American Academy of Child and Adolescent Psychiatry, 27*, 371-376.

Ryan, N. (1988b). MAOIs in adolescent major depression unresponsive to tricyclic antidepressants. *Journal of the American Academy of Child and Adolescent Psychiatry, 27*, 755-758.

Ryan, N., Puig-Antich, J., Cooper, T., Rabinovich, H., Ambrosini, P., Davies, M., King, J., Torres, D., & Fried, J. (1986). Imipramine in adolescent major depression: Plasma level and clinical response. *Acta Psychiatrica Scandinavica, 73*, 275-288.

Satterfield, J. H., Cantwell, D. P., Schell, A., & Blaschke, T. (1979). Growth of hyperactive children treated with methylphenidate. *Archives of General Psychiatry, 36*, 212-217.

Shaffer, D., Hedge, B., & Stephenson, J. (1978). Trial of an alpha-adrenolytic drug (indoramin) for nocturnal enuresis. *Developmental Medicine in Child Neurology, 20*, 183-188.

Shapiro, A. K., & Shapiro, E. (1984). Controlled study of pimozide vs. placebo in Tourette's

syndrome. *Journal of the American Academy of Child and Adolescent Psychiatry, 23*(2), 161–173.
Simeon, J. G. (1976). Pediatric psychopharmacology—a review of our findings and experience. In D. V. Siva Sankar (Ed.), *Psychopharmacology of childhood* (pp. 139–178). Westbury, New York: PJD Publications Limited.
Simeon, J. G. (1979). Biology and therapy of violent behavior in children. In J. Obiols, C. Ballus, E. G. Monclus, & J. Pujol (Eds.), *Biological psychiatry today* (pp. 1223–1228). Elsevier, North Holland: Biomedical Press.
Simeon, J. G., & Ferguson, H. B. (1985). Recent developments in the use of antidepressant and anxiolytic medications. *Psychiatric Clinics of North America, 8*, 893–907.
Simeon, J. G., & Ferguson, H. B. (1986, December). *Efficacy and safety of fluoxetine in the treatment of depressive disorders in adolescents.* Paper presented at the meeting of the American College of Neuropsychopharmacology, Washington, D.C.
Simeon, J. G., & Ferguson, H. B. (1987a). Alprazolam effects in children with anxiety disorders. *Canadian Journal of Psychiatry, 32*(7), 570–574.
Simeon, J. G. & Ferguson, H. B. (1987b). Treatment of sleep disturbances in children: Recent advances. In J. Noshpitz & S. Harrison (Eds.), *Basic handbook of child psychiatry* (pp. 470–478). New York: Basic Books Inc.
Simeon, J. G., Ferguson, H. B., Copping, W. M., & DiNicola, V. F. (1988, October). *Fluoxetine effects in adolescent depression.* Paper presented at the American Academy of Child and Adolescent Psychiatry, Seattle, Washington.
Simeon, J. G., Ferguson, H. B., & Van Wyck Fleet, J. (1986). Bupropion effects in attention deficit and conduct disorders. *Canadian Journal of Psychiatry, 31*(6), 581–585.
Simeon, J. G., Maguire, J., & Lawrence, S. (1981). Maprotiline effects in children with enuresis and behavioral disorders. *Progress in Neuro-Psychopharmacology, 5*, 495–498.
Simeon, J. G., & Saletu, B. (1979). Neurophysiology and child psychiatry. In B. Saletu, P. Berner, & L. Hollister (Eds.), *Proceedings of the 11th Congress of the Collegium Internationale Nuero-Psychopharmacologicum* (p. 313). New York: Pergamon Press.
Simeon, J. G., Utech, C., & Simeon, S., & Itil, T. M. (1974). Pediatric psychopharmacology outside the United States. *Diseases of the Nervous System, 35*(7), 37–47.
Sokol, M. S., Campbell, M., Goldstein, M., & Kriechman, A. M. (1987). Attention deficit disorder with hyperactivity and the dopamine hypothesis: Case presentations with theoretical background. *Journal of the American Academy of Child and Adolescent Psychiatry, 26*(3), 428–433.
Stephenson, J. D. (1979). Physiological and pharmacological basis for the chemotherapy of enuresis. *Psychological Medicine, 9*, 249–263.
Stores, G. (1978). Antiepileptics (anticonvulsants). In J. S. Werry (Ed.), *Pediatric psychopharmacology: The use of behavior modifying drugs in children* (pp. 274–315). New York: Brunner/Mazel.
Strober, M. (1984). Familial aspects of depressive disorder in early adolescence. In E. B. Weller & R. A. Weller (Eds.), *Current perspectives on major depressive disorders in children* (pp. 38–48). Washington, D.C.: American Psychiatric Press, Inc.
U.S. Department of Health. (1985). *Psychopharmacology Bulletin, 21*(4).
U.S. Department of Health. (1987). *Psychopharmacology Bulletin, 23*(1).
Volavka, J., Simeon, J., Simeon, S., Cho, D., & Reker, D. (1981). Effects of piracetam in dyslexia. *Psychopharmacology, 72*, 185–188.
Weiss, G. (1975). The natural history of hyperactivity in childhood and treatment with stimulant medication at different ages: A summary of research findings. *International Journal of Mental Health, 4*, 213–216.
Weizman, A., Tyano, S., Wijsenbeck, H., & Ben, D. M. (1984). High-dose diazepam treatment and its effect on prolactin in adolescent schizophrenic patients. *Psychopharmacology, 82*, 382–385.

Werry, J. S. (1977). The use of psychotropic drugs in children. *Journal of the American Academy of Child and Adolescent Psychiatry, 16*(3), 446–468.

Werry, J. S. (Ed.). (1978). *Pediatric psychopharmacology: The use of behavior modifying drugs in children.* New York: Brunner/Mazel.

Werry, J. S. (1982a). Advances in pediatric psychopharmacology, Part I: Introduction. *Journal of the American Academy of Child and Adolescent Psychiatry, 21*(1), 1–2.

Werry, J. S. (1982b). An overview of pediatric psychopharmacology. *Journal of the American Academy of Child and Adolescent Psychiatry, 21*(1), 3–9.

Werry, J. S. (1982c). Advances in pediatric psychopharmacology, Part II: Introduction. *Journal of the American Academy of Child and Adolescent Psychiatry, 21*(2), 105–106.

White, J. H. (1977). *Pediatric psychopharmacology: A practical guide to clinical application.* Baltimore: Williams and Wilkins Corporation.

Williams, D. T., Mehl, R., Yudofsky, S., Adams, D., & Roseman, B. (1982). The effect of propranolol on uncontrolled rage outbursts in children and adolescents with organic brain dysfunction. *Journal of the American Academy of Child and Adolescent Psychiatry, 21*(2), 129–135.

Wilsher, C. R. (1987). A brief review of studies of piracetam in dyslexia. *Journal of Psychopharmacology, 1*(2), 95–100.

Yager, J. (1988). The treatment of eating disorders. *The Journal of Clinical Psychiatry, 49*(Suppl. 9), 18–25.

Zametkin, A., Karoum, F., Linnoila, M., Rapoport, J., Brown, G., Chuang, L., & Wyatt, R. J. (1985). Stimulants, urinary catecholamines, and indoleamines in hyperactivity. A comparison of methylphenidate and dextroamphetamine. *Archives of General Psychiatry, 42*(3), 251–255.

Zametkin, A., & Rapoport, J. L. (1983). Tricyclic antidepressants and children. In G. Burrows, T. Norman, & B. Davies (Eds.), *Drugs in psychiatry, Volume 1: Antidepressants* (pp. 129–147). Amsterdam: Elsevier Science Publishers.

Zametkin, A., & Rapoport, J. L. (1987). Noradrenergic hypothesis of attention deficit disorder with hyperactivity: A critical review. In H. Y. Meltzer (Ed.), *Psychopharmacology: The third generation of progress* (pp. 837–842). New York: Raven Press.

Zametkin, A., Rapoport, J. L., Murphy, D. L., Linnoila, M., & Ismond, D. (1985). Treatment of childhood attention deficit disorder with hyperactivity with monoamine oxidase inhibitors. I. Clinical efficacy. *Archives of General Psychiatry, 42*(10), 962–966.

Zametkin, A., Rapoport, J. L., Murphy, D. L., Linnoila, M., Karoum, F., Potter, W. Z., & Ismond, D. (1985). Treatment of hyperactive children with monoamine oxidase inhibitors. II. Plasma and urinary monoamine findings after treatment. *Archives of General Psychiatry, 42*(10), 969–973.

# 9

# Recent Developments in Diet Therapy

## H. Bruce Ferguson

Proposals that food affects children's behaviors have surfaced sporadically in the clinical and research literature for over 50 years (Randolph, 1947; Rowe, 1931). In spite of this long-standing hypothetical association between food and behavior, it is only since 1970 that there has been widespread public and professional interest in altering diet as a therapeutic approach in dealing with disturbing behaviors and learning problems of children. Each food–behavior hypothesis developed a fervent public following in advance of appropriate controlled research testing. Indeed, much of the eventual experimental study of such hypotheses was in response to the widespread public acceptance of anecdotal reports of the effects of food on behavior. Also, in most cases, the food-related hypothesis was proposed as a general cause of behavior problems. Thus, the idea was not just that specific food substances could cause problem behaviors in children but that, in fact, they caused problem behaviors in large numbers of children.

In this chapter, the development and testing of three specific hypotheses relating food substances to behavior and learning problems in children will be reviewed. Such food-related explanations of children's disturbing behaviors are appealing to parents as well as to the professionals who have to treat these children. Unfortunately, these hypotheses are difficult to test directly and unambiguously. In addition, some of my own collaborative research will be presented to demonstrate the experimental strategies required to test food-related hypotheses and the difficulties inherent in using these methods.

---

*H. Bruce Ferguson*  Department of Psychology, Royal Ottawa Hospital, Ottawa, Ontario K1Z 7K4, Canada.

## Food Allergies and Behavior

As far as I am aware, the notion that food allergies could cause behavior problems was first suggested by Rowe (1931). Systematic examination of this hypothesis was probably delayed by a number of factors. One of the most important of these was the complexity of the field of allergy and the general disagreement over what constituted an accurate diagnostic test. Most of the literature consisted of clinical anecdotes, with the occasional open challenge in an uncontrolled setting. These anecdotes reported mainly physical allergic responses to a variety of food substances (e.g. Crook, Harrison, Crawford, & Emerson, 1961; Goldman et al., 1963). The possible effects of food allergies were examined in a large group of hyperactive and learning-disabled children (Trites, Tryphonas, & Ferguson, 1980). The objective of the study was to establish the incidence of food allergies in the sample and to determine whether behavior would be changed when the children were maintained on a diet free of foods to which they tested as allergic. The radioallergosorbent (RAST) test was used to test for elevated levels of serum IgE antibody to 42 different food extracts. Using a relatively liberal criterion, 47% of the 90 hyperactive children and 77% of the 22 learning-disabled (but not hyperactive) children showed positive reactions to at least one food. When a more conservative criterion was used, the figures were 31% of the hyperactive children and 32% of the learning-disabled children. The number of allergies per child ranged from 0 to 34. The average number was 1.84 in the hyperactive group and 1.77 in the learning-disabled group. There were no sex differences in the incidence of food allergy. The foods that most commonly provoked responses were meats and cereals.

Since the incidence of food allergies in these children was so high relative to the reported population incidence, the hypothesis that food allergies were related to behavior problems was then tested. Forty-eight children participated in a double-blind crossover diet-placebo study. The main dependent measures were the Conners ratings by teachers and parents. The experimental diets removed all foods to which the child showed an allergic response, while the placebo diet removed an equal number of foods that appeared to be consumed by the child and family with about the same frequency as the allergic foods. Neither experimental nor control diets were carefully monitored, but parents were asked to report diet infractions. Statistical analyses revealed no beneficial effects of the treatment versus the placebo diet. In addition, there were no diet order effects, no differences according to sex, and none according to the number or severity of allergies. Looking at the individual children's data, it was clear that there were a number of children who improved substantially on the treatment diet. However, approximately as many children showed similar improvements on the placebo diet. Thus, overall there was no evidence that these children's allergies to foods were contributing to their behavior or learning problems.

To examine parents' perceptions of the role of food allergies in their children's problems, an allergy questionnaire was developed and distributed to the parents of 190 child psychiatry patients and to 500 children in elementary schools (Simeon, Ferguson, Ralph, & Mistry, 1982). The most important finding was that the percentage of children perceived by parents to be showing an adverse or allergic response to food substances or other substances does not differ radically across the psychiatric and control groups. An interesting and suggestive finding, however, emerged from looking at the data of the school group alone. In this group, parents were asked if children had been referred for medical, emotional, or school problems, and the frequency of these referrals was examined as a function of reported allergic or adverse responses. The presence of perceived allergies to food plus other substances led to a significantly higher referral rate for all types of problems. It must be pointed out that it is not known if in fact these children did have allergies, because our data are parental reports of their perceptions of allergy and/or adverse response.

In general, it now appears to be more widely accepted that children do show adverse physical reactions to food. Bock (1986) reported testing 337 children with double-blind food challenges. It is of note that the "gold standard" in this area is at present double-blind food challenges rather than immunological testing. Of these children, 132 showed 165 positive food challenges. The only behavioral symptoms reported in this work are irritability and fussiness in conjunction with physical symptoms. Specifically, children with the so-called hyperactivity or "tension fatigue" syndrome were studied, but their symptoms could not be reproduced during the blind challenges. In this sense, these results were parallel to ours in our previous allergy study.

Finally, Eggar, Carter, Graham, Grumley, and Soothill (1985) treated 76 severely overactive children with what is termed an oligoantigenic diet. Twenty-five patients completed a double-blind placebo-controlled trial. Parent ratings of behavior were significantly improved on the diet relative to the placebo period; however, there were no differences on psychometric test results. There are few details on how the study was blinded and how the blind was maintained. It is difficult to maintain a double-blind in a diet study where parents are in fact aware of what the supposed offending substance is. Ultimately, since this study has produced results that are extremely interesting but contrary to past findings, it is important to withhold judgment until it has been carefully replicated. In fact, the authors themselves noted that "this trial clearly needs replication before results are widely applied to children with the hyperactive syndrome" (Eggar et al., 1985, p.544).

## Food Colors and Preservatives—The Feingold Hypothesis

Dr. Benjamin Feingold originated the claim that food colors and preservatives were, in fact, responsible for the hyperactive behavior and learning problems of large numbers of children in North America. To a great extent, it was Feingold's (1975) book that popularized the whole notion of diet effects on children's behavior. The so-called Feingold diet was adopted by thousands of parents as a treatment for their children's hyperactive behavior or learning problems. Subsequently, the effects of dyes and additives on children's behavior were tested carefully in double-blind placebo-controlled studies by Conners, Goyette, Southwick, Lees & Andrulonis (1976) and Harley, Ray, Tomas, et al. (1978). In these studies, elaborate attempts were made to maintain the blind. In general, the results were negative (Conners, 1980). In these studies, approximately half of the children showed improvements on the Feingold diet. However, about the same number of children showed improvements on the placebo diet. For this reason, the Feingold diet has been termed by some researchers to be a very effortful "placebo" treatment. While the collective results suggest that food colors and additives are not a general explanation of children's problems, a few comments are worthwhile. First, Weiss et al. (1980), in a detailed study of a number of children, identified one young girl who showed marked responses to dyes. In addition, in the Harley et al. study, behavior ratings of young children by adults discriminated between placebo and dye conditions. Therefore, it may be that in a small number of children (and perhaps younger children are more susceptible) dyes and additives do cause problems. A 10-year-old girl who was referred for hyperactivity, anxiety, and school failure showed a clear response to Red Dye No. 3. Using a double-blind challenge methodology, we observed repeatedly over a 4-month period deteriorations in behavior a few hours in duration following challenge with the red dye but not to placebo.

A widely cited study by supporters of the Feingold position is a report by Swanson and Kinsbourne (1980). They interpreted their findings as showing clear deleterious effects of food dyes on the learning performance of hyperactive children but no such effects on nonhyperactive children. Careful examination of their data has led others to suggest that the performance differences in their study are due to changes in the nonhyperactive rather than the hyperactive group (Ferguson, Rapoport, & Weingartner, 1980). Thus, the Swanson and Kinsbourne (1980) findings may not be so straightforward as was first thought.

A very recent study has presented the most supportive data yet for diet therapy (Kaplan, McNicol, Conte, & Moghadam, 1989). This was a double-blind crossover study of 24 hyperactive boys between the ages of 3 and 6. The boys were preselected to meet DSM-III criteria for attention deficit disorder with hyperactivity. In addition, they met entry criteria of showing sleep problems or having physical signs and symptoms associated with allergies. The study involved a 3-week baseline period, a placebo control of 3 weeks, and an experimental diet of 4 weeks. Order of experimental and placebo diets was counterbalanced. The experimental diet used was broader than any previously used. It eliminated not only artificial colors and flavors but also chocolate, monosodium glutamate, preservatives, caffeine, and any substance reported by families to affect their child. The evaluations of parental behavior ratings indicated that 10 children showed significant improvement (25%) on the experimental diet while 4 children showed mild (10%) responses. There were no children who improved on the placebo diet. In this study, elaborate precautions were taken to maintain the blind. In addition, the nutrient intake of the children was monitored, and it is significant to note that vitamin intake increased during the experimental diet while intake of calories, carbohydrates, and simple sugars decreased. Also, analysis of blood variables to assess nutritional status showed no differences between the groups. Finally, the nonbehavioral variables—for example, halitosis and sleep problems—tended to decrease but the change was not significant.

The design of the Kaplan et al. (1989) study is excellent, and while the results seem to conflict with previous reports, there are a number of important differences between this and previous studies. First, the subjects were younger and preselected for symptoms of allergy. Second, the actual diet used excluded a number of substances in addition to those excluded by the Feingold diet as well as decreasing carbohydrate and sugar intake and specific substances for the children. Thus, it is not possible to say which substances caused the changes observed. While conclusions regarding these dietary effects should perhaps remain guarded until replication is reported, Kaplan et al. should be applauded for the care with which the study was done, the inclusion of both physical and behavioral variables, and the careful monitoring of nutrient intake and nutritional status. This study provides a model of the type of study needed to make progress in this complex area.

## Sugar and Children's Behavior

Sugars represent the most recent alleged "culprit" as a food-related cause of children's behavioral problems. There are a number of reasons for its popularity as a hypothetical cause of "bad" behavior. First, almost all children consume a significant amount of refined sugar. Second, a number of animal studies have indicated that the relative amount of carbohydrate consumed could, in fact, have effects on brain transmitters (Fernstrom & Wurtman, 1972, 1974). Finally, the idea may have been given added impetus by a hypothesis relating abnormal glucose tolerance curves and hyperkinesis (Langseth &

Dowd, 1978). Prinz, Roberts, and Hartman (1980) reported significant positive correlations between the amount of sugar consumed and levels of destructive, aggressive, and restless behavior of hyperactive children. In nonhyperactive control children, increased sugar intake was significantly associated only with increased motor activity. Following this study, research interest in sugar effects increased rapidly. In a review article 6 years later, Milich, Wolraich, and Lindgren (1986) reviewed 2 additional correlational studies and 11 sugar challenge studies. Two of these challenge studies were carried out in our clinic (Ferguson, Stoddart, & Simeon, 1986). Since they are representative of the challenge method and many of its inherent problems, they will be reviewed briefly.

## Study 1

### Design

This study was a double-blind challenge with three administrations of sucrose and three of aspartame. Children came to the clinic for seven sessions during the same half-day period (i.e., morning or afternoon). The first visit was a baseline session and the remaining sessions were scheduled, two in each of 3 consecutive weeks. Test sessions were separated by a minimum of 48 hours to avoid possible carryover effects. Sucrose and aspartame (Nutrasweet-Searle) were dissolved in water and given at three "dosage" levels. Dosage levels were randomly assigned to weeks, and within weeks, sucrose and aspartame challenges were randomly assigned.

### Subjects

Eight volunteer subjects (6 boys, 2 girls) aged 5 to 13 (mean=112 months) were recruited by newspaper and television publicity. All were believed by parents to have adverse responses to sugar and were maintained on a low-sugar diet. Parents reported a variety of physical and behavioral symptoms with onset in all cases less than 1 hour after ingestion of sugar. At screening, all subjects were given a psychiatric evaluation and a medical history was obtained. The objectives and requirements of the study were explained and signed consents were obtained. Five children were diagnosed as attention deficit disorder with hyperactivity, one had a psychophysiological disorder, and two had no diagnosable disorder.

### Measures

The dependent measures included temperature and pulse recordings taken at the beginning and end of each session; activity levels monitored with wrist

# Diet Therapy

and ankle actometers; cognitive tests; observation measures of children's movements, verbalizations, on-task and off-task behavior during the cognitive testing; and behavior ratings by the examiner (Children's Psychiatric Rating Scale) and by the mother (Conners Parent Rating Scale).

The cognitive tests included the continuous performance test (CPT) of sustained attention, a paired-associated learning task, a memory task, and a variant of the 20 questions game.

*Procedure*

The procedure was identical for all sessions, which were approximately 2 hours in length. When the child arrived, vital signs were taken, the actometers placed on wrist and ankle, and the liquid drunk. Then the children completed the continuous performance task (CPT) to assess attention. One-half hour after consuming the liquid, the children completed the cognitive test battery to examine learning, memory, and problem solving. The CPT was completed once again, after which vital signs were measured and actometer readings were recorded. After the child had left the test situation, the examiner completed the Children's Psychiatric Rating Scale (CPRS) reflecting only the behavior during the test session. At the end of the day, the parent (mother) completed the Conners Parent Rating Scale and returned it to the clinic. At the baseline session all procedures were followed except for the ingestion of the challenge liquid.

*Results*

The data were examined in two ways. First, the results were analyzed as eight single-subject experiments. The data were examined for consistent sucrose–aspartame differences reflecting better or worse performance subsequent to the administration of either substance. There was no evidence of consistent change for any subject on any of the many variables recorded.

Subsequently, the data from all eight subjects were combined as a group, and *t*-test (correlated) comparisons were carried out for each variable contrasting sucrose versus aspartame at each "dosage" level, and sucrose versus aspartame, baseline versus sucrose, and baseline versus aspartame for the data averaged over the three dosage levels (sucrose and aspartame). Only 10 of 262 tests produced significant ($p < .05$) results. Not only is this fewer than would have been expected by chance, but 6 of these were on measures (Conners Parent Rating Scale and cognitive variables) that we have found in drug studies to change systematically with repeated administration independent of condition; i.e., they are due to "practice" effects. Thus, there was no evidence at all for a sucrose effect relative to aspartame, or of any change from baseline in either the sucrose or aspartame conditions.

## Study 2

### Design

The study was a double-blind challenge study with two administrations of sucrose and two of aspartame carried out on 9 days over 3 weeks. Baseline measures were collected on 2 days prior to the first challenge and between challenge days, which were separated by a minimum of 48 hours. Order of sucrose and aspartame was randomly assigned to each of the two pairs of challenge days. Psychometric measures were collected on the 2 baseline days prior to challenge and on each of the 4 challenge days.

Both sucrose and aspartame were given in 100 ml of apple juice, which naturally contained approximately 11 gm of fructose. Thirty grams of sucrose was added to the apple juice. Since aspartame is approximately 180 times as sweet as sugar, 167 mg of aspartame were added to the apple juice to produce a drink that was equivalent in sweetness.

### Subjects

Eighteen children (9 boys, 9 girls) from a preschool participated with parental consent and on a voluntary basis. No child had any known history of allergic reactions to sugar, of hypoglycemia, or of diabetes. They ranged in age from 3.5 to 5.3 years (mean = 4.2 years), with a mean IQ of 112 (Peabody Picture Vocabulary Test-Revised). All were right-handed.

### Measures

*Parent's Target Behavior Checklist.* Ten items were selected by the child's mother from the 93-item Conners Parent Rating Scale indicating behaviors most representative of her child on a "bad" day.

*Teacher's Target Behavior Checklist.* The preschool teacher responsible for each child selected 10 items from the 39-item Conners Teacher Rating Scale reflecting behaviors characteristic of that child on a "bad" day.

*Behavioral Observations.* An observational coding system was used. This system includes measures of peer interaction, of positive and negative verbal and nonverbal interaction, and of play categories. Observations were made for approximately 1 hour on groups of three study children playing within the same area of the preschool. An interval time-sampling observation method was used in which each child was observed for four consecutive 15-sec intervals before observation rotated to the next child. Interactions occurring during an interval

# Diet Therapy

were recorded, and when no interaction occurred, the child's play activity was recorded. Reliability observations were carried out for 32% of the observation sessions throughout the study. Overall interrater reliability for both interaction and play categories ranged from 86.9 to 95.8%, with a mean of 89.1%.

*Activity Levels.* These were monitored by wrist actometers.

*Test Measures.* The following were used:
1. Purdue Pegboard—Fine motor coordination was assessed by a version of the Purdue Pegboard adapted for use with preschoolers. The test was performed with the dominant (right) hand, nondominant (left) hand, and bimanually.
2. Developmental Drawings—This test consists of a series of simple drawings that become progressively more difficult and provides a measure of visuomotor coordination.
3. Standing on One Foot—This test was adapted from a subtest in the McCarthy Scales of Children's Abilities and was used as a measure of gross motor coordination.

## Procedure

To facilitate testing, children in the morning and afternoon preschool programs were studied in groups of three. The preschool routine included giving the children their juice in groups of three at 9:15 a.m. or 1:45 p.m. To minimize experimental error, all three children per group received the same challenge substance on each study day. After juice time, the actometers were placed on the children's wrists. Behavioral observations were coded for approximately 60 minutes of free-play activity in the preschool. The tests were administered individually in a quiet room 1 hour after the children had consumed the juice. Total testing time per child was approximately 10 minutes. The pegboard task was administered first because it was considered to be less demanding. This was followed with the drawing task, followed by the standing on one foot task. Not all children participated in the testing. Thirteen children completed the pegboard task while only 8 were able to carry out the developmental drawings, and 11 completed the standing on one foot task. Since 1 child would not wear the actometer, activity data were available for 17 children.

## Results

The data were examined as 18 single-subject experiments. Examination of the data plots revealed only two variables showing any consistent relationships between sucrose and aspartame challenge. Three children showed consistently poorer scores (by approximately 30%) on the Developmental Drawings on sucrose days than on aspartame or baseline days. In addition, three different children showed decreases (50%) in actometer scores on sucrose days relative to baseline or aspartame days.

Finally, the data available on each dependent measure were grouped and analyzed using SPSS MANOVA for repeated-measures designs. The results of these analyses revealed only one significant effect of challenge condition, and that was on the Developmental Drawings measure. This effect reflected the poorer performance on sugar days by three children, as noted above. There were no other main effects or interactions with challenge conditions. There were no differences between morning and afternoon groups.

Thus, in our two studies we have no evidence that sugars are responsible for behavior or learning disturbances in children. In fact, there are nine other double-blind challenge studies reported involving over 200 children (Milich et al., 1986). Many of these children were considered normal, others had received psychiatric diagnoses, and many were even selected specifically because their parents were convinced they showed adverse responses to sugar. The overall evidence is very much like ours, so it is clear that sugars are unlikely to be a causal factor in triggering disturbed behavior in large numbers of children. Furthermore, the results of the correlational studies are inconsistent and even where sugar intake has been associated with behavior, the effects are small and the nature of the causal relationship is indeterminate (Prinz et al., 1980; Wolraich, Stumbo, Milich, Chenard, & Schultz, 1988).

## *General Conclusions*

Over the past 15 years, there has been a series of claims of food-related general causes of children's disturbed behaviors. In each case, the hypothesis has gained enthusiastic support among the general public before proper scientific tests of the proposition have been undertaken. Subsequent controlled research has produced a data base that makes it clear that none of these food-related proposals is the cause for the behavior of large numbers of disturbed children. This does not mean that *no* child will show such responses. As our biochemical complexity becomes more obvious, it is clear that each of these hypotheses represents a possible physiological event for some children. Perhaps we will find children for whom sugar, food dyes, food additives, or some other food may cause idiosyncratic brain changes leading to disturbances in behavior and learning. Such hypotheses do not account for the high incidence of problems shown by children—for example, up to 20% of elementary school boys showing problems (Trites, Blouin, Ferguson, & Lynch, 1981).

The findings cited here do not mean that food substances cannot affect functioning. In fact, there are suggestions of effects of sugars on behavior, although these appear to be in the direction opposite to the original "Hallowe'em effect" hypothesis (Ferguson et al., 1987). In addition, subtle mood and performance effects of carbohydrate/protein meals (Spring, Chiodo, & Bowen, 1987) as well as behavioral effects of caffeine in children (Rapoport, Berg, Ismond, Zahn, & Neims, 1984) have been reported recently. We need to develop models within the context of nutritional effects on behavior (Conners, Caldwell, Caldwell, et al., 1984; Kaplan, 1988). Such elaborate models will be extremely difficult to test, but they represent an important first step toward placing the study of hypotheses, such as those considered here, in the proper context of possible associations between nutrition and behavior.

A final word about dealing with children and parents. On the basis of the research data, it may be concluded that food substances (dyes, additives, sugars) have no general adverse effects on behavior. Clinically, however, each child may be an individual exception to the general findings, so one must proceed with caution. In our experience, we have found parental opinions regarding food-related effects to be firmly entrenched and difficult to deal with. Children with problems frequently show variable and disturbing behavior, and, therefore, introducing particular foods can easily be associated with undesirable behavior. In the face of frequent spurious associations of suspected substances and "bad" behavior, parents need more than the opinions of skeptical professionals to change their beliefs. We have found carefully planned elimination diets and challenge testing involving the parents to be helpful in working with these cases. Such an approach takes time and effort but may be necessary to facilitate the adoption of more appropriate treatment strategies. Likewise, only time and systematic research and clinical strategies will properly educate parents and practitioners regarding potential diet effects.

## *References*

Bock, S. A. (1987). A critical evaluation of clinical trials in adverse reactions to foods in children. *Journal of Allergy and Clinical Immunology, 78*:165–174.

Conners, C. K. (1980). *Food additives and hyperactive children*. New York: Plenum Press.

Conners, C. K., Caldwell, J., Caldwell, L., Schwab, E., Kronsberg, S., Wells, K. C., Leong, N., & Blouin, A. G. (1985, February). *Experimental studies of sugar and aspartame on autonomic, cortical and behavioral responses of children*. Paper presented at a symposium, Diet and behavior: A multidisciplinary approach, sponsored by the American Medical Association and the International Life Sciences Institute, Arlington, Va.

Conners, C. K., Goyette, C. H., Southwick, D. A., Lees, J. M., & Andrulonis, P. A. (1976). Food additives and hyperkinesis: A controlled double-blind experiment. *Pediatrics, 58*, 154–166.

Crook, W. G., Harrison, W. W., Crawford, S. E., & Emerson, B. S. (1961). Systemic manifestations due to allergy. Report of fifty patients and a review of the literature on the subject. *Pediatrics, 27*, 790–799.

Eggar, J., Carter, C. M., Graham, P.J., Gumley, D., & Soothill, J. (1985). Controlled trial of oligoantigenic treatment of the hyperkinetic syndrome. *Lancet, 1*, (8428), 540–545.

Feingold, B. F. (1975). *Why is your child hyperactive?* New York: Random House.
Ferguson, H. B., Rapoport, J. L., & Weingartner, H. (1981). Technical comment: Food dyes impair performance of hyperactive children. *Science, 211*, 410.
Ferguson, H. B., Stoddart, C., & Simeon, J. G. (1986). Double-blind challenge studies of behavioral and cognitive effects of sucrose-aspartame ingestion in normal children. *Nutrition Reviews (Suppl.) 44*:144–150.
Fernstrom, J. D., & Wurtman, R. J. (1972). Brain serotonin content: Physiological regulation by plasma neutral amino acids. *Science, 178*, 414.
Fernstrom, J. D., & Wurtman, R. J. (1974). Nutrition and the brain. *Scientific American, 230*, 84.
Goldman, A. S., Anderson, D. W., Sellers, W. A., Saperstein, S., Kniken, W. T., Holpern, S. R., et al. (1963). Milk allergy: 1. Oral challenges with milk and isolated milk proteins in allergic children. *Pediatrics, 9*, 425–443.
Harley, J. P., Ray, R. S., Tomasi, L., Eichman, P. L., Mathews, C. G., Chun, R., Cleeland, C. S., & Traisman, E. (1978). Hyperkinesis and food additives: Testing and Feingold hypothesis. *Pediatrics, 61*, 818–828.
Kaplan, B. J. (1988). The relevance of food for children's cognitive and behavioral health. *Canadian Journal of Behavioral Science, 20*(4), 359–373.
Kaplan, B. J., McNicol, J., Conte, R. A., & Moghadam, H. K. (1989). Dietary replacement in preschool-aged hyperactive boys. *Pediatrics, 83*(1), 7–17.
Langseth, L., & Dowd, J. (1978). Glucose tolerance and hyperkinesis. *Food and Cosmetics Toxicology, 16*, 129–133.
Milich, R., Wolraich, M., & Lindgren, S. (1986). Sugar and hyperactivity: A critical review of empirical findings. *Clinical Psychology Review, 6*, 493–513.
Prinz, R. J., Roberts, W. A., & Hartman, E. (1980). Dietary correlates of hyperactivity in children. *Journal of Consulting and Clinical Psychology, 48*, 760–770.
Randolph, T. G. (1947). Allergy, a cause of fatigue, irritability and behavior problems in children. *Journal of Pediatrics, 31*, 560.
Rapoport, J. L., Berg, C. J., Ismond, D. R., Zahn, T. P., & Neims, A. (1984). Behavioral effects of caffeine in children. *Archives of General Psychiatry, 41*, 1073–1079.
Rowe, A. H. (1931). *Food allergy: Its manifestations, diagnosis and treatment.* Philadelphia: Lea and Febiger.
Simeon, J. G., Ferguson, H. B., Ralph, C., & Mistry, P. (1982). Parental reports of adverse responses to food substances in child psychiatry patients and controls. *Psychopharmacology Bulletin, 18*(4), 206–209.
Spring, B., Chiodo, J., & Bowen, D. J. (1987). Carbohydrates, tryptophan, and behavior: A methodological review. *Psychological Bulletin, 2*, 234–256.
Swanson, J. M., & Kinsbourne, M. (1980). Food dyes impair performance of hyperactive children on a laboratory learning test. *Science, 207*, 1485–1487.
Trites, R. L., Blouin, A. G. A., Ferguson, H. B., & Lynch, G. (1975). The Conners Teacher Rating Scale: An epidemiologic, inter-rater reliability and follow-up investigation. In K. D. Gadow & J. Loney (Eds.), *Psychosocial aspects of drug treatment for hyperactivity* (pp. 157–175). Washington, DC: American Academy for the Advancement of Sciences.
Trites, R. L., Tryphonas, H., & Ferguson, H. B. (1980). Diet treatment of hyperactivity in a child with food allergies. In R. M. Knights and D. Bakker (Eds.), *The rehabilitation, treatment, and management of learning disabilities*. Baltimore: University Park Press.
Weiss, B., Williams, J. H., Margen, S., Abrams, B., Caan, B., Citron, L. J., Cox, C., McKibben, J., Ogar, D., & Schultz, S. (1980). Behavioral responses to artificial food colors. *Science, 207*, 1487–1488.
Wolraich, M. L., Stumbo, P., Milich, R., Chenard, C., & Schultz, F. (1988). Dietary characteristics of hyperactive and control boys and their behavioral correlates. *Journal of the American Dietetic Association, 4*, 500–504.

# 10

# Treatment of Developmental Language Disorders

## Michel Dugas and Christophe Gérard

### Introduction

Any discussion on the treatment of language disorders raises nosological questions that are quite central to research in this area. We will focus on the treatment of specific developmental language disorders in the DSM-III sense of the term, and, more specifically, on developmental dysphasia as Bryan Woods (1985) defined it: "developmental dysphasia refers to a level of language function that is significantly below age norms, has always been so and is not adequately accounted for by general mental retardation, peripheral sensory or motor defects, severe emotional disturbance, or major environmental deprivation" (p. 139–144).

Excluding problems of stuttering and articulation disorders, there is little consensus on how to treat these children since there is no agreement yet on a clinical delineation of this group of disorders and on a way of dividing it. Most classification systems cannot operationally and differentially define profiles of evolution and therefore cannot identify those factors (especially therapeutic ones) that would specifically influence the course of the disorder.

On the surface, definitions of language disorders have become more reductionistic but have not necessarily become clinically more relevant. Specificity was associated with features that were intrinsic not to the disorders but to those exclusion criteria that were introduced for research reasons and purported to validate certain theoretical hypotheses. The search for etiological answers has led prematurely to putting aside the syndromic dimension of the disorder without making progress with regard to well-grounded therapeutic strategies. Unable to treat language diseases, we have to be satisfied with those

---

*Michel Dugas and Christophe Gérard*  Service de Psycho-Pathologie de l'Enfant et de l'Adolescent, Hôpital Robert Debre, 75935 Paris CEDEX 19, France.

decisions we can make regarding the syndrome on the basis of a physiopathological analysis. However, when we take this option, we stumble upon those objections that have been formulated by language fundamentalists, who have naturally come to be associated with the construction of theoretical models for the disorders.

There are cognitive, psycholinguistic, neuropsychological treatments, and the clinician, who cannot decide which of these camps to choose, has to settle for an integrated approach, a kind of patchwork of procedures imported from research. How can we reconcile these multiple approaches? We must accept the evidence of the lack of synchronization between research demands that aim to single out disorders and recognize their developmental factors of occurrence, on one hand, and the need to respond to therapeutic demands, on the other. The clinician cannot divorce himself from either approach and cannot attempt to use a consensual approach because it would alter the relevance of both approaches; he has to accept a dissociated approach, which necessarily leads to defining two types of developmental psychiatry: one that is independent from any model, the other that, on the contrary, is based on a fairly integrated model of the disorder.

The decision to implement a treatment plan for dysphasic children therefore requires that we make a number of choices regarding the problem and the theory of the disorder, the intervention strategies, the settings and skills to involve, the planning procedures, and the techniques. We intend to show how one can formalize these choices at the present time.

## Motivations for Treatment

Classification of motivations involved in treating the dysphasic child should help this progress of formalization. This can be reached only through an understanding of the evolution of those children with developmental language disorders.

It seems that the most severe linguistic deficits, those that are of interest to us according to our definition of dysphasia, are remarkably stable during the preschool age period (Silva, McGee, & Williams, 1983) as well as during adolescence (Paul, Cohen, & Caparulo, 1983); the stability seems particularly true for receptive dysphasia. The linguistic deficit appears to be associated, in both longitudinal and cross-sectional studies (Baker & Cantwell, 1987; Paul et al., 1983) with a higher risk of mental disorders, particularly emotional ones. These disorders, combined with massive academic difficulties, may jeopardize the social adjustment of the subjects as adults.

An evaluation of the short-term effects of any treatment on linguistic achievements is likely to be invalidated in its predictive value on social adjustment. Dysphasia has delayed deleterious effects on the type of cognitive development that is involved in acquiring formal operational thinking, pragmatic and metalinguistic abilities that characterize the social aspects of adolescent maturation (de Ajuriaguerra & Guignard, 1965; Wiig, 1987).

The treatment of the dysphasic child should not be restricted to the improvement of formal linguistic capacities. It should aim to modify the whole course of development to enable the child to (1) use a communication tool that allows an escape from concreteness, (2) use a tool of thinking that allows the expression of abstract abilities, (3) allow his or her taking pleasure in social exchange and its humorous manifestations, and (4) have access to modern means of communication without which children cannot play the social and professional roles to which their intellect entitles them.

## Conceptualization of Treatment

Language disorders are usually presented in terms of quantitative deviations from a norm concerning various psycholinguistic performances, deviations that are supposed to reflect an immediate deficit in communication. This conceptualization has little nosological and predictive value because it implies the use of intervention strategies geared toward normalization, without taking into account the dynamic characteristics of the dysphasic disorder, which seems to challenge all comparisons with normal development. Even if treatment allows us to objectify short-term changes, it has not been proven to modify developmental profiles in the long run. Our concept of the disorder implies that the currently noted stability of these deficits is linked to the structural impairment of the processes involved, with a cumulative effect, throughout the course of development, upon learning as well as on social and behavioral adjustment.

Such a concept has implications both in terms of symptom analysis and in terms of intervention strategies to be implemented. A clinical understanding of dysphasic disorders can be reached only by assuming that linguistic behaviors at a given time are the result of a stratification of functional disorders, of developmental lags and learning delays, of behavioral adjustments established by the subject and his or her environment. Therapeutic strategies are therefore necessarily multidimensional in their targets and objectives. Treatment goals must be both curative and preventative.

The conceptualization of the disorder directly affects the choices concerning modalities of intervention. The term *treatment* is inappropriate since the purpose is not to eradicate a factor of morbidity, as psychodynamic trends could lead us to believe. Nor is the term *management* suitable since it is not just a matter of compensating for the consequences of an intangible process. It is neither a matter of training, learning, or education, since the problem is not one of lack of content but rather lies in the manner in which this content is formed. We believe that the dynamic demands and the demands imposed by a multidimensional analysis go well with a rehabilitation approach.

To "rehabilitate" means that one starts with the individual knowledge of structural factors and then fits in those guides that will permit the adequate channeling of cognitive-linguistic development and the development of strategies of adjustment to the handicap and its consequences. In this sense, rehabilitation is of a neuropsychological and empirical nature. The therapeutic plan and the choice of procedures depend strictly on the characteristics of the dysphasic child when that child faces the verbal act.

## A Neuropsychological Model

Organizing the treatment of the dysphasic child represents another theoretical and practical choice: that of the concept we associate with the notion of structural deficit. Linguists and neurolinguists, whose impact on neuropsychology is well known, at this point have a different view and, in that sense, a different notion of the primary target (Prutting, 1987). Just as we do, they seem to think we should not be satisfied with a simple acknowledgment of formal deficits in the linguistic equipment and with a superficial patching-up approach. They assert that one can make sense out of these deficits through a process of systematization, in terms of a disorder of the linguistic structures that affects the manner in which coding is transculturally organized. Generally, this type of approach appears to be too theoretical and too functionalistic. Therapeutic programs that are derived from it are often purely experimental, their aim being limited to the validation of a fundamentalistic theoretical position. The intrinsic nature of the linguistic function, with its neurobiological and developmental corollaries, is no better defined, so that the choice of "modeling" of productions often remains as uncertain as it is with developmentalistic approaches. Finally, the link between the linguistic deficit and other deficits is ignored.

We believe that, at this level of formalization of primary therapeutic targets, it is also a clinical approach that must be defined on the basis of a real semiology, which describes linguistic deficits in terms of functional damage, but within an organizational model of language behaviors, taken as intentional voluntary acts. We will therefore use a traditional neuropsychological model, developed by Crosson (1985) in the light of our knowledge concerning the role of subcortical structures. This model is not based on a rigid sequence of operations that would link receptive and expressive aspects, taken as discrete systemic entities.

This model describes existing reciprocal relationships involving three groups of centers: (1) anterior cortical centers, locus of content programming for semantic and syntactic encoding, as well as the programming of motor sequences; (2) posterior cortical decoding centers; and (3) a group of subcortical centers that control the coherence of action of the above-mentioned centers, both at the time of programming and at the time of production of the language act. These relationships among these different centers allow us to describe several functional systems, and the specific damage of those systems leads one to describe several types of dysphasic disorders.

One type, called the "semantic-pragmatic syndrome," is defined by a deficit in formulation of the semantic and syntactic content. This disorder is characterized by expressive as well as receptive language impairment. In this respect Crosson had stressed the fact that anterior centers are involved in some receptive tasks, such as syntactic comprehension. The main features of this disorder include a language which superficially seems adequate but which deteriorates as soon as the subject has to use a code to fulfill a task with specific objectives. This is reflected in an absence of informational value, inadequate lexical or syntactic choices leading to semantic paraphasias on naming tasks, and incoherent speech, which resembles in some ways the psycholinguistic disorders of frontal subjects.

A second type, defined by a lack of control of semantic and syntactic encoding, is labeled according to Rapin's new terminology (Rapin & Allen, 1987) a "lexical syntactic syndrome," which we call amnesic dysphasia. The main characteristic of this disorder is a word-finding problem that is quite disabling and has little sensitivity to contextual or phonological props. Both receptively and expressively, there is an inability to use semantic categorization capacities that help maintain some cohesiveness between cognitive and language processes; lexical and syntactic choices become quite inadequate in their length. In contrast with the first type of disorder, subjects are here often acutely aware of their problem.

A third type, defined by a defective control of phonological encoding, is called the "phonological productive syndrome." It bears some resemblance with conduction aphasias in adults. The disorder is primarily expressive; expression is often fluent but marked by numerous phonemic distortions that are not systematically facilitative. Lexical encoding is also hampered by a major difficulty in controlling the phonemic sequence. We then observe word-finding difficulties for which the child tries to compensate through paraphonic approach behaviors. All situations of transposition, and more specifically repetition, are marked by this impairment in sequencing ability.

A fourth type is defined by the impairment of verbal comprehension; it leads us to describe receptive dysphasias, a more global and heterogeneous disorder than Rapin's auditory verbal agnosia (1987). These children appear to have a specific difficulty in creating and utilizing a verbal image on the basis of auditory modalities. The identification difficulty may be at a phonemic level, more or less associated with problems in identifying nonverbal noises. It may also be at the conceptual level of auditory segmentation, with an inability to recognize the guiding value of the word in the organization of the decoding process.

In the fifth and last type, "called dyspraxic dysphasia," the effective function of oral-motor command is defective. Depending on the severity of the impairment, Rapin and Allen (1987) distinguish (1) severe expressive disorders, real congenital aphemias, and (2) phonological syntactic syndrome, which is said to be the most frequent among dysphasic disorders. The main features are intact receptive capabilities, adequate lexical knowledge, a reduction in length of vocal utterances associated with difficulties in sequencing bucco-linguo-facial gestures, and the presence of syntactic encoding difficulties.

## Therapeutic Strategies

This neuropsychological approach, which attributes to the failure of one or several steps of the language act a central role in the manner the semiology of the disorder gets organized, leads us to recognize the structural heterogeneity of dysphasia, which is neglected in linguistic models.

We generally perform an initial analysis of linguistic behaviors, such as described by Rapin and Allen (1987). The neurological exam and neuropsychological data regarding other areas of information processing and of organization of the voluntary act allow us, using the above-mentioned model as a reference, to make physiopathological hypotheses that can then guide us, regarding ways of compensating for the deficits, and above all provide guidance without learning modalities.

An important problem, often brought up when rehabilitation strategies of neuropsychological disorders are discussed, is to decide whether deficits have to be directly worked on, or whether potentially existing compensatory skills should be developed. Answers vary according to the notion we have of cerebral plasticity. This notion of plasticity has encouraged the development of rehabilitation methods purporting to "train" the brain, as Rourke, Bakker, Fisk, and Strang (1983) say either through so-called sensory-motor methods, with the hope that the work of central processors will be facilitated by an optimization of the work of peripheral effectors and receptors, or through systematic but not necessarily specific stimulations of the central processors (Diller, 1976). This notion of a possible influence on neuronal plasticity remains purely speculative, at least with regard to congenital disorders. Geschwind and Galaburda's ideas

(1985) lead us to believe that plasticity is the result of a regulatory process involving neuronal death and synaptic reorganization, which are chronologically restricted to the first years of life. Plasticity is thus less organic than functional; it depends on the way information-processing systems are organized, predetermined at the time learning starts. As far as we are concerned, the choice of the therapeutic strategy is made on the basis of a situational observation, which determines whether or not one can act upon some of the deviant mechanisms that are at the source of the dysphasic disorder. Also, procedures are often mixed; that is, they attempt to correct deviant mechanisms and to develop means of going around them.

For instance, in disorders of the function of formulation, the rehabilitation process can focus, depending of the nature of the case, on the development of pragmatic capacities like integrating the role of speaker, taking into account the sequential nature of speech or of conversational language, developing the ability to utilize information given by the other person, so as to construct one's own responses, etc., or on a type of work leading to a better actualization of one's discourse in the face of those cognitive contingencies that triggered it (progressively controlling the level of concreteness and complexity of the context).

In those dysphasic disorders of a lexical-syntactic type, the primary target can be the retrieval function (using traditional techniques for the rehabilitation of memory disorders) or an optimization of categorization abilities leading to a better organization of semantic memory. In cases of verbal dyspraxia, one will try to integrate all facilitation mechanisms (e.g., tactile, visual, retroaction, automatic-intentional dissociation, melodic support) with work on the motivation to communicate, encouraging the subject's syntactic expansion capacities rather than the phonological qualities of his productions.

These vast technical principles do not summarize the rehabilitation process but constitute its backbone. Learning is organized around those principles and leads to a mastery of communication and to academic progress. Among the various suggested modalities of approach to structural disorders, one can see that these rehabilitation techniques are borrowed from very different fields. Depending on the case, they may be cognitive, psycholinguistic, perceptual or psychomotor; this reflects the interdisciplinary nature of clinical neuropsychology, a fact that seems to have been forgotten when applied to developmental disorders. This phenomenon is partially explained by the fact that those authors who have been interested in the therapeutic aspects of dysphasia have been concerned with the formalization of therapeutic progress and its evaluation. They suggest (Carrow-Woolfolk & Lynch, 1982) the use of treatment plan systems that are influenced by behavioral techniques, training objectives being distributed in discrete categories of psycholinguistic abilities: phonological, syntactic, semantic, pragmatic. These objectives are almost always reached through the use of modeling techniques. One of the recognized advantages of these efforts at planning ahead is that it is economical: the therapist's field of action is well delineated, techniques are simple, and interventions can be evaluated according to set objectives. But its major disadvantage is the inability to plan, in the same manner, generalization of progress to other areas of deficit and, more specifically to extralinguistic areas.

## Academic Acquisitions

For us, the generalization effect of the rehabilitation process is the result of an active approach based on an ongoing evaluation of existing interrelationships between structural deficits and their consequences on learning—linguistic, cognitive, or academic. These cannot be assessed according to a preestablished framework based on our knowledge of the development of a normal subject. This leads us to say that one must be cautious about the notion of prerequisites, often stressed in textbooks dealing with reading, for example. One must remember that the development of reading and spelling skills is one of the main objectives of the rehabilitation process for dysphasic subjects, an objective that is often neglected in standardized programs on the basis of psycholinguistic criteria. Yet a dysphasic subject cannot by definition master the written code as a normal or even a dyslexic subject would; the development of certain reading abilities is often a means of facilitating the rehabilitation process of oral language in cases of expressive dysphasias, and a means of compensating for the communicational handicap in some cases of receptive dysphasias. One sees here how therapeutic modalities and objectives are intertwined. We can hold the same type of reasoning regarding the development of math skills: The problems that dysphasic subjects face are linguistic, cognitive, and conceptual. Contingencies also vary from one subject to the other, and learning has to take into account other efforts made toward other objectives through integration of educational and rehabilitation endeavors. One should never take the process of generalization of the rehabilitation outcome to other areas as a logical consequence; instead this generalization process should constantly be induced.

## Organization of Treatment

These observations lead us to think about the organizational framework for this rehabilitation process. With regard to school integration, dysphasia seems to raise problems that are unique in comparison with other handicaps. Two requirements follow from these principles: first, that the approach be multidisciplinary, and second, that it be individualized. These requirements are valid for both the rehabilitation process and the educational one. In any case, these two processes are difficult to distinguish when we deal with dysphasic subjects. The way health care and schooling are organized in France does not allow us to meet these requirements. In many schools, there are special classrooms, but placement in these classrooms is made only on the basis of educational criteria that only take school failure into account, without really analyzing its reasons. The classrooms therefore regroup a very heterogeneous population of children who are failing to keep up with the normal learning rhythm and are not candidates for specialized institutions, which are currently reserved for subjects with mental or motor handicaps or with severe behavioral disorders. The essential feature of these classrooms is a slower pace of academic learning. Rehabilitation generally takes place outside of school, and it is provided either by a therapist after being referred by the family physician or by a psychoeducational public center. In the latter case, there is no liaison between school and therapeutic center; the various therapeutic plans are independently developed following the unique approach of the team that was selected by the family. Such inconsistencies led us to develop, within our unit, a rehabilitation clinic for language disorders.

We report below some of the characteristics of the population of 28 dysphasic children who stayed on our unit between 1983 and 1987. The length of stay varied between 3 and 20 months, with an average stay of 10 months; the children were between 7 and 13 years of age, the average age being 10 years; boys greatly outnumbered girls (25 boys out of 28). The reason for being admitted into the program was massive school failure in spite of adequate intellectual potential, as demonstrated by average Performance IQ figures on the WISC-R (Mean = 95). The marked difference between verbal and performance IQs (an average of 20 points) partially demonstrates the severity of the verbal handicap.

The different types of dysphasias observed in this population were 15 cases of expressive dysphasia, according to DSM-III terminology, distributed as follows: 5 cases of phonological-syntactical syndrome, 5 cases of lexical-syntactical syndrome, 5 cases of phonological production disorder. In addition to these cases of expressive dysphasia, we found 13 cases of receptive dysphasia. Language therapy occurred twice a day. This frequency is necessary to select and test strategies that are adapted to the estimated nature of those structural disorders, and to alter the learning process. Rehabilitation is provided by speech and language therapists on an individual basis.

Developmental learning and reading disorders were always present; developmental arithmetic disorders were not infrequent and were most often associated with expressive dysphasia; motor-coordination problems were mainly associated with phonological syntactical syndromes.

In this unit, language therapy is associated with more specific interventions targeting conceptual, cognitive, and psychomotor areas, but the various specialists articulate their interventions according to principles that are derived from a neuropsychological analysis. A physician specializing in developmental neuropsychology coordinates these various interventions, synchronizes these objectives with educational ones (which are also individualized and geared to prevent academic skills from lagging behind), and defines the best type of school placement upon discharge.

Coordination of the therapeutic program adjusts interventions to the emotional and behavioral status of the subjects, and involves the parents. Analysis of the subjects' behavioral reactions to the communicational impairment is complex since a multiplicity of factors are involved: age, type of dysphasic disorder, nature of associated cognitive disorders, environmental reactions. For interventions to be more efficient at this level, one has to understand that each type of dysphasic disorder has a unique way of impairing the child's relationships with the world at an early age. Dysphasic children conceptualize their relationship problems at different levels, depending on the nature and severity of those cognitive disorders that are associated with the linguistic disorders. Depending on the type of dysphasia, this leads to different behavioral adjustments to the relational handicap.

A neurodevelopmental analysis is a necessary prerequisite to choosing strategies of therapeutic intervention. For instance, expressive disorders are marked by very early verbal hypospontaneity, which is more severe than what is imposed by instrumental limitations. This observation is often explained in terms of a principle of economy, the child being said to prefer nonverbal modes of communication. The child becomes rapidly aware of the limitation imposed by this style of communication in the fulfillment of his wishes and in the responses he can give to an adult who expects him to grow up. The latter situation becomes particularly stressful when verbalization turns out to be the center of the adult's expectations, generally at the beginning of schooling. There is a marked discrepancy between the child's abilities to conceptualize his failure and what he can do to overcome it. This discrepancy is often magnified by the attitudes held by the educational team, which often attributes this expressive delay to a lack of emotional maturity; avoidance and separation anxiety then become logical maladjustments. The analysis that the child later makes of his various failures leads him to a type of conceptualization that is close to Seligman's model of "learned helplessness" (1975), with its emotional consequences, of which one possible manifestation is a real depressive syndrome. Children who primarily have a receptive disorder live a very different situation. The more pervasive impairment of the child's symbolization abilities cuts him off from the world of relationships. Relationship maladjustments are the result of anosognosia and of an impairment in the ability to apprehend reality. Withdrawal then becomes a necessity rather than a construction, and behavioral manifestations are so severe that these children are often thought to be psychotic. These observations allow us to distinguish two discrete modalities of approach to behavioral maladjustment. In the case of expressive disorders, interventions based on behavioristic techniques, with positive reinforcement, can be used, and as soon as the subject's development allows it, modified versions of cognitive therapies can be used as well. In the latter case, it is important to develop those semantic and pragmatic abilities that permit a better understanding of the relational reality, using sensory substitution and possibly codes of substitution. The fact that compensation is possible makes the relational disorders of these children more reversible than is generally the case for psychotic children.

In our population, at least one diagnosis of mental disorder was given to 21 out of our 28 cases. The disorders we observed were overanxious disorders (7 cases), affective disorders (4 cases), attention deficit disorders (4 cases), eating disorders (4 cases), conduct disorder (1 case), tics (1 case), and enuresis (2 cases).

The therapeutic process should include parents. Rehabilitation endeavors are often canceled out (1) if parents do not understand their child's pathology and the true nature of the child's adjustment disorders, or (2) if they do not adequately stimulate the child's linguistic abilities, because of lack of information on how the child can understand or express himself. It is clear that parents must be taught the basic principles of the rehabilitation process and that it is often beneficial to check at home the presence of generalization possibilities.

## *A Medical Model*

This way of conceptualizing the treatment of dysphasic disorders leads us to restore to favor the medical model, which has been accused (Ingram, 1987) of using a classification system of those disorders that was divorced from a linguistic theory and a developmental linguistic theory. Treatment does not aim for a laborious and chancy construction of linguistic skills in Chomsky's (1965) sense of the term, but for the optimal utilization and integration of potential linguistic performances, so as to prevent the whole sequence of developmental maladjustments that is increasingly well described in the clinical literature on dysphasic disorders. Patricia Howlin (1987) reviewed a number of studies that assessed various treatment programs with a specific target on linguistic deficits; she stressed that it is often difficult to separately evaluate the relevance of choices regarding psycholinguistic targets and regarding techniques. She shows how such learning programs, even the most sophisticated ones, do not hold in the face of a controlled evaluation of their impact on the development of linguistic skills, particularly when this evaluation is a long-term one, which is seldom the case. Treatment effects seem to concentrate primarily on behavioral variables; they depend on possibilities of immediate functional use of learning skills. Mainly, the various techniques must help the child improve the structuring of his linguistic environment for action purposes. Such observations are totally in accordance with our adaptive approach.

## Prospects

To these general considerations on treatment of dysphasia, we would like to add some comments on future prospects. We envision two main fields of investigation: prevention and imagery.

In view of our concept of treatment, which aims not only to have a specific impact on linguistic factors but to correct a deviant development as well, prevention goes through a better definition of high-risk populations. Recently, Robinson (1987) and Bishop (1987) reviewed the etiological factors of dysphasia. Their reviews pointed out that only the genetic factor had true predictive power. In addition, Robinson showed how the risk level can be calculated according to the sex of the child. To make progress in this area, predictive investigations have to take other variables into account—for instance, in the light of Geschwind and Galaburda's (1985) work—such as the stock of left-handed subjects, the morbid associations, and the familial association with learning disabilities. But the understanding of such predictive factors will be useless unless we have well-tested means of early intervention. In order to perfect them, one would have to apply them to subjects who are identifiable at birth. We have shown that children with congenital hemisyndromes would be good candidates for such evaluations (Gerard, Dugas, & Lacert, 1987).

In another area, progress achieved in functional imagery could compensate for the disadvantages that our empiricist notion of treatment of dysphasia implies for evaluation. Thanks to these developing procedures, one can directly objectify, on the basis of data provided by cerebral activity or cerebral metabolism studies, the impact of selected strategies, so as to act upon structural disorders. On the level of rehabilitation techniques, this would mean a replication of Lou's (1984) investigations designed to study the effect of methylphenidate on the distribution of cerebral blood flow. These research strategies should provide neurobiological arguments in favor of a cohesive formalized treatment of dysphasia. We have tried in this chapter to propose such a formalization on the basis of a neurodevelopmental model of language disorders.

ACKNOWLEDGMENTS. The authors thank Solange Cook, Ph.D., for linguistic assistance, Danièle Cambuzat for manuscript preparation, and Drs. Simeon and Ferguson for helpful suggestions regarding the manuscript.

## References

Baker, L., & Cantwell, D. P. (1987). A prospective psychiatric follow-up of children with speech/language disorders. *Journal of the American Academy of Child and Adolescent Psychiatry, 26*, 546–553.

Bishop, D. V. M. (1987). The causes of specific developmental language disorders ("developmental dysphasia"). *Journal of Child Psychology and Psychiatry, 28*, 1–8.

Carrow-Woolfolk, E., & Lynch, J. L. (1982). An integrative approach to language disorders in children. New York: Grune & Stratton.

Chomsky, N. (1965). Aspects of the theory of syntax. Cambridge, MA: M.I.T. Press.

Crosson, B. (1985) Sub-cortical functions in language: A working model. *Brain and Language, 25*, 257–292.

de Ajuriaguerra, J., & Guignard, F. (1965). Evolution et pronostic de la dysphasie de l'enfant. *Psychiatrie de l'Enfant, 8*, 391–453.

Diller, L. (1976). A model for cognitive retraining in rehabilitation. *Clinical Psychologist, 29*, 13–15.

Gerard, C., Dugas, M., & Lacert, P. (1987) *Dysphasia and early focal brain injury. Hypothesis for post-lesion cerebral reorganization*. Communication on the first international symposium on specific speech and language disorders in children, University of Reading.

Geschwind, N., & Galaburda, A. M. (1985) Cerebral lateralization. Biological mechanism, associations and pathology. I A hypothesis and a program for research. *Archives of Neurology, 42*, 428–459.

Howlin, P. (1987). Behavioural approaches to language. In W. Yule & M. Rutter (Eds.), *Language development and disorders* (pp. 367–390). Oxford: MacKeith Press.

Ingram, D. (1987). Categories of phonological disorders. *Proceedings of the first international symposium on specific speech and language disorders in children* (pp. 88–99). Reading, U.K.: University of Reading.

Lou, M. C., Henriksen, L., & Bruhn, P. (1984). Focal cerebral hypoperfusion in children with dysphasia and/or attention deficit disorders. *Archives of Neurology, 41*, 825–829.

Paul, R., Cohen, D. J., & Caparulo, B. K. (1983). A longitudinal study of patients with severe developmental disorders of language learning. *Journal of the American Academy of Child Psychiatry, 22*, 525–534.

Prutting, C. A. (1987). The pragmatic dimension: Discourse as a multilevel process. *Proceedings of the first international symposium on specific speech and language disorders in children* (pp. 114–134). Reading, U.K.: University of Reading.

Rapin, I., & Allen, D. A. (1987). Developmental dysphasia and autism in preschool children: Characteristics and subtypes. *Proceedings of the first international symposium on specific speech and language disorders in children* (pp. 20–35). Reading, U.K.: University of Reading.

Robinson, R. J. (1987). The causes of language disorder: Introduction and overview. *Proceedings of the first international symposium on specific speech and language disorders in children* (pp. 1–19). Reading, U.K.: University of Reading.

Rourke, B. P., Bakker, D. J., Fisk, J. L., & Strang, J. D. (1983). Child neuropsychology. An introduction to theory, research and clinical practice. New York: Guilford Press.

Seligman, M. E. P. (1975). *Helplessness: On depression development of abnormal psychology*. San Francisco: Freeman.

Silva, P. A., McGee, R., & Williams, S. M. (1983). Developmental language delay from three to seven years and its significance for low intelligence and reading difficulties at age seven. *Developmental Medicine and Child Neurology, 25*, 783–793.

Wiig, E. (1987). Strategic language use in adolescents with learning disabilities: Assessment and education. *Proceedings of the first international symposium on specific speech and language disorders in children* (pp. 181–200). Reading, U.K.: University of Reading.

Woods, B. T. (1985). Developmental dysphasia. In *Handbook of clinical neurology, Vol. 2: Neurobehavioral disorders* (pp. 139–144). Amsterdam: Elsevier Science Publishers.

# 11

# Child Psychotherapy

## Denis M. Donovan and Deborah McIntyre

### Introduction

#### Persistence of an Adult Model

The notion of conscious awareness as the clinical summum bonum dates from Freud and can be summed up succinctly in his famous *"Wo Es war, soll Ich werden"* (Where the Id was, the Ego shall be); (Freud, 1923). The idea of an "observing ego" is still very much alive in contemporary thinking about child psychotherapy. This can be seen in several examples from two child psychiatry tests.

> The ultimate aim [of therapy] is for the child to become freer within the experience, to gain a deeper awareness of himself and others, and to find a path to the reasonable expression of emotions....Attainment of any of these goals [of therapy] may become an end in itself along the way, but ordinarily they constitute intermediate points in a process that culminates in greater awareness....It is assumed that an expanded awareness of oneself and one's mode of relationship can be a powerful accompaniment of and, at times, the instigator of these psychological changes. (Carek, 1979, p. 36)

Carek notes, "What does happen in psychotherapy is in fact quite unspectacular." Given the spectacularly worrisome nature of much of the behavior that frequently occasions the entry of children into therapy, spectacular change would not seem an unreasonable goal. The expectation that little such change will actually occur in psychotherapy is not uncommon in psychiatric texts: "Psychotherapy aims to help but not to cure and it is an open question how much change should be expected" (Wilson & Hersov, 1985, p. 835). Wilson and Hersov also see the "observing ego" as a prerequisite for psychotherapy for they indicate that "children and adolescents should have all or some of the following capacities."

---

*Denis M. Donovan and Deborah McIntyre* • The Children's Center for Developmental Psychiatry, St. Petersburg, Florida 33710.

1. A sufficient degree of basic trust and ability to form and sustain a relationship with another person.
2. The capacity to distinguish sufficiently between fantasy and reality and to transfer feelings from one person to another.
3. The capacity to tolerate anxiety and intense emotions aroused in psychotherapy, without unmanageable loss of control.
4. The ability to recognize and verbalize thoughts and feelings.
5. The capacity for self-observation and reflection on the relationship between actions, thoughts and feelings. (1985, p. 834)

Are these reasonable requirements, especially if our population is to include the very young? They are, in fact, far too restrictive. Our first indication of this is the fact that the lack of those requisite capacities outlined above frequently constitutes the very reason the child is brought for treatment. Of more concern, however, is that these "capacities" do not correspond to how children think, interact, communicate, or change. This is especially true of the very young child and the mentally handicapped child—and neither age nor mental handicap need necessarily be a categorical barrier to effective psychotherapy. Furthermore, while the first three items above are reasonable goals of psychotherapy, they become unnecessarily exclusionary if viewed as prerequisites. However, both the fourth and the fifth would constitute ill-advised goals and unrealistic therapeutic preconditions in most cases of child psychotherapy.

## A Developmental–Contextual Approach

By shifting our perspective from one requiring that the child patient meet categorical criteria of treatability to one in which the clinical approach must adapt to the cognitive-developmental abilities and needs of the child, we can significantly increase the number of children and adolescents who can be successfully treated by psychotherapy. At the same time, we can significantly increase the efficacy of our psychotherapeutic interventions by appreciating what constitutes pragmatically successful child therapy. The effectiveness of child psychotherapy can be heightened by an understanding of (1) the ways in which children differ from adults in how they think, communicate, interact, and change; (2) the complexities of the "real worlds" in which children live; (3) how to structure and control the *therapeutic space* in which therapist and child interact; (4) how to assess and utilize *therapeutic aptness*; and finally, (5) by viewing psychotherapy within a *problem-solving* framework. When this is done, some of the traditional technical distinctions (e.g., between "behavior therapy" and "psychotherapy") begin to pale, as do some of the traditional structures of psychotherapy itself (such as the tripartite division of the process of therapy into beginning, middle, and end phases).

## How Children Think, Interact, Communicate, and Change

It is generally agreed that a stage-related model of psychotherapy with children not only is appropriate but is generally more successful (McDermott & Char, 1984). However, mental health professionals still tend to think of children as "concrete," immature, and incapable of complex abstract thought prior to the age of 12 or so (Fish-Murray, Koby, & van der Kolk, 1987; Tanguay 1985). This view, an outgrowth of Piagetian tradition (Piaget, 1970, 1972), places children in stages that do not actually correspond to their genuine cognitive abilities. In fact, evidence is accumulating which indicates that our traditional view of the perceptual and cognitive abilities of children is a gross underestimate of their real abilities. Much of this confusion is due to the fact that traditional *verbal* interview techniques, used regularly since Piaget's original pioneering studies, fail to elicit the child's true cognitive capabilities, especially in the early stages (Borke, 1971, 1973, 1975, 1978; Brainerd, 1978; Gardner, 1982). This failure to recognize the child's actual abilities and his or her stage-related cognitive style, owing largely to a widespread confusion of *speech* and *communication* (Mounin, 1970), can cause us grossly to underestimate both the complexity and the power of the child's actual lived experience. This, in turn, can blind us to the fascinating, complex, and sometimes horrifying world of the child.

If we leave the adult model of how children think and turn instead to recent findings in developmental psycholinguistics, we get a very different picture of early cognition. With the shift of emphasis in linguistics from form and structure to an intentional semantics inherent in the act of speaking, the way was paved for an ability to recognize, record, and analyze *intentional behavior* in the very young child (Greenfield, 1980).

Far from being "prelogical," children are, in fact, obligatory slaves of logic. We fail to understand this when we confuse reasonableness of thought and whether ideas and attitudes are "realistic" (i.e., correspond to how things "actually are") with logical thinking. Logic is simply a relatively closed system of interrelating propositions—which may or may not be true. Thus, the 2-1/2-year-old who states confidently that "germs come from Germany" is well within the bounds of a certain linguistic logic. Because logic is a necessary characteristic of any developing language (natural or artificial, as in computer languages), logical structures must first be constructed in order for the thinker ultimately to escape the very logic that was necessary to guide the development of the facilitating cognitive structures. Thus, we must all begin our cognitive development as incipient obligatory slaves of logic if we are to acquire the cognitive skills (structures) necessary to become "mature" thinkers—i.e., to escape the orbit of logic itself.

If this is understood, it becomes clear that it is not necessary to wait for a child to reach a given "stage" in order to be able to make an effective psychotherapeutic intervention. In fact, an understanding of the "logical binds" in which children unavoidably find themselves can allow the therapist to structure highly effective interventions at any stage of development. Consider the following example of one such "logical bind," and the strikingly simple intervention used to resolve it.

Christopher M. was a bright 7-year-old who was referred for evaluation by his school counselor because of escalating risk-taking behavior bordering on the suicidal, self-injurious acts such as banging his head on the outside of the school building and slamming his hand in a door or the school desktop on his head. Christopher's attention span had dwindled to practically nothing, his previously excellent grades had fallen, and he had become hard to handle and disruptive at school. He was also frequently putting his name under the "frowny face" on the blackboard.

What had happened to this previously well-adjusted academic achiever? Not long before the behavior change, Chris had looked both ways and then had ridden his bicycle into the path of a car that had just sped around the corner. He was thrown some 25 feet and ended up in the hospital unconscious for hours with five broken ribs, a collapsed right lung, hard-to-control internal bleeding, and a broken leg. He was in the hospital for 12 days.

But why the change and, specifically, why the development of *suicidal* behavior? Chris came from a family of Catholic converts. He, like the rest of his family, had undergone intensive instruction and continued to do so in his Catholic school. Chris was hit by the car on Holy Thursday. On Good Friday the chest tube was inserted and his mother was convinced that he was not going to survive. On Easter Sunday the tube was removed and Chris was pronounced "saved"—he would live.

During the initial therapeutic encounter Chris was asked where his name came from. "Chris comes from Christopher which comes from Christmas which comes from Christ," he replied. CHRISTopher = CHRISTmas = CHRIST. Chris's unconscious logic was pristine, clear, and tight: "I died and rose again; I can die and rise again." There was also considerable guilt over wishing that his younger brother had never been born and named a junior (the "one true Son of the Father"), but this had more to do with the self-punitive aspects of Chris's behavior change than with the potentially fatal risk taking. This guilt, moreover, might never have been actualized had it not been for the accident. But the core of what developed after the accident was his unconscious identification with the dead and risen Christ. In fact, Chris had gone to his mother one day with the family crucifix and had said, "Look at this," pointing to the red wound on the figure of Christ, "Christ had a chest tube—just like me!"

Chris's response to therapy was striking, and before long the worrisome behaviors and attitudes had changed. A few weeks before the first anniversary of the accident (Easter), however, Chris began to dart out from between parked cars in the school parking lot. It occurred to me (D.M.D.)

that we had left one logical link in the chain of meanings untouched. So, when Chris's mother repeated her renewed concerns about Chris's behavior at the beginning of the next session, I turned to Chris and said, "You know, if you run out in front of a car now and get killed—you'll go straight to Hell." Chris looked absolutely stunned and had to sit back on the couch. "What," he asked, shocked. "For Catholics, suicide is a sin, a mortal sin, Chris," I told him, "and if you run out in front of a car and get killed, you'll go straight to Hell—with no waiting!" Chris looked puzzled. "But when I got hit by that car last year," he said imploringly, "I wouldn't have gone to Hell then—if I'd died—would I?" "No," I told Chris, "not last year—but then you didn't *try* to get hit last year, did you?"

An even greater ease appeared in Chris's behavior and appearance after this session, and he got through the Easter anniversary comfortably. He finished the school year with good grades both in his subjects and in conduct.

This case illustrates graphically the strikingly self-referent nature of children's thinking in which the world is interpreted as if everything happens by them, to them, for them, and because of them.

## *The Interactive Style of Children*

Chris was a very verbal 7-year-old. Consequently, words could be used to undo, as it were, the logical bind in which he found himself as a result of the series of catastrophic coincidences that constituted his experience of the period of the accident. Another example from the very first encounter with this bright, verbal child, however, illustrates how interactive communication can be more effective than words as such.

> During his first session in the play therapy room, after the focus of activity had changed from the initial drawings on the table to play on the floor, Chris mentioned, almost in passing, that everyone was born with a penis, that half the population seemed to lose theirs—and he was very, very scared of losing his. Chris's therapist (D.M.) responded by picking up Mr. Kangaroo (a stuffed animal) and looking him over carefully. She then opened the roof of the large open-sided doll house to reveal the attic, put Mr. Kangaroo inside, and closed the roof. A moment later she took Mr. Kangaroo out. "Hmmm. Still the same," she said. She then repeated the process with Mr. Platypus, another stuffed animal.

Although they had not been presenting problems because they paled in seriousness when compared to Chris's suicidally risk-taking behavior, Chris— at 7 years of age—still sucked his thumb and wet the bed regularly. Both of these behaviors ceased as of the day of the intervention described above. It would have been a grievous technical error had Chris's therapist then pointed out to him (so that he would "understand" what had just transpired) that "not all babies are born with penises. Only boy babies are. And babies born with penises do not lose them." The need to "make the unconscious [or preconscious] conscious" often leads therapists to undo verbally what they have just accomplished symbolically and interactively. Such verbalizations are perceived by children as proof that the adult did not really believe in what he or she just did and, consequently, tend to kill the "magic" of the intervention. Because children are normative dissociators (Donovan & McIntyre, 1990; Putnam, 1987), mild dissociative phenomena being both ubiquitous and normal in childhood, it is only reasonable to capitalize on this "ability" whenever possible. Good child therapy, like hypnosis, utilizes and modifies *behavioral states of consciousness* (Putnam, 1987).

The more highly symbolic children are in their expressive behavior (often referred to as "acting-out"), the more receptive they are to symbolic interventions that *remain within the metaphor* and the more sensitive they are to anything that seems to indicate that the adult does not really believe in the efficacy of their interventions. Many otherwise superb child therapists negate the power and effectiveness of their therapeutic interventions by requiring that their child patients acknowledge a conscious awareness of the content and process of therapy. Only experience, however, can teach when to resolve verbally and when to resolve interactively. Generally, the younger the child, the more interactive and symbolic the interventions. With some children only experience can be calming. Another case example illustrates how dramatic such interventions can be.

> On the advice of her exasperated pediatrician, an enraged mother phoned the office. She was beside herself and wanted to sue because a "foreign" doctor had inadvertently given her 20-month-old son a double dose of antihistamine at the local emergency room when the child presented with a mild allergic rash. The toddler had an acute idiosyncratic hallucinatory psychotic reaction to the medication. He was terrified of the butterflies on his sheets, pillowcases, and curtains, which were all chasing him. At the time of the call, 3 days after the emergency room visit, the toddler was still terrified and would scream hysterically and thrash around as the family car approached the house. He had to be carried forcibly into his own home and could not be induced to set foot in his bedroom in spite of the fact that all of the butterfly material had been removed the first day.
>
> The boy's mother was told to go to the local hardware store and buy a cheap plastic plant sprayer. She was to fill it with several inches of water and add just enough perfume to give it a smell. She was then to put the sheets, pillowcases, and curtains back up and tell her son that she had a "magic potion that turns bad butterflies into good butterflies." She was instructed to spray the door frame to the bedroom very ceremoniously and then to spray each butterfly. She was to do this with great theatrical seriousness. The toddler slept in his bed that night, and the "bad butterflies" never returned.

No actual contact between therapist and child had taken place and yet the results were stunning, real, and lasting—as they often can be in good psychotherapy. The intervention was based on an understanding of the intensity and realness of the child's experience and the richness of the imagination of children, a richness than can bring both complications and resolutions to their lives.

*Communication and Speech*

Just as conscious awareness is often not a characteristic of the cognitive style of the child and does not play the preponderant role it does in adult life, so, too, with speech. Children love to talk, but their talk does not always serve the purpose observing adults may think. Similarly, "What if..." questions, which many conscientious parents attempt to answer with the certainty of the *Encyclopedia Britannica*, are frequently no more than *contact extenders* (Moskowitz, 1978), attempts on the part of the child to prolong the contact, a contact characterized by verbal exchange (Moskowitz, 1978). So, too, the incessant "Why?" which, like "What if's," tend to be characteristic of the years from 4 to 7, especially in boys.

Speech, then, does not always have the same significance and purpose in childhood that it does in later years. *Communication*, however, is a form of information exchange at any age. If the therapist recognizes in the child's productions (discrete behaviors) the behavioral equivalent of a *speech act* (Bruner, 1974; Searle, 1969, 1971), acts that express the *utterer's meaning* (Grice, 1967, cited in Bruner, 1974), then it will be seen that potential communication is occurring whenever children are behaving. This is all the more so when the moment has been primed (by interviews, history-taking, and the explicit statement of problems): What the therapist must look for are the behavioral equivalents of verbal utterances. The child's play (or just his or her behavior in the therapeutic setting) can constitute *behavioral speech acts* that are both potentially intelligible and potentially answerable. Without an awareness of this, the child's behavior may appear to constitute nothing more than "mere playing." Such behavioral speech acts must be viewed in serial fashion or the meaning-content of the behavior may be lost. Without the contextualization made possible by the therapist/observer's knowledge of the real-world circumstances of the individual's life, no communicative content may be recognized. (For a more detailed discussion, see Donovan & McIntyre, 1990.)

A professional friend recounted a visit that the late British child analyst D. W. Winnicott had made to a Danish colleague. After Winnicott's departure the colleague's children told their parents what a marvelous time they had had talking with the nice Englishman. "We talked and talked and he had the most marvelous stories," they said. This is a beautiful example of the potential intense power of communicative behavior, because Winnicott could not have "talked" to his colleague's children, and certainly not for several hours, for he spoke no Danish and the children spoke no English.

Children need not talk to be evaluated and/or treated psychotherapeutically. However, few children who experience the intense communicative potential of a genuinely *therapeutic space* (see below) will remain silent for long.

## The Real Worlds of Children

In order to understand the meaning of the presenting behavioral or affective symptoms, and to develop an effective interaction strategy, one must understand the real-life context in which the child lives. Such an understanding can often change the clinical picture radically, making it difficult to assign *arbitrary meanings* to symptom clusters. This runs counter to the prevailing approach to both diagnostics and therapeutics in which categorical treatments are increasingly applied to categorical diagnoses (and where third-party payments are often denied if such categorical diagnoses/treatments are not employed).

> Steve was a 15-year-old adoptee with a serious reading disability. Every year for the 9 years of his public school life since the first grade, Steve had been tested and retested by psychologists, psychoeducational experts, developmental pediatricians, neurologists, and psychiatrists. Consistently over the 9 years Steve's diagnosis of dyslexia remained the basis on which he was assigned to Specific Learning Disability classes. Apart from the cursory mention of his adoption after being removed from dangerously poor living conditions, only the scantiest reference to Steve's actual life was to be found in the many reports that accompanied him to his evaluation.

Steve's history, as reflected in all the school reports and psychologicals that accompanied him, certainly supported the diagnosis of dyslexia—and he did, in fact, have great difficulty when presented with graded readings. Steve seemed nervous when asked about reading and even more so when asked to read aloud. He smiled too much and maintained only the most fleeting eye contact. Yet the picture changed considerably when a more detailed history was taken.

> Before his adoption Steve had lived in numerous farm camps, following his migrant farmworker parents from job to job. At 6, just before entering the first grade, Steve accidentally overturned a large kerosene stove, burning his upper torso and arms so badly that it would later require five separate plastic surgeries for him to be able to move his arms normally at the shoulder. Steve's entire upper torso and arms were a confluent mass of scar tissue.

When Steve overturned the stove upon himself his mother, seated less than 5 feet away, *continued to read her book*. Even as his father scooped him up and placed him in the bathtub to put out the flames and cool him down, Steve's mother *never so much as looked up from her book*.

These were the circumstances under which this child entered first grade and began to learn to read. Shortly after the accident, Steve and his two sisters were taken away from their parents and separated, Steve going to medical foster care and his sisters to regular foster care. As minority children, they were not easy to place adoptively. Steve was even harder to place because of his newly scarred appearance and the daily nursing care he required. As a result, the children were placed separately and never reunited. Seen in this context, the meaning of *reading* itself is radically changed: No longer a "simple" developmental skill to be acquired with a certain sense of accomplishment, reading took on an "emotional charge," effectively signifying to Steve his mother's wish that he should die in flames. Once this context was established, the meaning of Steve's behavior, which had resulted in the referral for psychiatric evaluation, became evident: He had been caught setting fire to a woman's garden after stealing some of her vegetables. Did Steve have a genuine "neurodevelopmentally based" dyslexia? By this time the picture was greatly confused by years of failure. Had Steve's life been seen as relevant to his presenting problems at the time of the initial evaluation in first grade, the course of Steve's academic life might have been much different.

This case highlights the importance of a *contextual* approach to the diagnosis of child psychiatric disorders. A history of categorical "disorder" in the absence of a contextualizing life history provided Steve's teachers and counselors with a thoroughly misleading picture. It has become increasingly evident in the contemporary psychiatric literature that standard phenomenological approaches to clinical presentations can be most misleading and can result not only in misdiagnosis (Putnam, 1987), but also in potentially spurious research based on inaccurate diagnoses (Coles, 1987). The cost of not contextualizing disordered behavior can be extraordinarily high, in both human and economic terms (Coles 1987; Donovan 1987). This is especially true in cases of child physical and sexual abuse and gross neglect. Recent studies indicate an unusually high incidence of childhood abuse in the lives of chronically hospitalized psychotic women (Beck & van der Kolk, 1987). And it has been "only within the last five or six years that various studies have documented the long-term sequelae of child maltreatment which remain long after the cessation of abuse" (Green, 1986). These are not highly unusual occurrences in the lives of children but, rather, the brutal "tip" of an otherwise immense clinical "iceberg." Pynoos and Eth (1985, 1986), for example, point out that "the Sheriff's Homicide Division of Los Angeles County estimates that dependent children witness between 10 and 20% of the approximately 2000 annual homicides in their jurisdiction." Accidents, injuries, death, losses, and the many catastrophes that life inflicts in the lives of children—all play major roles in the response to experience. There is increasing evidence that such experience can have profound psychophysiologic effects, effects that can be formative, determining, and even lasting (van der Kolk, 1987).

If the clinician does not contextualize the presenting problems by viewing them within the real life experiences of the child patient, the otherwise obvious significance of the child's symptoms, interactional style, and production within the therapeutic evaluation may be lost. While we have become increasingly aware of the effect of gross man-made or natural catastrophic trauma because of the attention they are given in the media, the ubiquity of such experiences that do not receive media attention should not be underestimated. Nor should the role they play in the pathogenesis of "standard" psychiatric disorders (van der Kolk, 1987).

## The Therapeutic Process

The traditional tripartite division of the process of therapy into a beginning, middle, and end phases, with a diagnostic phase either preceding or incorporated into the beginning phase (Coppolillo, 1987; Loney, 1980), leads one to assume that a working relationship must be built over time, often before "therapeutic issues" can even be addressed, let alone resolved. While some children may, indeed, require a number of encounters in order to trust the therapist and the process of therapy enough to risk revelations or change, this is often not the case. Consequently, to work on "building a relationship" without addressing the problems (directly or indirectly, according the abilities and style of the child) can actually be a contradiction in terms.

Children generally come to therapy with some expectation of help. The initial interview with parents/custodians and child further primes the child's expectation of help and resolution by explicitly stating the problems. (It is technically self-defeating to interview parents without the child present because the process must then be reinitiated with the child. It also generally conveys to the child a sense of insecurity, collusiveness, or secret-keeping on the part of the therapist, making the development of trust harder.) If the therapist does not attempt to bring some sense of resolution to the child during the first encounter, the child may respond with either resistance or "empty" change, which does not generalize to the child's life outside the clinical setting. It is important for the child therapist to realize that most children do not share the typical adult view of psychotherapy. It rarely occurs to children that therapy has to be work, that it cannot be fun, that it has to cost money and take a long time, or that results cannot be instantaneous. These are adult expectations.

Children are also much more willing to "pretend" to be well without embarrassingly painful self-consciousness, thereby facilitating a transition to genuine wellness—a transition that, although relatively normal for children, can appear virtually miraculous to adults.

Thus, one cannot avoid establishing a relationship with the child from the very first encounter, be it in the waiting room or in one's office. It may also be diagnostically quite misleading to allow symptom behaviors to persist without an immediate attempt at resolution, since many children are capable of rapid change. And given the unusually high incidence (85%) of unilateral terminations (Novick, Benson, & Rembar, 1981), the therapeutic efficacy of the initial part of treatment may be crucial in the lives of many children.

## Therapeutic Space

The *therapeutic space* is the physical, temporal, and interpersonal space in which the child and the therapist interact. Because it is a virtual and potential space, it is constantly being elaborated. Its definition is entirely operational: It exists only as it is experienced by the child and the therapist. Every physical object it contains contributes to the nature of its structure, as does the way in which time is managed. Once this is realized, the evaluation–treatment dichotomy collapses immediately. If the concept of therapeutic space is meaningful, it dictates that the child's very first clinical encounter be structured therapeutically.

While psychotherapeutic interventions are possible in literally any context, most take place in an office or hospital setting. Such settings offer the possibility to exercise various degrees of control over the environment in which one works. There are a number of technical reasons why it is wise to do so. First, then therapeutic space constitutes the "ground" upon which to view the figure of the varying productions of the patient. If the ground is constantly changing, it becomes difficult or impossible to comprehend the changing figure. Second, children—even very small children—can be exquisitely perceptive of, and sensitive to, personal and environmental details. Children should perceive from the first contact that the very space they encounter "understands" them, that it is so firmly and consistently structured that (1) it is safe to be self-disclosing and (2) the space will make them feel secure.

As much as they may appear constantly to challenge them, children need, and are exquisitely responsive to, *structure, rules*, and *boundaries*. The intensity and power of the therapeutic space can be significantly enhanced if the following very simple premises upon which its structure must be built are accepted. (1) Structure, rules, and boundaries must be explicitly elaborated and implicitly maintained. (2) The therapeutic relationship and process should in no way collude with that which may have hurt the child (either intentionally or unintentionally): (3) While the therapeutic process may facilitate the child's expression of mistaken or negative self-perceptions, it should never allow them to stand. (4) This requires that harm to self, to others, or to property not be permissible within the therapeutic setting.

There are many operational "rules" that one can develop from these initial premises to help define the therapeutic space. They range from how one handles the difficult issues of confidentiality, to who and what is allowed (or not allowed) to enter the therapy room, to the contents of the room itself. While it is difficult to control the physical space of a shared therapy room, it is well worth the effort required to do so. Ideally, objects should have their own consistent place in the room. This simple consistency can reinforce a predictable continuity of experience, which may play a major, if subtle, role in the resolution of cognitive confusion or in the rebuilding of trust in the case of a hurt child. Similarly, allowing a child to leave a disordered therapy room is counter-therapeutic and undermines trust in adults who should be able to "hold the world together."

An appreciation of the concept of therapeutic space can also help the therapist to decide upon the actual contents of the therapy room (a room that should, ideally, be separate from one's office and from the space in which one meets with the child and his parents together). Unless one believes that feces-smearing is a productive and integrative behavior, there is no need to have excrementlike substances in the play therapy room. Clay, paint, and finger paints are not required for a child to be graphically expressive. Crayons, pencils, and possibly (washable) felt markers suffice. Similarly, to the logical mind of the child, broken or easily breakable toys signify, at best, that adults cannot hold the world together and, at worst, that adults allow children to be (symbolically) hurt or to have power they cannot possibly control. While this may have been the experience of the child in the lived world, real therapeutic progress is not possible unless the boundaries between the real (and often dangerous) world and the therapeutically integrative world are elaborated and maintained. For legal and clinical reasons it is wise not to have anatomically correct dolls (Donovan, 1988). It follows also that every session should have a sense of closure.

A number of other operational "rules" governing the therapeutic space can be defined. While, at first glance, they may give the impression of rigidity, they can actually be maintained with great subtlety when incorporated operationally into the interaction with the child. When comfortably and well followed, the rules are rarely perceived as such by outside observers, although children tend to become very protective of the complex structure that they define—often before they generalize to home, community, and school. Nonetheless, children will challenge these rules in all sorts of fascinating ways. The challenges can have both a communicative and a therapeutic content, which can, at times, be of crucial diagnostic significance. Abused children, for example, and children whose "space" has been similarly "invaded" (as in being hit by a car) will often challenge the integrity of the therapeutic space physically by trying to secrete objects into the play therapy room. This must be recognized by the therapist and the objects excluded from the space. Repeated attempts to "violate" the therapeutic space in this manner can be indicators of physical or sexual abuse when other indicators are absent. As such, they may constitute *behavioral memories*, especially in the younger child (Terr, 1988).

Often trust is not really established until the child learns that the structures, rules, and boundaries will be maintained consistently (in a totally nonpunitive manner), no matter how hard the child tries to break them. At this point, confidences about past experiences may be shared with the therapist which would otherwise have been kept secret, even confidences that may never have been shared with previous well-liked therapists.

## The Evaluation of Therapeutic Aptness

Dysfunction is easy to recognize and diagnose categorically. But it is all too easy to be mistaken with regard to the meaning of apparent pathology. This was strikingly obvious in the case of Steve above. It is much more fascinating, and certainly more clinically productive, to structure a first (evaluation) encounter to be maximally therapeutic. Such an encounter will, by its very nature, contain an assessment of the child's *therapeutic aptness*. Therapeutic aptness is the child's ability to utilize the therapeutic space in a creative manner: operationally to recognize in the therapeutic encounter real potential for communication and change. The key word here is *operational*: The child's ability to "recognize" the complex potentials of the therapeutic space is often expressed behaviorally—not discursively. Children, it must be remembered, are normatively dissociative beings.

## An Operational Assessment of "Play"

How children respond to the creative interventions presented to them can have powerful diagnostic and therapeutic implications. Presenting a room full of toys to a child is neither diagnostic nor therapeutic. The process must be structured. The first part of that structure is the intake interview in which the problems and history are reviewed. Part of the next phase of the *initial* encounter is the assessment of the child's ability to use a structured interactive encounter. How much structure is required of the therapist depends upon the native *therapeutic aptness* of the child. If the child does not initiate meaningful play (significant interaction with the contents of the room) within a few minutes, the child's activity and attention must be focused by the therapist.

Many children, however, will recognize the intense symbolic potential of the play therapy room immediately upon entering. This is easily seen in their almost reverent treatment of the space. Even so, one must still ask whether the child's play—even in a highly structured space—is *semic play* or *ludic play*.

Mark was the 7-year-old son of divorced parents; the father had been quite violent before abandoning the family. Mark had been expelled from several private schools because of bizarre and inappropriate behavior with peers and was now being considered for the Emotionally Handicapped class in his new public school. In the play therapy room, once the move had been made to the floor and the toys, Mark was presented with the family dolls. After Mark's therapist had the father doll terrorize the family, she sent the little boy off to school. "How does he feel?" she asked Mark. "Let's play Legos," he replied as he moved to empty out the box.

Mark's initial drawing of "a house" and "the people who live in that house" had been equally devoid of human narrative content. "I like to play cars," he said as he drew what appeared to be a gas station. Mark drew cars parked in front of the house in which the people were supposed to live, but there was no sign of human life either in the cars or in or around the house.

This child's response to a structured play interaction that paralleled real events from his own life was unusual: Most children begin to direct the play or take a responsive role within it soon after its initiation. In this child's case, his play remained empty for the duration of the evaluation, just as his discursive response to direct questions remained evasive and noncommittal.

*Ludic play* is "just playing. It is "empty" in that it contains no communicative content. Made up of multiple sentence-equivalents, it contains no *behavioral speech acts*. It is the play of playing house, playing cars, or playing teatime. It is not self-revelatory. In the several years that have passed since Mark was seen in evaluation, he has remained refractory to every therapeutic modality and setting—regardless of the clinician or the clinician's gender, training, or theoretical orientation. Chris, our first clinical example, represents the other end of the spectrum. *Semic play* is symbolic, communicative play.

In these two cases, the patient's first response to a structured communicative intervention had prognostic significance. Not all children, of course, are immediately responsive, even to the most competent and caring of interventions.

The "play algorithm" in Figure 1 illustrates graphically the variety of possible responses to such an approach.

The history prepares the therapist in advance with a rich armamentarium of potentially meaningful interventions. The history-taking process *contextualizes* the therapeutic encounter and marks it as relevant to the child, while providing the therapist with a life-context without which the productions of the child are difficult, if not impossible, to understand. (This is why "blind" interviews are just that: blind.) Children who have been in multiple prior failed

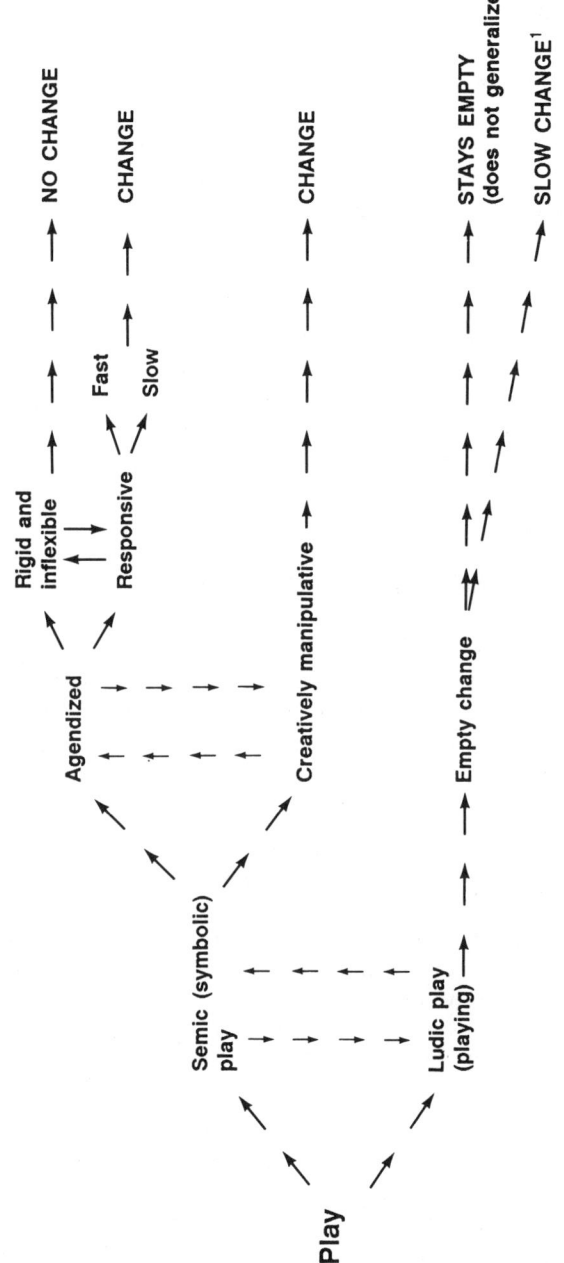

*Figure 1.* An operational assessment of "play."

[1] May be illusory

treatments are often particularly sensitive to such contextualized interventions in the first encounter and will frequently develop a working rapport much more rapidly than they had in the past. On the other hand, if there is no such life-relevant intervention and the child or adolescent feels that the therapist is simply adrift, the result can be an otherwise avoidable therapeutic nihilism on the part of the patient. If "rapport" develops under such circumstances, it is based on liking the therapist—not on feeling understood—and any resulting "change" is usually facetious and short-lived.

Such operational assessments are especially useful with children who have received "severe" diagnoses, such as psychosis, autism, major depression, or "central processing disorders." (See Coles, 1987 for a view of "learning disabilities" compatible with this therapeutic approach.) Often the response is quite rewarding. On the other hand, children who appear to be oblivious or out of touch may require great patience and sensitivity on the part of the therapist. When this approach is taken, even mentally handicapped children are often quite reachable because the techniques are geared to their cognitive style and ability.

### The "Ecology" of Child Psychotherapy

Children rarely seek out psychiatric treatment. For this reason alone parents or custodians need to be involved in the process. Because children are such exquisitely contextual beings, however, the term *individual psychotherapy* is either a misnomer or a sign that one has failed to realize the importance of the child's environment. This importance can be strikingly simple and strikingly obvious and yet escape everyone's attention.

> Simon was a 12-year-old seventh-grader who was referred for psychiatric evaluation and treatment because of long-standing academic underachievement, depression, and increasing hostility toward school personnel. He had been in therapy with public mental health services on and off since the first grade with no real change in his behavior. When this child's social history was reviewed, it was noted that Simon's mother had become pregnant with him in a conscious and purposeful attempt to save her deteriorating marriage. Simon's father abandoned the family the very week of Simon's birth, never to be heard from again.

It had never occurred to Simon's previous school counselors and psychologists, or to the many therapists who had previously treated him, that Simon's very birth was a "failure." He had been brought into the world literally to keep his father from leaving. In his own eyes he had clearly failed because his father had left. When this was reviewed with Simon and his mother, and the locus of responsibility was clearly seen to be in his father, Simon was able to put his anger and sadness where they belonged and stop punishing himself for having been a "congenital failure." With that process came a change in his relationship with the parent like figures of his school environment and a corresponding improvement in academic performance as his depression resolved. (Needless to say, Simon had no *conscious* notion of being a "categorical failure" because his birth did not save his parents' marriage. Although *explanations* are not *causes*, it is fascinating to see how often the operational modification of an explanation appears to have causal consequences.)

## *Parents and Teachers as Allies or Saboteurs of the Therapeutic Process*

> George was 3½ when his 23-year-old mother fell dead of a stroke at home just 9 days after giving birth 2 weeks prematurely to his brother, Billy. George, who had been a grossly overmothered, shy, and retiring child, simply withdrew. He was referred for psychiatric evaluation and treatment because the schools thought that he was either autistic or mentally handicapped, with a "central processing disorder." At the time of the initial evaluation, George was 6 years old, in a preschool class for 3-year-olds, noninteractive, blissfully uninvolved, and largely echolalic.
>
> George's first real coherent words in therapy were "I got mad at my mommy—and she died." Six months later George was mischievous and loquacious and in a class for the educationally handicapped. He was about to be mainstreamed into normal classes just prior to the anniversary of his mother's death. Fate was such that the anniversary of his mother's death effectively coincided with Halloween (the feast of ghosts and goblins). George's teacher, 7 months pregnant, offered him a small toy as a present, just as she did for her other pupils. She gave him a small parent skeleton with its arm around the shoulders of a child skeleton. George became acutely psychotic for a week and required three sessions to his normal one before regaining the ground that had been lost in an instant.

Child therapists cannot always count on colleagues to attend to details such as this. Unfortunately, such gross insensitivity to the *meaning* of obviously emotionally charged events in the lives of traumatized children may surprise—but is by no means unusual. Because the "therapeutic field" extends far beyond the office and the therapy room to include home, community, and school, to view "social" issues as ancillary is to deprive oneself of considerable therapeutic power. A good personal working relationship with the schools, social services, child protection teams, courts, and law enforcement can make therapeutic coordination much easier and more effective. Such an approach does, however, require considerable time—often uncompensated—beyond that usually spent in therapy. Even then, as we have seen, it cannot assure that disasters will not occur.

## Psychotherapy as a Problem-Solving Process

If one defines psychotherapy in terms of traditional theoretical models (Wilson & Hersov, 1985), then the effective scope of psychotherapy is, indeed, severely limited, and, as Carek notes, its outcome may, indeed, be "quite unspectacular." It may be limited to that which is verbally manageable within 45 or 50 minutes in an office setting. On the other hand, if one defines psychotherapy as a process of modification of mood, affect, and behavior that is based on an understanding of the real-world experiences of the patient and his current life-context as well as his cognitive and interaction style, then the effective potential of psychotherapy is seen to be immense.

> Jared R. was a 10-year-old biracial child who was referred for psychiatric evaluation by public health services because of self-destructive and self-injurious behavior (repeated attempts to stab his genitals with knives, scissors, and pencils, to scrape his skin off, and to jump out of moving vehicles), explosive crises, night terrors, and frequent auditory and visual hallucinations. Just prior to his appointment, Jared was hospitalized involuntarily on a psychiatric unit of a general hospital where he remained for 3 weeks. There he received medical psychotherapy, group therapy, milieu and activity therapies, and psychiatric medication. When his mother picked him up to take him home she was told by his attending psychiatrist, "I expect to see him back in the hospital shortly." There had been no behavioral change.
>
> When Jared was first seen following his discharge from the hospital, it was learned that his black father had horribly brutalized his white mother throughout Jared's early years. On one occasion, which Jared had witnessed at age 7, his father raped his mother, beat her, and attacked her so brutally with a knife that she subsequently required a hysterectomy.
>
> Was Jared psychotic—or was he caught in a horrible identity bind? The latter seemed to be the case, for he was constantly saying he hated himself because of his color and because he was attacking the same part of his body that he had seen his father use so brutally (in actuality and symbolically with the knife) on his mother. In light of this understanding, Jared was offered an opportunity to *disidentify* with his father (who was in prison and would no longer have contact with the family) while developing a respect for other black men. It was explained that violence did not "run in your blood," and, since he was a junior, he was asked if he would like to change his name. He agreed and changed it to J.R. His mother understood the importance of this and took him the following day for a new haircut, new glasses, and new clothes. J.R.'s explosive behavior, self-injuriousness, and oppositionalism (which had not changed with the hospitalization) immediately improved. He no longer needed to punish the father in himself and ceased trying to scrape off his skin. He began to like the black, as well as the white, in himself. However, his nightmares, in which he was pursued by his father or saw his father murder his mother, did not abate, and he was

still crawling in bed with his mother every night. J.R. was therefore given two big blue-and-white placebo capsules (called "Antinightmare Pills"), which were "so powerful that you can take only one a week." Two weeks later, when seen after the holidays, the mother reported that J.R. had slept well and in his own bed until the third day of the second week. She had asked J.R. if he had taken the second pill. He admitted that he had opened the capsule and had poured out "two-thirds" of it before taking it. "Antinightmare pills" were required for only 3 subsequent weeks, after which J.R. was able to sleep comfortably alone without "medication." Therapy was then able to proceed at a comfortable pace and to deal with less threatening issues of academic underachievement.

As mentioned, no behavioral changes had been noted during or after the hospitalization of this 10-year-old. The structured milieu of the hospital setting and the antipsychotic medication had not addressed the issues. J.R.'s psychiatrist concluded after 3 weeks that J.R. would be "returning soon" and told J.R.'s mother that his prognosis was "very poor." The clear advantage of a problem-solving *contextual* psychotherapeutic approach is that it can allow for a more accurate diagnosis in children, while immediately setting about to resolve the problems as defined. What may look *categorically* disastrous through the nosological lenses of instruments such as DSM may appear *contextually* quite treatable. Jared's behavioral memories and night terrors, for example, suggested a behavioral response to lived experience (Donovan & McIntyre, 1990) likely to respond to an intensely experienced *behavioral intervention*. One can then structure the therapy, in terms of both content and length, on the basis of the needs, strengths, and responses of the individual child or adolescent patient. Had such an approach been used initially with Jared, 3 weeks and 6000 Medicaid dollars would have been saved. The course of some therapies will be found to follow a traditional tripartite sequence. Others will terminate quickly. In the case of extremely difficult patients, the utilization of such a therapeutically optimistic approach will make it easier to face the painful fact that some children do not change whether in or out of the hospital. If one has facilitated the transfer of trust from the therapist to the child's environment, then termination need not be a difficult process.

## *References*

Beck, J. C. & van der Kolk, B. (1987). Reports of childhood incest and current behavior of chronically hospitalized psychotic women. *American Journal of Psychiatry, 144,11*:1474–1476.

Borke, H. (1971). Interpersonal perception of young children: Ego-centrism or empathy? *Developmental Psychology, 5*, 263–269.

Borke, H. (1973). The development of empathy in Chinese and American children between three and six years of age: A cross-cultural study. *Developmental Psychology, 9*, 102–108.

Borke, H. (1975). Piaget's mountains revisited: Changes in the egocentric landscape. *Developmental Psychology, 11*, 240–143.
Borke, H. (1978). Piaget's view of social interaction and the theoretical construct of empathy. In L. S. Siegel & C. J. Brainerd (Eds.), *Alternatives to Piaget: Critical essays on the theory*. New York: Academic Press.
Brainerd, C. J. (1978). Learning research and Piagetian theory. In L. S. Siegel & C. J. Brainerd (Eds.), *Alternatives to Piaget: Critical essays on the theory*. New York: Academic Press.
Bruner, J. S. (1974). The ontogenesis of speech acts. *Journal of Child Language, 1*(2), 1–19.
Bryant, P. (1974). *Perception and understanding in young children*. New York: Basic Books.
Carek, D. J. (1979). Individual psychodynamically oriented psychotherapy. In S. I. Harrison (Ed.), *Basic handbook of child psychiatry* (Vol. 3). New York: Basic Books.
Coles, G. (1987). *The learning mystique. A critical look at "learning disabilities."* New York: Pantheon.
Coppolillo, H. P. (1987). *Psychodynamic psychotherapy of children*. Madison: International Universities Press.
Donovan, D. M. (1987). Costs of factitious illness. *Hospital and Community Psychiatry, 38*(6), 571–572.
Donovan, D. M. (1988). Anatomically correct dolls: Research vs. clinical practice. *Journal of the American Academy of Child and Adolescent Psychiatry, 27*, 662.
Donovan, D. M. (1989). The paraconscious. *Journal of the American Academy of Psychoanalysis, 17*(2), 223–252.
Donovan, D. M., & McIntyre, D. (1990). *Healing the hurt child: A developmental-contextual approach*. New York: W. W. Norton.
Fish-Murray, C. C., Koby, E. V., & van der Kolk, B. A. (1987). Evolving ideas: The effect of abuse on children's thought. In B. A. van der Kolk (Ed.), *Psychological trauma*. Washington, DC: American Psychiatric Press.
Freud, S. (1923), *The Ego and The Id, The Standard Edition of The Complete Psychological Works, Vol. 14*. W. W. Norton & Co.
Gardner, H. (1982). *Developmental psychology* (2nd ed.) Boston: Little, Brown.
Green, A. (1986). True and false allegations of sexual abuse in child custody disputes. *Journal of the American Academy of Child and Adolescent Psychiatry, 25*(4), 449–456.
Greenfield, P. M. (1980). Towards an operational and logical analysis of intentionality. In D. Olson (Ed.), *The social foundations of language: Essays in honor of Jerome S. Bruner*. New York: W. W. Norton.
Looney, J. (1980). Treatment planning in child psychiatry. *Journal of the American Academy of Child Psychiatry, 23*, 529–536.
McDermott, J. F., & Char, W. F. (1984). Stage-related models of psychotherapy with children. *Journal of the American Academy of Child and Adolescent Psychiatry, 23*, 537–543.
Moskowitz, B. A. (1978). The acquisition of language. *Scientific American, November*, 92–108.
Mounin, G. (1970). *Introduction à la sémiologie*. Paris: Les Editions de Minuit.
Novick, J., Benson, R., & Rembar, J. (1981). Patterns of termination in an outpatient clinic for children and adolescents. *Journal of the American Academy of Child Psychiatry, 20*, 834–844.
Piaget, J. (1970). *Structuralism*. New York: Basic Books.
Piaget, J. (1972). *The child and reality: Problems of genetic psychology*. New York: Penguin Books.
Putnam, F. (1978, October 22). *Dissociative disorders: A developmental perspective*. Paper presented at the symposium Long Term Effects of Childhood Sexual Abuse, Annual Meeting of the American Academy of Child and Adolescent Psychiatry, Washington, DC.
Pynoos, R. S., & Eth, S. (1985). Children traumatized by witnessing acts of violence: Homicide, rape or suicidal behavior. In S. Eth & R. S. Pynoos, (Eds.), *Post-traumatic stress disorder in children*. Washington, DC: American Psychiatric Press.
Pynoos, R. S., & Eth, S. (1986). Witness to violence: The child interview. *Journal of the American Academy of Child Psychiatry, 25*, 306–319.

Searle, J. R. (1969). *Speech acts: An essay in the philosophy of language*. London: Oxford University Press.
Searle, J. R. (1971). What is a speech act? In J. R. Searle (Ed.), *The philosophy of language*. London: Cambridge University Press.
Tanguay, P. (1985). Piaget: New and improved. *Newsletter of the American Academy of Child Psychiatry, Fall*, 10–12.
Terr, L. (1988). What happens to early memories of trauma? A study of twenty children under age five at the time of documented traumatic events. *Journal of the American Academy of Child and Adolescent Psychiatry, 27*, 96–104.
van der Kolk, B. (Ed.). (1987). *Psychological trauma*. Washington, DC: American Psychiatric Press.
Wilson, P., & Hersov, L. (1985). Individual and group psychotherapy. In M. Rutter & L. Hersov (Eds.), *Textbook of child and adolescent psychiatry*. Oxford: Blackwell.

# 12

# Family Therapy
## A Context for Child Psychiatry

### Vincenzo F. DiNicola

> If we take a transpersonal view of the family, all forms of mental illness must be considered logical adaptations to a deviant and illogical transpersonal system.
> Selvini Palazzoli (1963/1978, p. 193)

*Family therapist* is not a euphonious term; Janet Malcolm (1978) complained that it sounded like a job description for a funeral home director. It does not have an authoritative sound; neither does it conjure up the impressive academic and research aura associated with such cognate disciplines as clinical psychology and psychiatry. Indeed, practitioners of this approach are always redefining themselves as structural or strategic therapists, systemic consultants, and constructivists, to name a few aliases. What this indicates is a tension in the field about what is central to the activity of family therapy: Is it united by a broad concern with the *family* (in all its social, cultural, and historical dimensions, and its clinical and developmental aspects) or divided by competing methods of *therapy* (with their diverse interviewing techniques and interventions, and their disparate views of the nature of the family, of change, and of therapy)?

To call oneself a family therapist in dealing with children's psychiatric problems is, among other things, to make a number of strategic choices about how one defines the nature of children's psychiatric problems, how to approach the treatment of such problems, and at what level to aim one's interventions. Defining the family and defining family therapy is a complex, multidisciplinary task. No definitive answer is available for this unfinished task, but one may

---

**Vincenzo F. DiNicola**   Division of Child and Adolescent Psychiatry, University of Ottawa; and Family Psychiatry Service and Adolescent Day Care Program, Royal Ottawa Hospital, Ottawa, Ontario, K1Z 7K4, Canada.

draw a *map* of the territory, make a personal *construction*, or offer a new syntax or *punctuation*, as family therapists say. In this chapter, I offer one map of the family field, review the evolution of family therapy, its major approaches, and examine current trends and problems. Along the way, I offer five propositions (numbered, in italics) that may serve as building blocks for a comprehensive family approach to child psychiatry.

## Mapping the Family Field

### The Family

1. *Families are organized around extragenetic programs or blueprints for the governance of behavior (games, myths, and scripts) that elaborate both family process and larger social and cultural roles and rules, customs and conventions.* This approach to the family was inspired by anthropologist Clifford Geertz's (1973) definition of culture. "Both systems, family and culture, are best described in terms of the programmes and rules that operate within them, rather than by any immanent features they are perceived to contain" (DiNicola, 1985, p. 85). This implies the transgenerational transmission of these blueprints or programs in the manner of myths and scripts that organize family life into a kind of game or drama. Practically, this means that the patterns and contents of what is transmitted may not be apparent on one generational plane (say, the parental couple) or even between two generations (parents and children) but may need to be examined across three generations.

This approach also takes a position on the issue of the relationship between biology and culture. Sociobiology (Wilson, 1978) has put forth a model for complex family, social and cultural behaviors that follow from biological considerations. This model, however, is controversial, and biology and culture are best treated as separate domains, linked in ways yet to be explored. An instructive analogy from cognitive psychology states that the music we hear from a record is of a different order from the apparatus that produces it. The music we hear (culture, family life) reveals little about the apparatus (biology) beyond the clarity of the recording, and the apparatus tells us little about the music played on it, except that if it is not functioning, it may not be "true" to the possibilities of the recording.

### Family Therapy

Family studies is a rich and broad field, encompassing many disciplines. In an attempt to forge a common identity for the disciplines that study the family, the overarching term *famology* was coined (Burr & Leigh, 1983). Family therapy as a mental health movement, however, is clearly identified as a clinical or therapeutic enterprise whose common concern is the family as a treatment context. The activities of the family therapy field can be divided into three areas—family theory, family therapy, and family research. Most people in the field are clinicians concerned with therapeutic aspects, including training, treatment, and evaluation. Family therapy has made an impact on the three professions that practice it most (social work, clinical psychology, and child psychiatry), although Minuchin's claim (Malcolm, 1978) that family therapy would take over psychiatry in a couple of decades was overstated.

Family therapy developed as a distinct therapeutic approach in the United States in the 1950s (Kaslow, 1980). Its origins and development there are well documented (Hoffman, 1981), and its spread to other parts of the world continues. Reviews of family therapy's growth are technical and practical, recounting the frustrations with individually oriented therapies, especially in treating severe pathology such as anorexia nervosa and schizophrenic disorders. A few writers have attempted to relate the family therapy movement to trends within child psychiatry (Malone, 1979) or to sociological considerations (Lasch, 1979).

## A Relational Context

Psychotherapies may be characterized in a few key words that highlight their features. Owing to its emphasis on the patient's intrapsychic changes in the evolution of therapy, dynamic psychotherapy is best summed up as an intrapsychic *process* therapy. This led to an elaboration of mental mechanisms as determinants of behavior. For behavior therapy, the switch from mind to behavior meant a switch from process to *outcome*. Behavior therapy is contextual in a limited way, acknowledging that the individual lives in an environment that shapes him. Family therapy is almost uniquely a *context* approach. The progression from mind to behavior is extended to *relations*, with an increasing degree of observability and verifiability. This is a progression since both mind and behavior make up experience, but family therapy attempts the greater task of placing the acquisition, development, and evolution of these components in a *relational context*. It is this overall process that produces what we call experience. The family, as the most significant relational context, is the crucible for experience. Experience is examined in the relations among components—mind to behavior, person to surround, part to whole. Accordingly, family therapy admits a new language of therapy. However, "The language of family therapy (some theorists argue that even therapy itself) is not so much a new vocabulary of therapy as a new syntax or *punctuation* of these relations" (DiNicola, 1985, p. 84).

2. *Family therapy, like family conflict, is the continuation of family process*

*by other means.* This was inspired by Von Clausewitz's (1982) definition of war ("continuation of policy by other means"), which radically redefined war as a political event, thereby placing it in the context of international relations. One of the implications of this definition of family therapy is to "normalize" the nature of family conflicts (continuation of family process) and to highlight the fact that family therapists see family conflicts cut from the same cloth as other aspects of family functioning. Accordingly, family therapy is not about some superadded disease process visited upon the family or some other factor that can be bracketed as external to the family, but rather about family process itself. Does this imply that mental disorders are emergent from family process?

## Family Therapy Models of Mental Disorders

Three models of the relation between family process and mental disorders may be distinguished:

### Relational Disorders

Mental disorders as *emergent* from family process is the strong position of some family therapy theorists and applies to some disorders. Disorders that serve as models for this position are conduct disorders and encopresis. Selvini Palazzoli (1963/1978) holds the strong view that "if we take a transpersonal view of the family, *all forms of mental illness must be considered logical adaptations to a deviant and illogical transpersonal system*" (p. 193, italics in original). In this view, mental disorders are *relational disorders*. This does not mean, however, that families "cause" mental disorders. Such mechanistic notions about the association of events, relevant for classical physics and other natural sciences, have diminishing meaning for the human sciences. Family therapists distinguish between *lineal* versus *circular causality* (Simon, Stierlin, & Wynne, 1985). Lineality describes a relation among a series of events such that the sequence does not come back to the starting point, whereas in circularity, the initial events are also affected by the progression of events, in a recursive process.

### Triggering Events

For other disorders, *family conflicts are triggering events* for underlying (individual vulnerability, be it biological or psychological) or supraordinate (social and cultural) risk factors. Disorders that serve as models for this approach are anorexia nervosa and elective mutism. Given a vulnerability that may have its roots in temperament, biological substrates, early experiences, or confounding interactions within the family and other highly valued emotional relationships, a particular child may become sensitized to the family environment, which may lead him to be perceived as disturbed/disturbing.

## Maladaptive Responses

For still other disorders, the family process becomes distorted and distorting, growing around the problem or event, as a *maladaptive response* to it. These patterns of parental behavior serve as a model for this view: protectiveness in asthma; inconsistent or inadequate limit-setting in attention-deficit hyperactivity disorder; and hostile, critical, and intrusive attitudes and behavior in schizophrenic disorders. One or both parents may display these patterns, but it is important to view them individually, each with a separate personal history, different attitudes toward his or her spouse, and toward the child. Selvini Palazzoli (personal communication, July 16, 1989) argues that each of the parents interacts with the child in a way that depends directly on the type of relationship with the partner; for example, a father will be hostile toward the very child whom the mother favors.

In all three cases, the family becomes organized around certain scripts, games, or myths (see Andolfi, Angelo, & de Nichilo, 1987/1989; Selvini Palazzoli, Cirillo, Selvini, & Sorrentino, 1988/1989) that become blueprints for elaborating behavior patterns, creating a kind of unique subculture within each family. Such patterns develop over time and are transmitted from one generation to the next as games or myths. To make sense of a given family's script in the here and now, therefore, implies looking at "family" across at least three generations.

3. *Family therapy places children, their development, and their relational problems into a natural and meaningful context.* Many such natural, social, and cultural contexts may be useful for child psychiatry, such as family, school, peer groups, caste, class, ethnic, or religious communities. However, the family is the only universal social and biological human context across cultures and through time. As a universal human context, the family is an especially fruitful portal of entry for the child psychiatrist whenever other variables are in flux — for example, working across cultures, across social class barriers, religious and ethnic differences. Only the family can provide the contextual cues of the child's natural and meaningful world. "A phenomenon remains unintelligible as long as the range of observation is not wide enough to include the context in which the phenomenon occurs" (Watzlawick, Beavin, & Jackson, 1967, pp. 20–21). Using this conceptual tool, "family therapy," according to Selvini Palazzoli (1963/1978), "is the starting point for the study of ever wider social units" (p. 241).

## Tools of the Trade

Most family therapy is done with ambulatory patients who visit family centers for treatment. A good deal of family therapy takes place in children's hospitals and agencies where the *child* may be hospitalized or attending a day treatment program for concurrent investigation or treatment; anorexia nervosa is a chief example. Usually, whole families are sent—i.e., all who live together under one roof. There are variations. Some do "family therapy" (Wcakland, 1983), especially "family of origin" work with individuals (Bowen, 1978); others involve three or more generations and other significant actors in the family drama. Another variation is a combination of family and group techniques in multiple family groups (Strelnick, 1977).

The question of concurrent therapy (pharmacotherapy, therapy for individual family members or for the parental couple, ongoing contact with the referring person) receives disparate answers. Most institutions work comfortably with a team approach where multiple modalities are easily coordinated. Some see family therapy as a first step that clarifies the nature of the problems and prepares the way for individual or marital therapy. However, boundary problems between referring sources and therapists exist both at the outset and as an ongoing irritant to therapy. These problems between systems have been addressed most explicitly by the strategic-systemic therapists, especially by the Milan associates who consider all such questions as part of the treatment context and potential "snares in family therapy," obscuring who the real patient is and what the family game is really about (Selvini Palazzoli & Prata, 1982).

Key indications for family therapy are families with symptomatic children, adolescent separation problems, psychosomatic illness, couple conflicts, family violence, threatened or actual parental separation and divorce, and problems with blended or reconstituted families (see McDermott, 1981). In many children's centers, a family assessment with or without ensuing family therapy has become the rule. Symptoms treated in family therapy range from school refusal to more serious psychotic states and life-threatening anorexia nervosa. Despite family therapy's disavowal of psychiatric diagnosis, some of its techniques have been developed to work with specific disorders, such as anorexia nervosa and schizophrenic disorders. These techniques have been applied to other children's problems as they dealt with generic issues about family structure and boundaries (in Minuchin's structural family therapy, see below) or paradoxical communications (in Milan systemic family therapy, see below). Few contraindications have been reported (Guttman, 1973), although doubts are held by clinicians about coping with acute psychotic behavior, incest, and violence without resorting to other measures, such as psychoactive drugs, hospitalization or placement, or a legal mandate for the protection of children or other family members.

Basic tools of the trade now include the use of the *one-way mirror*, with an *observing team* watching one or more therapists interact with the family. *Videotaping* and *live supervision* are now standard not only for training but for working treatment teams. The notion of a *family map* is not only a rich metaphor, it has been made into a clinical tool with the refinement of Bowen's (1978) work on family genograms by McGoldrick and Gerson (1985). A basic vocabulary of family therapy has evolved (Gerson & Barsky, 1979; Simon et al., 1985) as part of its conceptual tools. Perhaps the two most basic terms are *identified patient* and *family system*. Their implications are instructive and provocative. "Identified patient" implies that the consultant feels free to redefine the problem, to find the appropriate context for examining it, and even to question who is really the patient. To refer to a "family system" is to imply an interconnection of family members and to throw the notion of "identifying the patient" into even greater relief and doubt—all of which makes for provocation to families and fellow professionals.

4. *Family therapy is a tool for observation and for change.* "To understand how anything works, we must first try to change its function" (Kurt Lewin, cited in Selvini Palazzoli, 1963/1978, p. 201). Family therapy is often compared to anthropology because of the common feeling of the therapist being an outsider to the family's private culture. Yet anthropologists are not asked to intervene in cultures to change them, as family therapists are asked to change families. This yields different and deeper insights along with greater responsibilities. Why? Listening to the clockmaker talk about his work (anthropology) is different from taking the clock apart to fix it (family therapy). Family therapists observe and, in the act of observing, attempt changes.

## Major Family Therapy Approaches

A comprehensive review of the many current practitioners and theorists of family therapy yields an encyclopedic array of theories and methods (see Gurman & Kniskern, 1981), which includes as a broad classification (a) psychodynamic approaches, (b) behavioral and cognitive approaches, (c) intergenerational (including existential and symbolic-experiential) approaches, (d) systems theory (including structural, strategic, and systemic) approaches, and (e) the psychoeducational model. What a critical review needs, however, is a minimal map charting key notions and practices. At present, therefore, three overarching schools may be distinguished: (1) the structural schools, (2) the strategic approach, and (3) the systemic model.

### The Structural School

This is identified with psychiatrist Salvador Minuchin and the Philadelphia Child Guidance Clinic, which he directed for many years. Minuchin's first project with New York slum families led to the development of his family therapy approach, delineating now classic concepts about family structure (Minuchin, Montalvo, Guerney, Rosman, & Schumer, 1967). Structural family therapy emphasizes hierarchical relationships between parents and children, labeled parental and sibling subsystems. Observations of families led to the delineation of alliances and boundaries within and between these subsystems. Dysfunctional boundaries are understood to produce two family interaction styles. *Enmeshed* families have diffuse and poorly defined boundaries; in such families, individuals are seen as poorly differentiated, shown by individuals' inability to articulate their own thoughts, feelings, and needs. *Disengaged* families have inappropriately rigid boundaries, expressed in a lack of parental functioning, leaving young children unguided and uncared for. Alliances are relationships between family members that serve a function in the structure and attempt to redefine it. Therapeutic techniques follow from this view of the family.

Minuchin's approach to engaging the family is to unbalance the structure by affiliating or *joining* with one of the subsystems (Minuchin & Fishman, 1981). By emphasizing interactions, structural therapy bypasses what family members merely say to each other, getting them to *enact* their problems. The structural therapist is active and directive, and the restructuring work of the family happens largely within the sessions. A famous example is the "family lunch session" in the therapist's first meeting with families with an anorectic member (Rosman, Minuchin, & Liebman, 1975).

Minuchin offers two things—a clear theory of therapy that is based on an explicit theory of the family, and a technique of family therapy that follows cogently and consistently from his theory. Furthermore, he has trained many leading clinicians and his work has gained widespread acceptance. Outcome studies on his work show a high and persistent response rate (86% for anorexia nervosa; Minuchin, Rosman, & Baker, 1978). One problem may be that his school is so neatly consistent that he has painted himself into a corner. Minuchin has no heir apparent or successor to continue his work. Structural family therapy sometimes has the same ineluctable logic and self-confirming approach as psychoanalysis, leading to some of the same circular problems. To construct new therapeutic tools for different problems, one has to step away from this school altogether. For example, it is hard to import structural family therapy into cultures that do not accept active intervention with family members. A traditional Moslem family, with clear religious proscriptions about social contact between the sexes, would find it very hard to enact family dramas in front of strangers. Furthermore, such central structural notions as "enmeshment" lack specificity and appear generic when applied beyond a narrow range of North American families. Many Greek and Italian immigrant families, for example, appear enmeshed to the structural therapist when they display *familism*, a shared concern for the good of the whole family (see DiNicola, 1985, 1986).

## The Strategic Approach

This approach has more complex origins and outgrowths. Its origin is with a diverse group of social scientists in Palo Alto, California, in the 1950s. Two research groups working on similar problems spawned (1) the Brief Therapy Model associated with the Mental Research Institute (MRI) — the purest example of the strategic approach, and (2) the structural-strategic model of Jay Haley and Cloé Madanes. Haley was a member of Gregory Bateson's double-bind project, one of the two Palo Alto groups. In addition, the Palo Alto groups and the strategic therapies they developed later inspired the systemic model of the Milan associates (Selvini Palazzoli, Boscolo, Cecchin, & Prata, 1975/1978), which retained many features of the strategic approach. More on this below.

Bateson's double-bind project began at Palo Alto in 1952. This produced the most famous paper in the field of family therapy, "Toward a Theory of Schizophrenia" (Bateson, Jackson, Haley, & Weakland, 1956), an attempt to understand the paradoxical elements of communication that lead to disturbed/disturbing family behavior. Bateson, who was an anthropologist, had done earlier work in New Guinea. Bateson saw in the *Naven* ritual of the Iatmul culture a kind of balancing act in order to harmonize the relations between a child and relatives on both sides of his family, a process he called *schismogenesis* — symmetrical and complementary behavior. These and other notions of his have become basic conceptual tools, and Bateson is rightly considered one of the intellectual founders of the field. Bateson was rather laconic on clinical questions, remaining a theorist. Of his students, Haley made the greatest impact, having developed a consistent approach that may be labeled structural-strategic. Like the structural school, Haley's work highlights hierarchies, although Haley emphasizes the authority and power invested in families even more. Therapy is aimed at developing strategies that will put parents in charge of solving the problem (Haley, 1980). Assuming a confused family hierarchy, the therapist aligns with the parents *against* the problematic child, since siding with the child will aggravate the hierarchy problem. Haley's work shares with Minuchin's the technique of *reframing* — i.e., casting the behavior in a new, usually positive, light. The strategic approach also employs paradoxical techniques, directives in which the therapist "wants the [family] member to resist him so that they will change" (Haley, 1987, p. 76). Again like Minuchin, Haley is active and directive, working in the here and now, oriented to the family, and aimed at symptomatic behavior. Strategic differs from structural therapy in giving directives and setting tasks that are carried out between sessions. Strategic therapists do not articulate a theory of the family, focusing instead on devising strategies for symptom resolution.

Haley is a skillful writer whose early essays are brilliant jabs at then-current theories and therapies. He uses the same masterful control of irony and paradox with the reader ("The art of being a failure as a therapist," Haley,

1986) that he presumably uses in therapy, with powerful effects. This has understandably led to concerns about the value choices strategic therapists make, about the ethics of prescribing provocative tasks in volatile family situations, and the means/ends trade-off that is implied. On another level, beyond pragmatics (or what works), there is concern about the sincerity and authenticity of the therapist's presence (DiNicola, 1988). Another problem for child psychiatry is whether it is wise to display such verbal wizardry (sometimes perceived as manipulative) with children and adolescents who are struggling with their own sense of identity, integrity, and sincerity.

## The Systemic Model

Bateson's ideas were further developed in a clinical context by the Milan associates (Selvini Palazzoli et al., 1975/1978). Mara Selvini Palazzoli did much of the early work on anorexia nervosa, making individual dynamic and family interactional observations. After abandoning the psychoanalytic approach in the face of its meager results with this disorder, she switched to family therapy, establishing the Center for Family Studies in Milan in 1967. Adopting the systemic model, Selvini Palazzoli's group creatively translated Bateson's ideas into family therapy. Most family therapists invoke a *systemic approach* to the family, in the sense of family life as an interaction within a defined field with a rich interplay among members, rather than isolating independent events. The Milan associates founded their systemic model on a triad of influences: general system theory (Bertalanffy, 1968), the communications approach (Watzlawick et al., 1967), and especially the work of Bateson (1972) — yielding a much wider scope to their scrutiny of variables.

Some contrasts bring the defining characteristics of the Milan systemic model into focus. Haley presents the family as a hierarchy and invokes a clear structure he considers functional; the Milan model was much more concerned with the process of communication, the nature of its changing complexity (rather than a static structure). Haley's hierarchical approach implies ideas of power and control (not cybernetic metaphors), while the Milan model stressed *reflexivity* — a kind of domino theory of the family, with each member affecting every other member. Both Haley and the MRI model hold repetitive behavior as most important (focus on these patterns follows from a concern with structure); the Milan model, following Bateson, considers information primary. In this latter view, behavior is a message about the current knowledge the family holds about itself and the rest of the world, and is therefore information. Above all, the Milan therapist constructs maps that chart the family's knowledge and relations (or myths and rules).

While strategies for resolving dysfunctional interactions were adapted from strategic therapies with their emphasis on the here and now, the Milan model eschewed directiveness for *neutrality* and aimed its therapeutic interventions at the family game or construction of reality. Most fundamentally, whereas in the Milan model, "the therapists' main interest was family, not therapy," as Selvini Palazzoli et al. (1988/1989) present it, "strategic therapists tend to place therapy itself at the center of their scrutiny—one needs only to glance through the titles of some major work in the field to confirm this" (p. 7; cf. Haley, 1963, 1987).

The Milan model is the most comprehensive approach to family therapy to date, attempting to employ a systemic approach to every aspect of therapy—recording the referral, interactions with the referring person, and meeting the family. Key therapeutic tools include their method of interviewing, called *circular questioning* (Penn, 1982); *hypothesizing*, the formulation of a hypothesis based on the interview; and *neutrality*, the attempt by the therapists not to enter into alliances or coalitions with family members (Selvini Palazzoli, Boscolo, Cecchin, & Prata, 1980). Unlike Minuchin, who joins the family by unbalancing the system, the Milan associates attempted to stay out of such involvements, trying instead to guess the family game in order to construct interventions to be carried out between sessions. A guiding principle in making interventions is *positive connotation*—understanding the meaning of the system in context. The Milan associates became noted for their creative construction of *prescriptions* delivered to the family in the form of *rituals, tasks*, or *messages* from the treatment team. If the family was thought to be involved in a *paradoxical communication* holding them in an unproductive stalemate, a prescription was aimed as a *counterparadox* in order to amplify the game into checkmate, freeing the family members to change (Selvini Palazzoli et al., 1975/1978).

Such prescriptions are highly provocative and shock the system into change when well aimed. This example is from my family treatment of a young anorectic girl using Milan systemic therapy. Meeting the family for an evening appointment to accommodate the father who was an out-of-town laborer, I was confronted with his question: "What time did you get up this morning? I've been up since 5:00 a.m." I understood him to mean that he worked hard to feed his family. But his words also conveyed a paradox. In the face of such hard work, the family's food practically dipped in his blood, how dare his daughter refuse to eat? On the other hand, how could she eat food bought at such a cost? My message was to thank him for his comment, which helped me understand how frustrating it was for him to come to sessions after working hard all day to feed his family. I turned to the daughter and said I understood now what a selfless sacrifice she was making to show everybody that she would not eat more than her share, since food was such a precious commodity. I congratulated then *cautioned her not to start eating too much* or she would seem greedy and ungrateful. The whole family, furthermore, ought to thank her for her selflessness, which highlighted her father's hard work. The anorectic scenario in the family could not continue, thus reframed. The parents either had to accept my explanation for their behavior (very unlikely) or resist it and become defiant by insisting that she eat. After some reflection, the girl was bound to defy my explanation that she was selfless toward her family since she was seething with resentment and was starving herself to gain some control. I put her in a "positive bind" whereby defiance toward me would lead to healthy behavior (by eating). It is a counterparadox because my message did not suggest what the anorectic girl should do, it simply made the paradoxical family game much harder to play.

The Milan associates have now split into different teams. Boscolo and Cecchin (Boscolo, Cecchin, Hoffman, & Penn, 1987) continued their work on the circular interviewing process itself as the mainstay of therapy and are very involved in training. They are concerned in part with epistemological problems of *the family's construction of reality*, which may be characterized as neocognitivism, and partly with pragmatic issues of refining their interviewing style. Selvini Palazzoli formed a new team, continuing her clinical research with a new method she calls the *invariant prescription* and a new metaphor for family interactions she calls *family games* (Selvini Palazzoli et al., 1988/1989). With her most recent work, Selvini Palazzoli is again at the cutting edge of the field. It has generated controversy, and perhaps it is still too experimental for broad application. Nonetheless, Selvini Palazzoli has attempted a herculean task—the construction of a general model of family games involved in psychotic processes, "an effort to extract from the 'noise' of the psychotic family some recognizable recurring points" (Selvini Palazzoli, personal communication, July 16, 1989), what she has called her "road-map to schizo-land" (DiNicola, 1984).

## How Family Therapy Functions

5. *Family therapy functions by processing information, or by the method of differences.* Family therapy, unlike other therapies, is based on general system theory, cybernetics, and information theory. A key idea is from Bateson (1980), who defines information as "news of a difference." Family therapy is not only behavioral, cognitive, or interactive, but deals with an information-based view of human systems. First, the very process of meeting families is an information exchange, in which differences (in language, culture, values, and definitions of self, family, and health) yield data. This information processing involves contrasts and comparisons by the method of differences. Circular questioning (Penn, 1982), a form of metacommunication about the behavior of others in the family, is a specific application of the method of differences: "Who is most

# Family Therapy

concerned about Johnny? Who gets most upset? Who can comfort him better, mother or father?"—such questions are addressed to each family member in turn.

The interventions of family therapy can be understood as ways of feeding back, transmitting, or transforming the information obtained. Accordingly, family therapists do three things:

*Enhance Uncertainty.* Past and present information is reflected back to the family; information from inside the system is released. This is aimed at unfreezing rigidity. This may be done by circular questioning with an emphasis on neutrality (Milan style), by unbalancing the family system by joining one subsystem (Minuchin's technique), or by a more intense provocation (Andolfi et al., 1987/1989).

*Introduce Novelty.* Information is offered from the outside. Within the session, structural interventions may be enacted (Minuchin's approach). Beyond the session, rituals and tasks may be prescribed (the strategic and systemic approaches). This is aimed at providing new skills and a different view of family relationships.

*Encourage Diversity.* Diverse possibilities are imagined, old information is perceived as new (i.e., transformed), or new information is received into the system by its members. Within the session, different possibilities are explored (Minuchin gets the family to enact new scenarios; the Milan associates ask *future questions*—Penn, 1985). Beyond the session, the family is encouraged to experiment with alternative interactions. This is aimed at the family's discovering new solutions for itself.

There is a progression here from pathology to health ("rigidity" to "new solutions") and from active involvement of the therapist to his withdrawing from center stage and the family's taking over without him.

## Maturity of Family Therapy

After some 30 years, the field of family therapy has achieved a degree of maturity. Family therapy is accepted in the therapeutic tool kits of the mental health professions. Institutes of family therapy are thriving in many large cities in North America and Europe. Numerous marital and family therapy journals with original clinical and research papers in most European languages are well established. A chapter on family therapy routinely appears in review texts of child psychiatry (e.g., Dare, 1985).

Furthermore, the field now has numerous integrative overviews (e.g.,

Hoffman, 1981) and handbooks of techniques. The handbook of family therapy (Gurman & Kniskern, 1981) and the handbook of marital therapy (Jacobson & Gurman, 1985) are solid and competent overviews of both theory and technique. A handbook of measurements for marriage and family therapy (Fredman & Sherman, 1987) critically reviews the available measurements of family assessment, marital communication and intimacy scales, marital satisfaction and adjustment, and family inventories. Another important marker of theoretical maturity is the appearance of a basic vocabulary of family terms (Gerson & Barsky, 1979) and a book-length treatment of the language of family therapy (Simon et al., 1985). Books on practical issues abound (see Gurman, 1981).

Supervision (Whiffen & Byng-Hall, 1982) is increasingly the topic at meetings and in journals. The major approaches have their own models of training (e.g., Andolfi & Menghi, 1980; Boscolo & Cecchin, 1982). Training techniques that are very specific to the problems of treating families have emerged; for example, the "family of origin technique" (Braverman, 1982) has become a kind of analogue to the training analysis.

Two other topics that signal family therapy's development are reports of failures and increasing concern with ethical issues. Family therapy failures received a full-length multiauthored treatment (Coleman, 1985). This raises the larger questions of the indications and contraindications of family therapy and the hope for family therapy to take its place in the differential therapeutics of child psychiatry rather than to act as a competing approach (Malone, 1979). Within mainstream psychiatry, two trends that are hallmarks of its maturity are (1) the evolution of a comprehensive, reliable diagnostic schema (DSM-III-R) with widespread acceptance, and (2) differential therapeutics (Frances, Clarkin, & Perry, 1984). In its attempt to construe mental illness in relational terms, has family therapy refused to deal with the disease process and its impact on family process? This raises two related problems in family therapy: (1) problems in diagnosis and classification and (2) indications (McDermott, 1981) and contraindications (Guttman, 1973).

In general, family therapy has attempted to redefine issues in psychiatric diagnosis as issues about the classification of family interactional styles (e.g., Minuchin's notions of enmeshment and disengagement), or to find interactional patterns for specific disorders (e.g., Selvini Palazzoli's typology of family games in psychotic disorders). However, other workers are developing specialized techniques by diagnosis (or differential therapeutics). Recent examples are family work with affective disorders (Clarkin, Haas, & Glick, 1988a; DiNicola, 1989), eating disorders (Sargent, Liebman, & Silver, 1985; Schwartz, Barrett, & Saba, 1985), and schizophrenia (Anderson, Reiss, & Hogarty, 1986). Evaluating the outcome of family therapy parallels the problems of evaluating the psychotherapies and has special problems of its own. A sound (though dated) review is available in Gurman and Kniskern (1981). There is unquestionably more work to be done on outcome in light of family therapy's maturing approach to diagnosis and differential therapeutics.

Another trend in recent years has been serious attention to the integration of disparate family therapy models (Fraser, 1984; Rakoff, 1984; Roberts, 1984) and family therapy's relationships with other psychotherapies, such as marital therapy and individual therapy (Martin, 1977). There has also been a "rediscovery" of the individual (Minuchin, 1985). While family therapy may have always been practiced in an eclectic way, it is now being actively integrated with other therapeutic modalities, such as psychopharmacology (Epstein, Keitner, Bishop, & Miller, 1988) and inpatient treatment (Clarkin, Haas, & Glick, 1988b).

Family therapists have also examined the problems of building family therapy teams within eclectic institutions (see Boscolo & Cecchin, 1982) and problems of how different systems get in the way of family treatment. Interagency problems, problems of complex systems, and working with larger systems such as school boards are difficult but rewarding issues being examined (Selvini Palazzoli et al., 1981/1986). Family therapy's relationship to child psychiatry, once declared a war (McDermott & Char, 1974), has now achieved a productive coexistence (Malone, 1979), and the issue is now what family therapy and child psychiatry have to learn from each other (Grunebaum & Belfer, 1986).

Ethical problems with family therapy have been raised by practitioners themselves (DiNicola, 1988; Walrond-Skinner & Watson, 1987) as well as by critics (Maranhão, 1984). Family therapy also addresses larger social issues concerning the family within the wider social network (Foulks, 1981), values (Stein, 1985), and family therapy's response to the social forces that shape violence within the family (S. Minuchin, 1984). Problems in providing service to different ethnic groups (McGoldrick, Pearce, & Giordano, 1982) and other cross-cultural issues (Falicov, 1983), including its applicability in other cultures (DiNicola, 1985, 1986), are now fruitfully addressed.

There is a recent coalescence of themes among senior family therapists around the notion of family life as a narrative. Some earlier concepts were family rules, family myths, family rituals. Later, theorists commented on family scripts and the family drama. Recently, the family story or narrative and family games are commonly used metaphors for family life. The progression is from a series of concepts in which family patterns are seen as rigidly encoded, like the genetic code, to a more complex and less deterministic notion of the family story as a narrative that may be read, edited, and interpreted in various ways. This offers the family an opportunity to take charge of its own fate, making the therapist less active and directive. There is also a progression from the neobehavioral "here and now" of the strategic therapists to the "system-with-a-history" of Selvini Palazzoli's recent work on family games, and Andolfi's three-generational model of family myths.

## Controversies

From the early work on schizophrenia and the family in the 1950s to the present, the schizophrenic disorders have been at the center of family therapy activity. The Bateson group's (1956) paper on the double-bind theory of schizophrenia received enormous clinical and research attention. And while that theory is now discredited, there is no doubt that it generated a family approach to the disorders. Critics are likely to forget that antipsychotic drugs came on the scene at the very same time and took years to establish their clinical efficacy (and dangers). After decades of research, there are still only two clinically relevant aspects of treatment: antipsychotic drugs, which are the mainstay for stabilization and maintenance, and family interactions, which may be more or less beneficial to individuals with schizophrenic disorders. Current research suggests that appropriate management should include specialized attention to both aspects.

The research on expressed emotion (EE) in families with schizophrenic patients (Vaughn & Leff, 1976), along with the psychoeducational model (Anderson et al., 1986), has provided some proven and widely accepted tools for family management. This work is not squarely in the family therapy tradition, although it is welcome because it is research-based and compatible with mainstream family therapy since it emphasizes the family as an adaptive and resourceful system. Selvini Palazzoli's latest family work is also on psychotic disorders, and a controversy has arisen between her totally family-oriented approach and the more eclectic models of Anderson and the EE researchers. Nonetheless, all workers agree on the importance of family factors. Manfred Bleuler (1982), perhaps the leading authority on the schizophrenias and son of the psychiatrist who coined the term, has said, "It is certain that many life experiences, particularly those connected with the patient's family, play a role in the development of schizophrenia" (p. 11).

Other critiques have examined family therapy's expansion into wider, cultural aspects of the family. Maranhão (1984), an anthropologist, offered a cogent and biting review of the McGoldrick et al. (1982) volume on ethnicity and family therapy. He lamented the use of short ethnic vignettes as "cultural snapshots," concluding that family therapy lacked seriousness when addressing such aspects. In a critique of the "workshop circuit" (McLean, 1986), in which prominent family therapists present their work and do live consultations with families, concern was expressed about the mechanistic features of the treatment model, packaged as marketable commodities (workshops, training tapes), and the dispassionate distance it created between the therapist and the family. While these points apply to other therapies, they are more cogent for family therapists, who argue (as I do) that this approach emphasizes the social and contextual nature of mental illness.

Finally, to date no one profession "owns" family therapy, although social workers are the most numerous practitioners. There are problems with setting appropriate standards for training, supervision, and standards of practice that apply across professions. Efforts to establish marital and family therapy as a separate profession are evident, though not welcome to all. A trenchant critique of family therapy's professionalization is offered by Treacher (1986), who fears that it will become a "disabling profession" by gaining higher status for its practitioners while restricting access to and dissemination of its knowledge. The history of the helping professions, including psychiatry, suggests that the enshrinement of specific treatment approaches, such as psychoanalysis, into separate institutes leads to decreased communication with other practitioners, while increasing their insularity.

## Conclusion

The contextual approach of family therapy admits the study of "ever wider social units" in an era of increasing atomization of children's psychiatric disorders down to their "biological roots." While the biological approach holds promise to produce valuable insights with clinical implications, its data about children out of context sometimes have a disembodied quality. A family approach may help to give the more isolated data of biological research a natural context for clinical applications.

These five propositions, developed in the foregoing overview of the field of family therapy, may serve as building blocks for a comprehensive family approach to child psychiatry:

1. Families are organized around extragenetic programs or blueprints for the governance of behavior (games, myths, and scripts) that elaborate both family process and larger social and cultural roles and rules, customs and conventions.
2. Family therapy, like family conflict, is the continuation of family process by other means.
3. Family therapy places children, their development, and their relational problems into a natural and meaningful context.
4. Family therapy is a tool for both observation and for change.
5. Family therapy functions by processing information, or by the method of differences.

ACKNOWLEDGMENTS. I wish to thank Professor Mara Selvini Palazzoli, M.D., for her critical review of this chapter, and Professor Raymond Prince, M.D., editor-in-chief of *Transcultural Psychiatric Research Review*, for permission to expand and update some material that first appeared in an overview in Volume XXII, Issue 2 (1985), on family therapy and transcultural psychiatry.

## References

Anderson, C. M., Reiss, D. J., & Hogarty, G. E. (1986). *Schizophrenia and the family: A practitioner's guide to psychoeducation and management*. New York: Guilford Press.

Andolfi, M., Angelo, M., & de Nichilo, M. (1989). *The myth of Atlas: Families and the therapeutic story* (V. F. DiNicola, Ed. & Trans.). New York: Brunner/Mazel. (Original work published 1987)

Andolfi, M., & Menghi, P. (1980). A model for training in family therapy. In M. Andolfi & I. Zwerling (Eds.), *Dimensions of family therapy* (pp. 239–259). New York: Guilford Press.

Bateson, G. (1972). *Steps to an ecology of mind*. New York: Ballantine Books.

Bateson, G. (1980). *Mind and nature: A necessary unity*. New York: Ballantine Books.

Bateson, G., Jackson, D. D., Haley, J., & Weakland, J. H. (1956). Toward a theory of schizophrenia. *Behavioral Science, 1*, 251–264.

Bertalanffy, L. von. (1968). *General system theory*. New York: George Braziller.

Bleuler, M. (1982). Manfred Bleuler. In M. Shepherd (Ed.), *Psychiatrists on psychiatry* (pp. 1–13). Cambridge: Cambridge University Press.

Boscolo, L., & Cecchin, G. (1982). Training in systemic therapy at the Milan centre. In R. Whiffen & J. Byng-Hall (Eds.), *Family therapy supervision: Recent developments in practice* (pp. 153–165). New York: Grune & Stratton.

Boscolo, L., Cecchin, G., Hoffman, L., & Penn, P. (1987). *Milan systemic family therapy: Conversations in theory and practice*. New York: Basic Books.

Bowen, M. (1978). *Family therapy in clinical practice*. New York: Jason Aronson.

Braverman, S. (1982). Family of origin as a training resource for family therapists. *Canadian Journal of Psychiatry, 27*, 629–633.

Burr, W. R., & Leigh, G. K. (1983). Famology: A new discipline. *Journal of Marriage and the Family, 45*, 467–480.

Clarkin, J. F., Haas, G. L., & Glick, I. D. (Eds.). (1988a). *Affective disorders and the family: Assessment and treatment*. New York: Guilford Press.

Clarkin, J. F., Haas, G. L., & Glick, I. D. (1988b). Inpatient family intervention. In J. F. Clarkin, G. L. Haas, & I. D. Glick (Eds.), *Affective disorders and the family: Assessment and treatment* (pp. 134–152). New York: Guilford Press.

Coleman, S. B. (Ed.). (1985). *Failures in family therapy*. New York: Guilford Press.

Dare, C. (1985). Family therapy. In M. Rutter & L. Hersov (Eds.), *Child and adolescent psychiatry: Modern approaches* (2nd ed., pp. 809–825). Oxford: Blackwell Scientific Publications.

DiNicola, V. F. (1984). Road-map to schizo-land: Mara Selvini Palazzoli and the Milan model of systemic family therapy. *Journal of Strategic and Systemic Therapies, 3*(2), 50–62.

DiNicola, V. F. (1985). Family therapy and transcultural psychiatry: An emerging synthesis. *Transcultural Psychiatric Research Review, 22*(2 & 3), 81–113; 151–180.

DiNicola, V. F. (1986). Beyond Babel: Family therapy as cultural translation. *International Journal of Family Psychiatry, 7*, 179–191.

DiNicola, V. F. (1988). Saying it and meaning it: Forging an ethic for family therapy. *Journal of Strategic and Systemic Therapies, 7*(4), 1–7.

DiNicola, V. F. (1989). The child's predicament in families with a mood disorder: Research findings and family interventions. *Psychiatric Clinics of North America, 12*(4), 933–949.

Epstein, N. B., Keitner, G. I., Bishop, D. S., & Miller, I. W. (1988). Combined use of pharmacological and family therapy. In J. F. Clarkin, G. L. Haas, & I. D. Glick (Eds.), *Affective disorders and the family: Assessment and treatment* (pp. 153–172). New York: Guilford Press.

Falicov, C. J. (Ed.). (1983). *Cultural perspectives in family therapy*. Rockville, MD: Aspen Systems Corporation.

Foulks, E. F. (1981). Social network therapies and society: An overview. *International Journal of Family Therapy, 3*, 316–320.

Frances, A., Clarkin, J. F., & Perry, S. (1984). *Differential therapeutics in psychiatry: The art and science of treatment selection*. New York: Brunner/Mazel.
Fraser, J. S. (Ed.). (1984). Two issues on integrating the models. Part one: Special issue on integration/disintegration. *Journal of Strategic and Systemic Therapies, 3*(3).
Fredman, N., & Sherman, R. (1987). *Handbook of measurements for marriage and family therapy*. New York: Brunner/Mazel.
Geertz, C. (1973). The impact of the concept of culture on the concept of man. In *The interpretation of cultures* (pp. 33–54). New York: Basic Books.
Gerson, M. J., & Barsky, M. (1979). For the new family therapist: A glossary of terms. *American Journal of Family Therapy, 7*, 15–30.
Grunebaum, H., & Belfer, M. L. (1986). What family therapists might learn from child psychiatry. *Journal of Marital and Family Therapy, 12*, 415–423.
Gurman, A. S. (Ed.). (1981). *Questions and answers in the practice of family therapy*. New York: Brunner/Mazel.
Gurman, A. S., & Kniskern, D. P. (Eds.). (1981). *Handbook of family therapy*. New York: Brunner/Mazel.
Guttman, H. (1973). A contraindication for family therapy. *Archives of General Psychiatry, 29*, 352–355.
Haley, J. (1963). *Strategies of psychotherapy*. New York: Grune & Stratton.
Haley, J. (1980). *Leaving home*. New York: McGraw-Hill.
Haley, J. (1986). *The power tactics of Jesus Christ and other essays* (2nd ed.). Rockville, MD: Triangle Press.
Haley, J. (1987). *Problem-solving therapy* (2nd ed.). San Francisco: Jossey-Bass.
Hoffman, L. (1981). *Foundations of family therapy, a conceptual framework for systems change*. New York: Basic Books.
Jacobson, N. S., & Gurman, A. S. (Eds.). (1985). *Clinical handbook of marital therapy*. New York: Guilford Press.
Kaslow, F. W. (1980). History of family therapy in the United States. *Marriage and Family Review, 3*, 77–111.
Lasch, C. (1979). *Haven in a heartless world: The family besieged*. New York: Basic Books.
Malcolm, J. (1978). A reporter at large: The one-way mirror. *New Yorker*, May 15, 39–114.
Malone, C. A. (1979). Child psychiatry and family therapy. *Journal of the American Academy of Child Psychiatry, 18*, 4–21.
Maranhão, T. (1984). Family therapy and anthropology. *Culture, Medicine and Psychiatry, 8*, 255–279.
Martin, F. (1977). Some implications from the theory and practice of family therapy for individual therapy (and vice versa). *British Journal of Medical Psychology, 50*, 53–64.
McDermott, J. F., Jr. (1981). Indications for family therapy. *Journal of the American Academy of Child Psychiatry, 20*, 409–419.
McDermott, J. F., Jr., & Char, W. F. (1974). The undeclared war between child and family therapy. *Journal of the American Academy of Child Psychiatry, 13*, 422–436.
McGoldrick, M., & Gerson, R. (1985). *Genograms in family assessment*. New York: W. W. Norton.
McGoldrick, M., Pearce, J. K., & Giordano, J. (Eds.). (1982). *Ethnicity and family therapy*. New York: Guilford Press.
McLean, A. (1986). Family therapy workshops in the United States: Potential abuses in the production of therapy in an advanced capitalist society. *Social Science and Medicine, 23*, 179–189.
Minuchin, P. (1985). Families and individual development: Provocations from the field of family therapy. *Child Development, 56*, 289–302.

Minuchin, S. (1984). *Family kaleidoscope: Images of violence and healing*. Cambridge, MA: Harvard University Press.
Minuchin, S., & Fishman, H. C. (1981). *Family therapy techniques*. Cambridge, MA: Harvard University Press.
Minuchin, S., Montalvo, B., Guerney, B. G., Rosman, B. L., & Schumer, F. (1967). *Families of the slums: An exploration of their structure and treatment*. New York: Basic Books.
Minuchin, S., Rosman, B. L., & Baker, L. (1978). *Psychosomatic families: Anorexia nervosa in context*. Cambridge, MA: Harvard University Press.
Penn, P. (1982). Circular questioning. *Family Process, 21*, 267–280.
Penn, P. (1985). Feed forward: Future questions, future maps. *Family Process, 24*, 299–311.
Rakoff, V. (1984). The necessity for multiple models in family therapy. *Journal of Family Therapy, 6*, 199–210.
Roberts, J. (Ed.). (1984). Two issues on integrating the models. Part two—Special issue on integration—Case studies: Mixing and switching models in clinical practice. *Journal of Strategic and Systemic Therapies, 3*(4).
Rosman, B. L., Minuchin, S., & Liebman, R. (1975). Family lunch session: An introduction to family therapy in anorexia nervosa. *American Journal of Orthopsychiatry, 45*, 846–853.
Sargent, J., Liebman, R., & Silver, M. (1985). Family therapy for anorexia nervosa. In D. M. Garner & P. E. Garfinkel (Eds.), *Handbook of psychotherapy for anorexia nervosa and bulimia* (pp. 257–279). New York: Guilford Press.
Schwartz, R. C., Barrett, M. J., & Saba, G. (1985). Family therapy for bulimia. In D. M. Garner & P. E. Garfinkel (Eds.), *Handbook of psychotherapy for anorexia nervosa and bulimia* (pp. 280–307). New York: Guilford Press.
Selvini Palazzoli, M. (1978). *Self-starvation: From individual to family therapy in the treatment of anorexia nervosa* (A. Pomerans, Trans.). New York: Jason Aronson. (Original work published 1963)
Selvini Palazzoli, M., Anolli, L., DiBlasio, P., Giossi, L., Pisano, I., Ricci., C., Sacchi, & Ugazio, V. (1986). *The hidden games of organizations* (A. Pomerans, Trans.). New York: Pantheon. (Original work published 1981)
Selvini Palazzoli, M., Boscolo, L., Cecchin, G., & Prata, G. (1978). *Paradox and counterparadox: A new model in the therapy of the family in schizophrenic transaction* (E. V. Burt, Trans.). New York: Jason Aronson. (Original work published 1975)
Selvini Palazzoli, M., Boscolo, L., Cecchin, G., & Prata, G. (1980). Hypothesizing—circularity—neutrality: Three guidelines for the conductor of the session. *Family Process, 19*, 3–12.
Selvini Palazzoli, M., Cirillo, S., Selvini, M., & Sorrentino, A. M. (1989). *Family games: General models of psychotic processes in the family* (V. Kleiber, Trans.). New York: W. W. Norton. (Original work published 1988)
Selvini Palazzoli, M., & Prata, G. (1982). Snares in family therapy. *Journal of Marital and Family Therapy, 8*, 443–450.
Simon, F. B., Stierlin, H., & Wynne, L. C. (1985). *The language of family therapy: A systemic vocabulary and sourcebook*. New York: Family Process Press.
Stein, H. F. (1985). Values and family therapy. In J. Schwartzman (Ed.), *Families and other systems* (pp. 201–243). New York: Guilford Press.
Strelnick, A. H. (1977). Multiple family group therapy: A review of the literature. *Family Process, 16*, 307–325.
Treacher, A. (1986). Invisible patients, invisible families—A critical exploration of some technocratic trends in family therapy. *Journal of Family Therapy, 8*, 267–306.
Vaughn, C. E., & Leff, J. P. (1976). The influence of family and social factors on the course of psychiatric illness. *British Journal of Psychiatry, 129*, 125–137.
Von Clausewitz, C. (1982). *On war*. New York: Penguin.

Walrond-Skinner, S., & Watson, D. (Eds.). (1987). *Ethical issues in family therapy*. New York: Routledge & Kegan Paul.
Watzlawick, P., Beavin, J. H., & Jackson, D. D. (1967). *Pragmatics of human communication*. New York: Norton.
Weakland, J. H. (1983). "Family therapy" with individuals. *Journal of Strategic and Systemic Therapies, 2*(4), 1–9.
Wilson, E. O. (1978). *On human nature*. Cambridge, MA: Harvard University Press.

# Index

Aberrant Behavior Checklist, 85
Abnormal Involuntary Movement Scale, 81
Acting-out, 183
Adolescents, depression treatment, 19–29
　adult-oriented treatment, 19–20
　biological therapies, 23–26
　combined treatment, 26
　psychological therapies, 20–23
Affective disorders
　anxiety disorder and, 33–34
　dysphasia and, 173, 173
　familial, 139
　family therapy, 212
Aggression; *see also* Self-injurious behavior
　anorexia nervosa and, 124
　antisocial, 5
　　characteristics, 9–10
　assessment, 85
　associated features, 10
　attentional deficit hyperactivity disorder and, 85–86
　conduct disorders and, 9–10
　hyperactivity and, 1, 2
　mental retardation and, 83
　oppositional disorders and, 9–10
　prevalence, 11
　prognosis, 10–11
　sex ratio, 11
　treatment, 11–14, 85–86
　　hospitalization, 83, 85
　　pharmacological, 13–14, 85–91, 144
Agnosia, auditory verbal, 167
Agoraphobia, 34, 35
Al-Anon, 106
AlaTeen, 106
Alcoholics Anonymous, 102, 106
Alcoholism
　attention deficit hyperactivity disorder and, 5

Alcoholism (*Cont.*)
　complications, 102
　depression and, 34, 36
　symptoms, 103
　treatment
　　legislation regarding, 101
　　pharmacological, 134
　　WHO report, 99
　withdrawal, 104, 105, 107–110
Alexithymic personality disorder, 120
Alpha-blockers, 105
Alprazolam
　as obsessive-compulsive disorder therapy, 64
　as school phobia therapy, 41–43, 139
　as separation anxiety therapy, 143
Amitriptyline, 24, 63
Amphetamine, abuse, 99
d-Amphetamine
　as attention deficit hyperactivity disorder therapy, 6, 7, 86, 135–136
　dopamine interaction, 137
　norepinephrine interaction, 137
　as stereotypy cause, 86
Anorexia nervosa
　bulimia and, 18, 128
　chronicity, 118, 130
　definition, 117–118
　denial in, 120
　as family therapy model, 202
　incidence, 129
　in males, 124
　mental illness and, 127, 128
　mortality due to, 127
　personality disorders and, 120, 124
　prevention, 130
　relapse, 118, 127
　spontaneous cure, 118
　treatment, 115–132

Anorexia nervosa (*Cont.*)
  treatment (*Cont.*)
    art therapy, 123
    choice of, 128–129
    core therapy, 121, 124, 125, 129
    factors affecting, 116
    family therapy, 121, 122–123, 204
    group therapy, 122–123, 128
    hospitalization, 124–127
    indications for, 128–129
    informational aspect, 118
    integrated model, 117–128
    milieu therapy, 124–125, 128
    movement therapy, 123–124, 128–129
    outcome, 127–128, 130–131
    outpatient treatment, 118
    pharmacological therapy, 124, 129, 134, 140–141
    psychotherapy, 120–121
    self-supporting therapy, 120–121
    supportive therapy, 119
    therapist's qualities, 117
    weight gain, 120, 124, 125
Anosognosia, 172
Antiaggressive drugs, 144; *see also* Aggression, treatment, pharmacological
Antiandrogenic therapy, 64
Anticonvulsants
  as conduct disorder-related epilepsy therapy, 14
  as psychotropic agents, 144
  withdrawal applications, 105, 109
Antidepressants, 137–138; *see also* Tricyclic antidepressants
  as depression therapy, 13, 23–25
  as bulimia therapy, 124
  as eating disorder therapy, 140–141
Antihistamines, as anxiolytics, 143
Antipsychotics, 141–142
  as aggression therapy, 144
  as anxiolytics, 143
  as autism therapy, 142
  withdrawal, 141–142
Antisocial behavior
  aggression and, 5, 9–10
  hyperactivity and, 2
Antisocial personality, parental, 5
Anxiety
  affective disorder and, 33–34
  depression and, 33

Anxiety (*Cont.*)
  drug abuse and, 36, 104
  dysphasia and, 173
  obsessive–compulsive disorder and, 55
  pharmacological treatment, 40, 143
  prevalence, 35
  school phobia and, 32–33, 42
    familial factors, 34–36
Anxiolytics, 143
Aptness, therapeutic, 189–192
Arousal, 55–56
Art therapy, 123, 128
Aspartame, 156–160
Atenolol, 89
Attention deficit disorders
  differential diagnosis, 4
  *DSM–III* classification, 1, 2–3
  pharmacological treatment, 8, 138–139
Attention deficit hyperactivity disorder
  alcoholism and, 5
  associated features, 3
  conduct disorders and, 1–2
  diagnosis, 2–6
  diet therapy, 154–155
  differential diagnosis, 4
  etiology, 5–6, 137
  familial factors, 5, 6, 7
  hyperactivity and, 1, 2–3, 8–9
  impulsivity and, 2, 3, 8, 9, 13
  onset age, 5
  oppositional disorder and, 2
  prevalence, 4–5
  sex ratio, 4–5
  treatment, 6–9
    behavior therapy, 8–9
    pharmacological, 6–8, 14, 15, 85- 86, 135–137, 138–139
Autism, 77–98
  assessment, 78
  *DSM–III* classification, 78
  early infantile, 77–78
  history, 77–78
  intelligence quotient, 78
  onset age, 77
  prevalence, 78
  seizures and, 78
  self-injurious behavior and, 83
  sex ratio, 78
  stereotypy and, 80–81, 82, 83

# Index

Autism (*Cont.*)
  treatment
    behavior therapy, 79
    pharmacological, 78, 79–83, 84, 90, 142

Barbiturates
  abuse, 99
  as anxiolytics, 143
  withdrawal, 105, 110–111
Bateson, Gregory, 207
Beck Depression Inventory, 21, 35
Behavior, communicative, 183–184
Behavioral Observation System, 78
Behavior therapy
  for anorexia nervosa, 128
  for attention deficit hyperactivity disorder, 8–9
  for autism, 79
  for conduct disorders, 11–12
  contextual approach, 201
  for hyperactivity, 8–9
  for obsessive–compulsive disorder, 52–60, 68–69
    behavioral models and, 54–56
  for oppositional defiant disorders, 11–12
Bellevue Index of Depression, 21
Benadryl: *see* Diphenhydramine
Benzodiazepines
  adverse effects, 143
  as anxiety therapy, 40
  efficacy, 143
  as obsessive–compulsive disorder therapy, 63–64
  withdrawal from, 143
  in withdrawal therapy, 105
Beta-blockers
  as aggression therapy, 89
  as autism therapy, 89
  as self-injurious behavior therapy, 89
  withdrawal applications, 105
Bipolar disorder, 13, 144
Borderline conditions, 134
Borderline personality disorder, 124
Brief Therapy Model, 207
Bulimia nervosa, 115
  anorexia nervosa and, 118, 125, 128
  pharmacological treatment, 124, 134, 137, 140–141
Bupropion, 138
Buspirone, 105

Carbamazepine
  as aggression therapy, 88–89, 90, 91, 144
  as conduct disorder therapy, 14
  withdrawal applications, 105
Child abuse, 185, 189
Childhood Autism Rating Scale, 78
Children's Depression Index, 33
Children's Depression Rating Scale, 33, 36
Children's Depression Scale, 32
Children's Manifest Anxiety Scale, 33, 35, 36, 42
Children's Psychiatric Rating Scale, 78, 85, 157
Chloral hydrate, 105, 109
Chlordiazepoxide
  as obsessive–compulsive disorder therapy, 63
  as school phobia therapy, 39–40
  withdrawal applications, 105
Chloroprothixene, 63
Chlorpromazine
  as attention deficit hyperactivity disorder therapy, 8
  as autism therapy, 79
  contraindications in epilepsy, 141
  as obsessive–compulsive disorder therapy, 63
  seizure threshold effects, 78, 79
  withdrawal applications, 104, 108, 112
Clinical Global Impressions, 78
Clomipramine
  as behavior disorder therapy, 138
  as obsessive–compulsive disorder therapy, 61–63, 65, 66, 67, 140
  as school phobia therapy, 40–41, 139
Clonidine
  as attention deficit hyperactivty disorder therapy, 8, 137
  as conduct disorder therapy, 14
  as obsessive–compulsive disorder therapy, 64
  as Tourette's syndrome therapy, 142
  withdrawal applications, 105, 111–112
Clorgyline, 62, 63
Cocaine
  abuse, 100
  withdrawal, 105
Cognitive–behavioral therapy
  for attention deficit hyperactivity disorder, 9

Cognitive–behavioral therapy (*Cont.*)
  for depression, 21–22
  for school phobia, 44
Cognitive development, in dysphasia, 165
Cognitive function
  dietary factors, 157–160
  psychoactive drug effects, 78
Cognitive processes, 179–181
Communication
  with children, 179, 181–184
  paradoxical, 209
Comprehensive Psychiatric Rating Scale–Obsessive Compulsive Subscale, 51
Conditioning
  aversive/avoidance, 54, 57
  instrumental, 54
  operant, 60
Conduct disorders
  aggression and, 9–10, 144
    hospitalization effects, 83, 85
  attention deficit hyperactivity disorder and, 1–2
  definition, 10
  diagnostic work-up, 15
  differential diagnosis, 4
  *DSM–III* classification, 1, 2, 10
  dysphasia and, 173
  as family therapy model, 202
  prevalence, 11
  prognosis, 10–11
  school phobia and, 33
  sex ratio, 11
  treatment, 11–14
    pharmacological, 13–14, 138–139
Conners Parent Rating Scale, 157
Conners Parent–Teacher Questionnaire, 78
Connotation, positive, 209
Consciousness, behavioral states of, 182
Cortisol, 139
Culture, 200

Defiant disorder, school phobia and, 33
Denial
  in anorexia nervosa, 117, 120
  in obsessive–compulsive disorder, 51
Depression
  alcoholism and, 34, 36
  anxiety disorder and, 33
  factors associated with, 19

Depression (*Cont.*)
  panic disorder and, 34
  school phobia and, 32, 42
    familial factors, 34–36
  symptoms, 139
  treatment, 19–29
    adult-oriented treatment, 19–20
    biological therapies, 23–26
    combined treatment, 26
    family therapy, 140
    pharmacological, 134, 137, 139–140
    psychological therapies, 20–23
Desensitization, systemic, 56, 57
Desipramine
  as attention deficit hyperactivity disorder therapy, 7, 8
  as depression therapy, 24, 25, 140
  as eating disorder therapy, 141
  as obsessive–compulsive disorder therapy, 62
Detoxification, 104–106; *see also* Withdrawal
Dexamethasone suppression test, 139
Dextroamphetamine, 6
*Diagnostic and Statistical Manual–III*, diagnostic criteria
  attention deficit disorders, 1, 2–3
  autism, 78
  conduct disorders, 2, 10
  disruptive behavior, 1
  hyperactivity, 2
Diazepam
  as obsessive–compulsive disorder therapy, 63
  as schizophrenia therapy, 143
  withdrawal applications, 105, 108, 110, 112
Diet therapy, 151–162
  for attention deficit hyperactivity disorder, 8
  Feingold, 154, 155
  oligoantigenic, 153
  for withdrawal, 109–110
Diphenhydramine, 104, 108
L-Dopa, 8
Dopamine, 137
Doubting, in obsessive–compulsive disorder, 51
Doxepin, 63
Drug abuse
  anxiety and, 36
  effects, 100
  HIV infection and, 106

Drug abuse (*Cont.*)
  legislation regarding treatment, 101
  trends, 99–100
  WHO survey, 99
Dyskinesia
  antipsychotics-related, 8, 141
  neuroleptics-related, 87
    stereotypy and, 80–81
  oro-buccal-lingual, 80
  tardive, 8
Dyslexia, 136
Dysphasia, developmental
  amnesic, 167
  associated disorders, 164, 171, 172–173
  cognitive development effects, 165
  conduction, 167
  definition, 163
  dyspraxic, 168
  etiology, 174
  lexical syntactic syndrome, 167, 169
  phonological productive syndrome, 167
  prevention, 174
  receptive, 167–168, 172–173
  semantic pragmatic syndrome, 167, 168
  treatment
    academic acquisitions, 170
    conceptualization of, 165–166
    imagery, 174
    medical model, 173–174
    motivations for, 164–165
    neuropsychological model, 166–168
    organization of, 170–173
    therapeutic strategies, 168–170
Dyspraxia, verbal, 169
Dysthymia, 134

Eating disorders; *see also* Anorexia nervosa; Bulimia nervosa
  diagnosistic criteria, 115
  pharmacological treatment, 140–141
Ego, observing, 177
Electroconvulsive therapy, for depression, 26
Enuresis
  dysphasia and, 173
  pharmacological treatment, 137, 138
Epilepsy, 14, 141; *see also* Seizures
Exposure, as obsessive–compulsive disorder therapy, 57, 58–59

Familism, 206
Family games, 210, 213
Family therapist, 199
Family therapy, 199–219
  for anorexia nervosa, 121, 122–123, 204
  approaches, 205–210
    strategic, 207–208
    structural, 205–206
    systemic, 208–210
  concurrent therapy, 204
  for depression, 23, 140
  development of, 211–213
  ethical problems, 213
  family field mapping, 200–202, 205
  functioning of, 210–211
  indications for, 204
  mental disorder models in, 202–203
  for obsessive–compulsive disorder, 53, 69
  problems in, 212
  for schizophrenia, 212, 214
  for school phobia, 44
  techniques, 204–205
  terminology, 205, 212
Famology, 200
Feingold diet, 154, 155
Fenfluramine, as autism therapy, 81–82, 84, 90, 142
Flooding, cognitive, 56–57
Fluoxetine, 140
Fluoxetine
  as depression therapy, 140
  as eating disorder therapy, 141
  as obsessive–compulsive disorder therapy, 64, 65, 67, 69
Fluphenazine, 141
  efficacy, 141
Flurazepam, 108
Fluvoxamine, as obsessive–compulsive disorder therapy, 67, 69, 140
Food additives, 6, 154–155
Food allergy, 152–153
Food dye, 154–155
Freud, Sigmund, 177

Genogram, 23
Group therapy
  for anorexia nervosa, 122–124, 128
  for obsessive–compulsive disorder, 69
Growth hormone, 139

Growth suppression, psychostimulant-related, 137

Haley, Jay, 207
Hallucinogens
  abuse, 99, 100
  complications, 102
Haloperidol
  as aggression therapy, 86–87, 90, 91
  as autism therapy, 79–80, 81, 84, 91, 142
  as dyskinesia cause, 81
  efficacy, 141
  as hyperactivity therapy, 86
  as obsessive–compulsive disorder therapy, 63
  as Tourette's syndrome therapy, 142
  withdrawal from, 142
  in withdrawal procedures, 104, 108
Helplessness, learned, 172
Homicide, children as witnesses of, 185–186
Hospitalization
  for aggression, 83, 85
  for anorexia nervosa, 124–127
    discharge, 125–127
Human immunodeficiency virus (HIV) infection, 106
Hyperactivity
  aggression and, 1, 2
  anorexia nervosa and, 124, 128
  antisocial behavior and, 2
  attention deficit hyperactivity disorder and, 1, 2–3, 8–9
  DSM–III classification, 2
  food allergy and, 152–153
  prevalence, 4–5
  sugar and, 156
  treatment
    behavior therapy, 8–9
    diet therapy, 154–155
    pharmacological, 8–9, 83, 86, 87
    psychotherapy, 9
Hyperserotonemia, autism and, 81
Hypospontaneity, verbal, 172
Hypothesizing, 209
Hysterical personality, parental, 5

Id, 177
Imagery, 174

Imipramine
  adverse effects, 138
  as attention deficit hyperactivity disorder therapy, 7, 8
  as behavior disorder therapy, 24, 138, 139–140
  dosage guidelines, 138
  as eating disorder therapy, 141
  as obsessive–compulsive disorder therapy, 62, 63, 64
  as school phobia therapy, 40, 41–43, 139, 143
  seizure threshold effects, 78
Immersion therapy, 57
Impulsivity
  in attention deficit hyperactivity disorder, 2, 3, 8, 9, 13
  treatment, 9, 13
Indecision, in obsessive–compulsive disorder, 51
Insomnia, 137, 143
Intellectualization, in obsessive–compulsive disorder, 51, 52
Intelligence quotient, in autism, 78
Interpersonal Psychotherapy model, 23
Isolation, in obsessive–compulsive disorder, 51

Korsakoff syndrome, 101

Language disorders, developmental; see also Dysphasia, developmental
  definition, 163
  treatment, 163–164
Lead chelating agents, 8
Learning disability
  dysphasia and, 171, 174
  food allergy and, 152–153
Leyton Obsessional Inventory–Child Version, 51
Lithium
  as aggression therapy, 87–88, 91, 144
  as attention deficit hyperactivity disorder therapy, 8
  as conduct disorder therapy, 13
  as depression therapy, 25, 140
  as obsessive–compulsive disorder therapy, 64
  as self-injurious behavior therapy, 87–88
Liver failure, substance abuse and, 101

# Index

Logic, of children, 179–181
Lorazepam, withdrawal applications, 105, 108, 110
Loxapine, 63
LSD, 99

Magical thinking, 51, 52
Magnesium pemoline
  as attention deficit hyperactivity disorder therapy, 7, 136, 137
  dopamine interaction, 137
  norepinephrine interaction, 137
Maprotiline, 138
Marijuana, 99–100
Memory, behavioral, 189
Mental disorder models, in family therapy, 202–205
Mental Research Institute, 207, 208
Mental retardation, aggression and, 83
Meprobamate, 143
Metachlorophenylpiperazine, 67
Methadone
  overdose, 105
  withdrawal applications, 111
Methylphenidate
  as attention deficit hyperactivity disorder therapy, 6–7, 86, 135, 136–137
  as depression therapy, 26
  dopamine interaction, 137
  as hyperactivity therapy, 83
  norepinephrine interaction, 137
  as stereotypy cause, 86
Mianserin, 64
Milieu therapy
  for anorexia nervosa, 124–125, 128
  for obsessive–compulsive disorder, 53, 69
Minuchin, Salvador, 205–206, 207
Monoamine oxidase inhibitors
  as anxiety therapy, 40
  as depression therapy, 24–25, 140
  as obsessive–compulsive disorder therapy, 63, 64
Mood disturbance, 144
Mother–child relationship, in school phobia, 32, 37
Movement therapy, for anorexia nervosa, 123–124, 128–129
Mutism, 202

Nadolol, 89

Naloxone
  as self-injurious behavior therapy, 89
  withdrawal applications, 105, 111
Naltrexone
  as autism therapy, 82, 84
  as self-injurious behavior therapy, 89–90, 91
Narcissistic personality disorder, 120
Narcotics
  abuse, 99, 102
  withdrawal, 105, 111–112
Narcotics Anonymous, 102, 106
National Institute of Mental Health–Obsessive Compulsive Scale, 51
Neuroleptics
  as aggression therapy, 13–14, 86–87, 90
  as anorexia nervosa therapy, 124
  as autism therapy, 79–81, 142
  as dyskinesia cause, 80–81, 87
  as eating disorder therapy, 141
  as obsessive-compulsive disorder therapy, 63
  withdrawal applications, 104
Neutrality, 209
Nialamide, 63
Norepinephrine, 137
Nortriptyline
  as depression therapy, 24, 25
  as obsessive–compulsive disorder therapy, 62

Obesity, as eating disorder, 115
Obsessive–compulsive disorder
  in adolescence, 50
  behavioral models, 54–56
  diagnosis, 50–51
  incidence, 49, 50
  onset age, 49–50
  serotonin hypothesis, 66–68
  symptoms, 50–51
    severity, 51
  treatment
    behavioral, 53–60, 68–69
    pharmacological, 61–68, 69, 137, 140
    psychotherapy, 51–53, 69
Obsessive Compulsive Rating Scale, 51
Opiate antagonists
  as autism therapy, 82
  as self-injurious behavior therapy, 89–90
Opioids, abuse, 103

Oppositional defiant disorder, 2
   aggression and, 9–10
   attention deficit hyperactivity disorder and, 2
   differential diagnosis, 4
   DSM–III classification, 1
   treatment, 11–12, 14
Oxazepam, 63

Palazzoli, Mara Selvini, 208, 210, 213
Panic attack/disorder
   depression and, 34
   obsessive–compulsive disorder and, 63
   prevalence, 35
   separation anxiety and, 34
   pharmacological treatment, 137
Paradoxical interventions, for depression, 23
Parasomnia, 137
Parents
   personality disorders, 5
   therapeutic process involvement, 193
      for anorexia nervosa, 122–123
      for attention deficit hyperactivity disorder, 9
      for conduct disorder, 12–13
Parents Target Behavior Checklist, 158
Pentobarbital, withdrawal applications, 105, 110–111
Pharmacological therapy: see Psychopharmacology
Phenelzine
   as eating disorder therapy, 141
   as obsessive–compulsive disorder therapy, 63
   as school phobia therapy, 39–40
Phenobarbital
   as school phobia therapy, 39–40
   withdrawal applications, 105, 111, 112
Phenytoin, 144
Phobic behavior, 54, 63
Phototherapy, 26
Physician, substance abuse treatment role, 100–112
   attitudes towards, 100–101
   detoxification, 104–106
   diagnosis, 102–103
   emergency treatment, 103–104
   rehabilitation, 106
   training for, 101
   withdrawal procedures, 107–112

Piaget, Jean, 179
Pimozide
   as aggression therapy, 86–87, 90, 91
      with haloperidol, 86–87
   as autism therapy, 79, 80, 84
   efficacy, 141
   as hyperactivity therapy, 87
   as Tourette's syndrome therapy, 142
Piracetam, 136
Plasticity, neuronal, 168–169
Play
   as behavioral speech act, 183
   therapeutic implications, 189–192
Practolol, 64
Problem-focused therapy, 52
Problem-solving, therapeutic, 194–195
Propranolol
   as aggression therapy, 89, 91, 144
   as conduct disorder therapy, 14
   withdrawal applications, 105
Psychiatric disorders; see also specific psychiatric disorders
   food allergy and, 153
   pharmacological treatment, 137
Psychoanalytic treatment; see also Psychotherapy, child
   of obsessive–compulsive disorder, 51–52, 69
Psychodynamic approach
   in depression therapy, 22–23
   in obsessive–compulsive disorder therapy, 51–52, 69
Psychopharmacology, child and adolescent, 133–150; see also names of individual drugs
   for aggression, 13–14, 85–91, 144
   for alcohol abuse, 134
   for anorexia nervosa, 124, 129, 134, 140–141
   antiaggressive drugs, 144
   antidepressants, 137–138
   antipsychotics, 141–142
   anxiolytics, 143
   for attention deficit disorders, 6–8, 14, 15, 85–86, 135–137, 138–139
   for autism, 78, 79–83, 84, 90, 142
   for borderline conditions, 134
   for bulimia nervosa, 124, 134, 137, 140–141
   for conduct disorders, 13–14, 138–139

# Index

Psychopharmacology, child and adolescent (*Cont.*)
  for depression, 134, 139–140
  for detoxification, 104–106
  for dysthymia, 134
  for eating disorders, 140–141
  for enuresis, 137, 138
  for obsessive–compulsive disorder, 61-68, 69, 137, 140
  prescription guidelines, 134–135
  for school phobia, 31–32, 39–43, 45, 137, 139
  for separation anxiety, 139, 143
  stimulants, 135–137
  for substance abuse, 134
  for Tourette's syndrome, 142
Psychosis
  alcoholic, 99
  drug abuse-related, 102, 104
  pharmacological treatment, 141
  psychostimulant-related, 136–137
Psychostimulants, 135–137
  abuse, 99, 102, 103
  adverse effects, 136–137
  as aggression therapy, 85–86, 144
  as attention deficit hyperactivity disorder therapy, 6–7, 13, 137
  as autism therapy, 83, 84
  as conduct disorder therapy, 13
  as hyperactivity therapy, 8–9
  as stereotypy cause, 86
Psychotherapy, child, 177–197
  for anorexia nervosa, 120–121
  children's capacities and, 177–178
  children's cognitive processes and, 179–181
  children's interactive style and, 181–183
  communication and, 179, 181–184
  conscious awareness and, 177
  for depression, 20–23
  developmental/contextual approach, 178, 184–186, 195
  "ecology" of, 192–193
  for hyperactivity, 9
  for obsessive–compulsive disorder, 51–53
  parents'/teachers' roles, 193
  play assessment, 189–192
  as problem-solving process, 194–195
  for school phobia, 39
  stage-related model, 179–181

Psychotherapy, child (*Cont.*)
  therapeutic process, 186–187, 188
  therapeutic space, 187–189
Punishment, as conduct disorder therapy, 12

Questioning, circular, 209, 210–211

Radioallergosorbent test(RAST), 152
Rationalization, 51
Reaction formation, 51
Reading disability
  in dyslexia, 136
  in dysphasia, 171
  pharmacological therapy, 136
Reality, family's construction of, 210
Reflexivity, 208
Reframing, 207
Regression, 51
Reinforcement, positive, as conduct disorder therapy, 11–12
Relaxation therapy, 21–22
Repression, 51
Response prevention, as obsessive–compulsive disorder therapy, 58–59, 60
Reynolds Adolescent Depression Scale, 21
Rimland E–2 checklist, 78
Rituals, in obsessive–compulsive disorder, 54, 55
  behavioral treatment, 56–60, 68–69

Schismogenesis, 207
Schizophrenia, treatment
  family therapy, 212, 214
  pharmacological, 143
School phobia
  anxiety and, 32–33, 42
  familial factors, 34–36
  conduct disorders and, 33
  defiant disorders and, 33
  depression and, 31, 32, 42
  familial factors, 34–36
  diagnosis, 32–34
  evaluation, 36–37
  mother–child relationship in, 32, 37
  parental factors, 34–36, 37–39, 44–45
    treatment implications, 38–39
  separation anxiety and, 31, 38
  severity rating, 33
  symptoms, 31

School phobia (*Cont.*)
  treatment
    pharmacological, 31–32, 39–43, 45, 137, 139
    school reentry program, 43–44
School refusal, 31, 32–34
Sedatives/hypnotics
  complications, 102
  symptoms, 103
  withdrawal, 105, 110–111
Seizures
  autism and, 78
  pharmacological treatment, 143
  tricyclic antidepressants-related, 138
Self-control therapy, 12
Self-help groups, for anorexics, 122
Self-injurious behavior
  assessment, 85
  autism and, 83
  mental retardation and, 83
  treatment, 86, 87, 89–90
Self-statements, 9
Self-supporting therapy, 120–121
Separation anxiety
  panic disorder and, 34
  pharmacological treatment, 139, 143
  school phobia and, 31, 38
Serotonin hypothesis, of obsessive–compulsive disorder, 66–68
Sex ratio
  in aggression, 11
  in attention deficit hyperactivity disorder, 4–5
  in autism, 78
  in conduct disorders, 11
Sleep deprivation, 26
Sleeping medications, withdrawal applications, 105, 108–109
Social therapy, 23
Sociobiology, 200
Sodium valproate, 144
Solvents, abuse, 102
Space, therapeutic, 187–189
Speech; *see also* Communication
  behavioral, 183, 190
State–Trait Anxiety Scale–Revised, 36
Stereotypy
  autism and, 80–81, 82, 83
  psychostimulants and, 86, 137
Stimulants: *see* Psychostimulants

Substance abuse disorders, 99–113; *see also* Alcoholism; Drug abuse
  diagnosis, 102–103
  prevention, 100
  support groups, 102, 106
  treatment
    detoxification, 104–106
    pharmacological, 134
    professional training for, 101
    professional attitudes and, 100–101
    rehabilitation, 106
    withdrawal procedures, 106–112
Sugar, behavior problems and, 155–160
Sulpiride, 40
Sulthiam, 144
Support groups, for substance abusers, 102, 106
Supportive therapy
  for anorexia nervosa, 119
  for obsessive–compulsive disorder, 53

Teacher(s), therapeutic process involvement, 193
Teachers Target Behavior Checklist, 158
Thioridazine, 8, 86
Thiothixene, 141
Thorazine: *see* Chlorpromazine
Thought processes, of children, 179–181
Thought stopping, as obsessive–compulsive disorder therapy, 57–58, 60
Thyroid hormone, as depression therapy, 25
Tic
  attention deficit hyperactivity disorder and, 8
  dysphasia and, 173
  psychostimulants and, 137
  transient disorder, 142
Timed Objective Rating Scale for Aggression, 85
"Time out," 12
Tourette's syndrome, 137, 142
Tranquilizers, withdrawal applications, 104–105, 108, 110
Tranylcypromine, 63
Trazodone, 65, 67
Triazolam, 105, 109

# Index

Tricyclic antidepressants
  adverse effects, 138
  as anorexia nervosa therapy, 124
  as anxiety therapy, 40
  as attention deficit hyperactivity disorder therapy, 7–8
  as conduct disorder therapy, 13
  as depression therapy, 13, 23–25
  efficacy, 139–140
  patient monitoring and, 140
  as school phobia therapy, 41
  withdrawal applications, 105
Trifluperazine, 63
Trimipramine, 63
L-Tryptophan, 64, 65
Two-factor learning theory, 54
Tybamate, 143

Undoing, in obsessive–compulsive disorder, 51

Unsocialized aggressive conduct disorder, 10, 13, 14
Urine drug testing, 106

Valproic acid, 14, 144
Visual Analogue Scale, for anxiety, 33, 36–37
Vitamins, in withdrawal therapy, 106, 107–108

Winnicott, D. W., 183–184
Withdrawal, 106–112
  alcohol, 104, 105, 107–110
  antipsychotics, 141, 141–142
  benzodiazepines, 143
  narcotics, 105, 111–112
  sedatives/hypnotics, 105, 110–111
World Health Organization, 99

Zimelidine, as obsessive-compulsive therapy, 64–65, 67

# *About the Editors*

*Dr. Jovan Simeon* is a Professor of Psychiatry at the Department of Psychiatry, School of Medicine, University of Ottawa, and Director of Child Psychiatry Research at the Royal Ottawa Hospital. He obtained his M.D. at Zagreb University in Yugoslavia and did his training in psychiatry and child psychiatry at Edinburgh University in Scotland. He is a Fellow of the Royal College of Psychiatrists in Great Britain, the American Psychiatric Association, and the Royal College of Physicians in Canada. Dr. Simeon is a diplomate of the American Board of Psychiatry and Child Psychiatry and has held University appointments at New York Medical College and Missouri University in St. Louis, Missouri. His main research interests have been the diagnostic evaluation and treatment of psychiatric disorders in children and adolescents and especially the psychopharmacology of hyperactivity, depression, and anxiety. He has published extensively in these areas.

*Dr. Bruce Ferguson* is Director of Psychology at the Royal Ottawa Hospital, Adjunct Professor of Psychiatry at the University of Ottawa, and Adjunct Research Professor of Psychology at Carleton University. He studied at Queen's University in Kingston, Canada and obtained his doctorate from Monash University in Melbourne, Australia. He has held research appointments at Queen's University, the National Institute of Mental Health in Bethesda, Maryland, and has taught developmental psychology at Carleton University. His main research interests have been in the diagnosis, treatment, and mechanisms underlying childhood behavior and learning disorders. He has published in the areas of hyperactivity and learning disorders.